Enabling Recovery

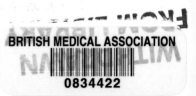

This book is dedicated to the memory of Paul Wolfson, who died while it was being written. Paul was a long-standing member of the Executive Committee of the Faculty of Rehabilitation and Social Psychiatry of the Royal College of Psychiatrists and latterly its vice-chair. He was an inspirational leader within rehabilitation psychiatry and brought important lived experience into his work. Most importantly he was a very nice and very funny man. He is much missed.

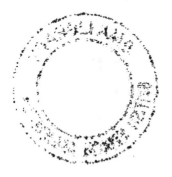

Enabling Recovery

The principles and practice of rehabilitation psychiatry

Second edition

Edited by Frank Holloway, Sridevi Kalidindi, Helen Killaspy and Glenn Roberts

RCPsych Publications

RCPsych Publications is an imprint of the Royal College of Psychiatrists,
21 Prescot Street, London E1 8BB, UK
http://www.rcpsych.ac.uk

British Library Cataloguing-in-Publication Data.
A catalogue record for this book is available from the British Library.
ISBN 978-1-909726-33-8

Distributed in North America by Publishers Storage and Shipping Company.

The views presented in this book do not necessarily reflect those of the Royal College of
Psychiatrists, and the publishers are not responsible for any error of omission or fact.

Printed by Bell & Bain Limited, Glasgow, UK.

Contents

Contributors

Ryan Aguiar Consultant Clinical Neuropsychologist, Ashworth Hospital, Mersey Care NHS Trust

Elina Baker Clinical Psychologist, Devon Partnership NHS Trust, Exeter

Dinesh Bhugra Professor of Mental Health and Cultural Diversity, Institute of Psychiatry, King's College London

Jed Boardman Consultant/Senior Lecturer in Social Psychiatry, South London and Maudsley NHS Foundation Trust, Maudlsey Hospital, Denmark Hill, London

Georgina Boon Highly Specialist Pharmacist, Pharmacy Department, South London and Maudsley NHS Foundation Trust, London

Jerome Carson School of Education Psychology, University of Bolton

Tom K. J. Craig Professor of Social and Community Psychiatry, Health Services Research, Institute of Psychiatry, London

Steffan Davies Consultant Forensic and Rehabilitation Psychiatrist, Northamptonshire Healthcare NHS Foundation Trust, Northampton

Tom Edwards Consultant Psychiatrist, Dudley and Walsall Assertive Outreach and Recovery Team, Dorothy Pattison Hospital, Walsall, West Midlands

Matthew Erlich New York State Office of Mental Health and Division of Psychiatry, Columbia University College of Physicians and Surgeons, New York

Gráinne Fadden Consultant Clinical Psychologist, Birmingham and Solihull Mental Health NHS Foundation Trust; Honorary Senior Research Fellow, University of Birmingham; Director, Meriden Family Programme, Birmingham

Daniel De La Harpe Golden Clinical Research Worker, Institute of Psychiatry, London

Joseph Hayes Medical Research Council Fellow, Division of Psychiatry, University College London; Camden and Islington NHS Foundation Trust, London

Frank Holloway Emeritus Consultant Psychiatrist, South London and Maudsley NHS Foundation Trust

Thérèse Jenkins Occupational Therapist, Rehabilitation and Recovery Team, Complex Care, Psychosis Clinical Academic Group, South London and Maudsley NHS Foundation Trust, King's Health Partners, London

Sridevi Kalidindi Consultant Psychiatrist in Rehabilitation, Clinical Lead for Local Contracts, South London and Maudsley NHS Foundation Trust; Chair, Faculty of Rehabilitation and Social Psychiatry, Royal College of Psychiatrists, Co-Chair, Joint Commissioning Panel for Mental Health

Sanjith Kamath Consultant Psychiatrist, St Andrew's Healthcare, Northampton

Helen Killaspy Professor of Rehabilitation Psychiatry, Mental Health Sciences Unit, University College London

Cheryl Kipping Consultant Nurse (Dual Diagnosis), South London and Maudsley NHS Foundation Trust, London

Czarina Kirk Guild Lodge Secure Acquired Brain Injury Service, Lancashirecare NHS Foundation Trust, Preston

Kevin Lewis Kevin Lewis Consulting, Director of the Personalisation Programme at the National Mental Health Development Unit, Department of Health 2009–2011

James MacCabe Senior Clinical Lecturer, Department of Psychosis Studies, Institute of Psychiatry, King's College London; Honorary Consultant Psychiatrist, National Psychosis Unit

Alan Meaden Consultant Lead Psychologist for Adult Services (South and East Central), Psychology Lead for Rehabilitation Services, Birmingham and Solihull Mental Health NHS Trust, Birmingham

Shawn Mitchell Consultant Psychiatrist, St Andrew's Healthcare, Northampton

David Osborn Professor and Consultant Psychiatrist, Division of Psychiatry, University College London; Camden and Islington NHS Foundation Trust, London

Stefan Priebe Professor of Social and Community Psychiatry, Newham Centre for Mental Health, London

Simon Procter Programme Director, Master of Music Therapy training programme, Nordoff Robbins, London

Julie Repper Recovery Lead, Nottinghamshire Healthcare NHS Trust; Associate Professor of Recovery and Social Inclusion, University of Nottingham

Glenn Roberts Consultant in independent practice, Devon

Dene Robertson Consultant Psychiatrist, Service Lead for Developmental Disorders, Bethlem Royal Hospital, Beckenham, Kent

Frank Röhricht Consultant Psychiatrist, East London NHS Foundation Trust, and Honorary Professor, University of Essex

Lloyd I. Sederer Medical Director, New York State Office of Mental Health and Columbia University's Mailman School of Public Health, New York

Geoff Shepherd Professor of Psychology, Senior Policy Advisor, Centre for Mental Health, London

Craig Steel Psychology Department, University of Reading

Melinda Sweeting Consultant Psychiatrist, High Support Rehabilitation Team (Southwark); Associate Clinical Director, Complex Care Pathway, Psychosis CAG, South London and Maudsley NHS Foundation Trust

Rumina Taylor Department of Psychology, Institute of Psychiatry, King's College London

Rangaswamy Thara Director, Schizophrenia Research Foundation, Chennai, India

Simon Tobitt Clinical Psychologist, Rehabilitation and Recovery Team, Complex Care, Psychosis Clinical Academic Group, South London and Maudsley NHS Foundation Trust, King's Health Partners, London

Emma Watson Peer Support Worker, Nottinghamshire Healthcare NHSTrust and Peer Trainer, Insitute of Mental Health, Nottingham

Stuart Webster Director, blueSCI, Manchester

Paul Wolfson (deceased) formerly Consultant Rehabilitation Psychiatrist, Oxleas NHS Foundation Trust, Pinewood House, Pinewood Place, Dartford

Til Wykes Professor of Clinical Psychology and Rehabilitation and Vice Dean for Research, Institute of Psychiatry, Psychology & Neuroscience, King's College London

Figures, tables and boxes

Preface

This book aims to provide a comprehensive account of contemporary practice within psychiatric rehabilitation services and indeed beyond mental health services that have a specific rehabilitation badge. As the second edition of a book first published in 2006, it is a celebration of significant progress in the specialty of rehabilitation and in our broader understanding of how people experiencing severe mental health problems can be supported (or not) in their personal recovery journeys. It is also a celebration of diversity: our authors come from diverse backgrounds and use a wide range of theoretical and practical approaches in their work. Throughout you will read a range of terms to describe the people with whom the services work: 'patients', 'clients', 'service users' (the most popular term), 'sufferers' and 'experts by experience' are all used by different authors in different contexts. What unites our authors is a passion to support service users in recovering a sense of agency, to allow them to get back control over their lives.

There is no 'magic bullet' in rehabilitation practice akin to an antibiotic used early in the course of a bacterial infection. Inevitably, practitioners need to be pragmatic and eclectic in their day-to-day work. This pragmatism rightly involves of being aware of the evidence base, but, given the limitations, conflicts and complexities surrounding that evidence base, rehabilitation practice must also reflect the values of the practitioner and others, notably the service user (Adshead, 2009). Values-based practice is a dynamic process that requires constant reflection – it is a toolkit that can be used to guide decision-making rather than a set of rigid, protocolised rules (Woodbridge & Fulford, 2004; Fulford, 2009). Mental health practice continually presents situations where values conflict – the most obvious example being the use of compulsion to deprive people of their liberty and treat them against their will. More subtle is when the rehabilitation practitioner seeks to improve a person's functional skills or personal hygiene in the face of indifference or even hostility. Practitioners can at times be guilty of not seeing the wood for the trees as they concentrate on eliminating symptoms at the expense of a person's desire to live as good a life as possible on his or her own terms. Balancing societal values and individual wishes is always a tricky business, rendered all the more complex in a diverse, multicultural context.

Organisation of the book

Each chapter seeks to cover a topic comprehensively, so readers can readily dip into the book as their interest takes them. However, we do have a structure to the book. Part 1, 'Setting the scene', addresses key conceptual issues surrounding rehabilitation practice. Part 2, 'Treatment approaches', describes the wide range of therapeutic options that are available. Part 3, 'Key elements of a rehabilitation service', reviews the building blocks of an effective service that addresses the rehabilitation needs of service users, encompassing both hospital and community care. Part 4, 'Special topics in psychiatric rehabilitation', covers a range of issues, including specific disorders that are important to rehabilitation practice (acquired brain injury and autism spectrum disorder), the complex issue of risk management, international perspectives on rehabilitation and, importantly, how to expand the evidence base. Parts 2–4 of the book have brief introductory chapters that offer an overview of the issues covered. Part 5 ends the main text with two chapters looking at future directions in policy and practice.

Why a second edition and what has changed?

Any second edition of a textbook requires justification. Readers familiar with the first edition will notice some continuity in editorship and authorship but also very significant change. In broad terms, the first edition was seeking to (re-)establish the credibility of psychiatric rehabilitation as a discipline and integrate it with then relatively novel concepts derived from what was called the Recovery Movement. Psychiatric rehabilitation was a marginal aspect of the 'modernised' mental health system that was introduced in the UK during the first years of the new millennium (Holloway, 2005). The recovery approach is now very much in the mental health mainstream (Roberts & Hollins, 2007; and see Chapter 3, 'Rehabilitation as a values-led practice: the contribution of recovery, social inclusion and personalisation'). Psychiatric rehabilitation as a discipline, its practices and the core services have moved from marginalisation to acceptance (Joint Commissioning Panel for Mental Health, 2012).

The second edition has been completely revised and reflects the increasing confidence and maturity of the discipline. As the evidence base evolves, there is a need to provide an update on approaches to treatment relevant to rehabilitation practice. These are described in Part 2 of the book ('Treatment approaches'). Developments in cognitive therapy, family interventions, the management of challenging behaviour and medication are presented. We provide an update on the physical healthcare of people living with severe mental illness, an issue that has rightly gained increasing prominence since *Enabling Recovery* was first published. Reflecting the increased confidence of practitioners, a new chapter, 'Rehabilitation at the coalface' (Chapter 8), provides some practical advice on working with service users that is underpinned by psychological theory. Other new chapters address the complexities surrounding working with comorbid substance misuse and the role of creative therapies and creativity in rehabilitation and recovery (Chapters 12 and 13).

In Part 3 ('Key elements of a rehabilitation service') there is a new chapter on rehabilitation in hospital settings (Chapter 17), in retrospect a surprising omission from the first edition of the book. Importantly, there is a chapter on the role of the peer support worker, which includes a contribution from someone working in that role (Chapter 21). Chapters on other elements of the rehabilitation service system have been revised to reflect changes in the evidence base and current practice.

In Part 4 of the book ('Special topics in psychiatric rehabilitation') new chapters provide updates on the complex issues surrounding acquired brain injury (Chapter 24) and autism spectrum disorders (Chapter 25), both of which are regularly encountered within mainstream rehabilitation practice. The first edition included a chapter on forensic rehabilitation, which anticipated an understanding within forensic services that their client group has rehabilitation needs that go beyond the management of offending behaviour. Increasingly mainstream rehabilitation services are working with patients who have been convicted of offences and this change of emphasis is captured in the present edition in Chapter 26, on 'Risk management in rehabilitation practice'. Two new chapters provide an international perspective on rehabilitation (Chapter 27) and, importantly, rehabilitation in low- and middle-income countries (Chapter 28), where non-governmental organisations play a particularly prominent role.

In revising *Enabling Recovery*, the editors have had to make difficult decisions about what to include and what to omit. When the first edition was published, there was a need to link rehabilitation with services providing early intervention in psychosis (EIP), which were then a new component of mainstream mental health services. The practices of EIP services were and remain fully consistent with those outlined in this book: what has become increasingly clear is that EIP, valuable though it is, does not abolish the need for specialist long-term support for some people experiencing an initial episode of psychosis.

Setting the scene – overview

In Part 1 we have a series of introductory chapters that attempt to set later contributions in context. It begins with an account of the 'pre-history' of psychiatric rehabilitation (Chapter 1). In the UK, rehabilitation practitioners are proud to look back on the opening of The Retreat in York, which ushered in 'moral treatment' as a humane and effective response to people experiencing severe mental illness. In reality, humane (and inhumane) responses to mental illness appear early in recorded history and the advances of the early 19th century were soon lost as the expanding asylum system entered what has been described as its 'long sleep'. The deinstitutionalisation movement that began in the 1950s ushered in an era where rehabilitation was both fashionable and markedly effective. However, in later decades the rhetoric of community care led to denial of the reality that some people experience.

Subsequent chapters explore core concepts in contemporary practice – psychiatric rehabilitation, recovery, social inclusion and personalisation (Chapters 2 and 3). Chapter 2 discusses rather unfashionable concepts such as the disability, impairment and handicap associated with severe mental illness. It also offers a contemporary definition of psychiatric rehabilitation, developed from the responses of practitioners:

> A whole system approach to recovery from mental ill health which maximizes an individual's quality of life and social inclusion by encouraging their skills, promoting independence and autonomy in order to give them hope for the future and which leads to successful community living through appropriate support. (Killaspy *et al*, 2005: p. 163)

This definition has been drawn upon by many of our contributors.

The complexities surrounding the relationship between the recovery approach and rehabilitation practice are explored in Chapter 3, which also describes in some detail the social exclusion that people with mental illness experience and how this might be addressed. There is an evolving personalisation agenda aimed at restoring authority through choice and control – its full implications for service users and practice are yet to be understood.

Any intervention provided by mental health services must be based on an appropriate assessment of the person's problems and needs. A range of approaches to assessment in rehabilitation is described in Chapter 4, which emphasises the importance of using structured methods without losing sight of the patient as a person. Structured assessment is particularly important in the measurement of the outcome of an intervention. Part 1 ends with two contributions looking at ways of understanding the experience of people with severe mental health problems, both of which emphasise the importance of narrative and listening to the person's story (Chapters 5 and 6).

Taken together, these introductory chapters provide a vital account of the intellectual underpinnings of practice and the complexities surrounding contemporary psychiatric rehabilitation.

References

Adshead G (2009) Systemic thinking and values-based practice. *Advances in Psychiatric Treatment*, **15**: 470–8.

Fulford KWM (2009) Values, science and society. In *Psychiatric Ethics* (4th edn) (eds S Bloch, SA Green): 61–84. Oxford University Press.

Holloway F (2005) *The Forgotten Need for Psychiatric Rehabilitation. A Position Statement from the Faculty of Rehabilitation and Social Psychiatry*. Royal College of Psychiatrists.

Joint Commissioning Panel for Mental Health (2012) *Guidance for Commissioners of Rehabilitation Services for People with Complex Mental Health Needs*. Royal College of Psychiatrists.

Killaspy H, Harden C, Holloway F, *et al* (2005) What do mental health rehabilitation services do and what are they for? A national survey in England. *Journal of Mental Health*, **14**: 157–66.

Roberts G, Hollins S (2007) Recovery: our common purpose? Editorial. *Advances in Psychiatric Treatment*, **13**: 397–9.

Woodbridge K, Fulford KWM (2004) *Whose Values? A Workbook for Values-Based Practice in Mental Health Care*. Sainsbury Centre for Mental Health.

Part 1

Setting the scene

CHAPTER 1

Rehabilitation in a historical context

Paul Wolfson and Frank Holloway

> Those who cannot remember the past are condemned to repeat it.
> George Santayana

Introduction

'Rehabilitation psychiatry' is a relatively new term. It combines a word that is quite old – rehabilitation (which initially related to restoring one's title or place in society, and which gained its current meaning only in the early 20th century) – with a word – psychiatry – first coined in the early 19th century (from the Greek 'healing the mind'). Specific rehabilitation departments were developed in UK mental hospitals only in the 1950s, since when rehabilitation services have flourished, declined and then re-emerged as a core element of mental healthcare, albeit often rebranded under various fashionable rubrics.

This chapter looks at the 'pre-history' of psychiatric rehabilitation and its development since the 1950s, when it was first identified as a specialty. The story is inevitably highly selective, given the range of material available. Some important themes, for example the voice of the patient (or service user, or survivor), which was first influential during the 19th century, and the Recovery Movement and its precursors, are discussed in detail elsewhere in this book (see Chapters 6 and 3, respectively). The present chapter draws largely but not exclusively on the evolution of ideas and practice in England: very similar though subtly different stories could be told for France, Germany and the USA (Stone, 1998).

The difficulties of any historical analysis of psychiatry were well described by Berrios & Freeman (1991) in their introduction to *150 Years of British Psychiatry*. One problem is 'presentism' – seeing the past from a perspective that takes no account of the intellectual, social and cultural context of the times. A further potential pitfall is developing a story of uninterrupted progress (in historical jargon, the Whiggish interpretation of history[1]): in reality, progress in what we would now call psychiatric

---

1. Whigs were a political faction opposed to Tories in the English Parliament from the 1680s: they became the Liberal Party and the Tories became the Conservative Party. Whigs were identified as believing in progress, Tories as believing in the status quo.

rehabilitation has ebbed and flowed. Another problem with any attempt at understanding the past, not mentioned by Berrios & Freeman, is that historical sources overwhelmingly represent the experiences of a privileged and literate elite.

Understandings of mental disorder

Abnormal mental states and aberrant behaviour are described in some of the earliest written records (Stone, 1998). Historians of psychiatry identify three common ways of understanding mental disorder. The first is a religious perspective, which can be positive, in terms of accessing a higher level of consciousness, or negative, relating to possession by evil spirits. The second is somatic and describes physical causes – though the proposed nature of these causes has varied since the time of Hippocrates (Brown, 1997). The third explanatory framework involves psychological and socio-environmental causation: grief, passion, stress, association of ideas, unconscious mental processes, life events and cognitive distortions.

These alternative ways of understanding have had practical effects. A belief in somatic causation suggests the use of physical treatments, which in the past have included dieting, purging and bloodletting. The psychological approach suggests that understanding the causes of the person's problems and attention to the person's social environment should lead to resolution of the problem. Religious understandings have led to both acceptance and inclusion and very marked exclusion from society.

Ancient ideas on madness and its treatment

There are numerous descriptions of abnormal mental states in the Old Testament. Saul, the first King of Israel, is generally accepted as suffering from an affective disorder, with episodes of depression and possibly mania (Stein, 2011). His affliction is described in religious terms: 'The spirit of the Lord had forsaken Saul, and at times an evil spirit from the Lord would seize him suddenly' (1 Samuel 16: 14). Treatment, however, was psychological: 'And whenever a spirit from God came upon Saul, David would take his harp and play on it, so that Saul found relief: he recovered and the evil spirit left him alone' (I Samuel 16: 23).

A number of familiar mental disorders are described in the writings ascribed to Hippocrates (c.450–370 BCE): mania, paranoia, hysteria and melancholia. The Hippocratic corpus provides a physical account of mental states: 'from the brain, and from the brain only, arise our pleasures, joys … as well as our sorrows, pain, grief and tears. It is the same organ that makes us mad or delirious, inspires us with dread and fear, brings sleeplessness … and aimless anxiety' (quoted in Stone, 1998: p. 10). Disease in general was attributed to an imbalance of humours or elements, which are variously described. Mania was thought to be caused by an accumulation of yellow bile heating and drying the brain, while melancholia was thought to be caused by an accumulation of black bile.

Humoralism was the dominant explanatory framework for disease in Graeco-Roman times and remained so well into the early modern period (Brown, 1997). A range of treatments were advocated by the humoralists, aimed at restoring the balance of the humours. These included bloodletting, enemas, induced vomiting and starvation. Plato, in *The Republic*, advocated that people whose psychological constitution is 'warped' (understood here to mean people who are chronically mentally ill) be put to death (Book III 410) – anticipating eugenic policies by more than 2000 years.

Another tradition is linked to the philosopher Epicurus (341–270 BCE), who taught that the right philosophy, which is based on scientific knowledge, cures the anxieties of the soul in the same way that the right medicine cures the pains of the body. The philosopher and physician Asclepiades (*c.*24–40 BCE), a follower of Epicurus, rejected humoralism and was sceptical about harsh physical treatments. He recommended instead mild therapeutic methods, such as healthy diet, exposure to light, massage, physical exercise, the use of medicinal herbs and, in some cases, wine. Asclepiades described delusions and hallucinations and 'was a pioneer of the humane treatment of mental disorders ... free[ing] insane persons from confinement in the dark and treat[ing] them using labor and music therapy, in addition to healthy diet and massages' (Yapijakis, 2009).

Epicureans believed in a psychological approach to the treatment of mental disorder and also identified psychological causes. Soranus of Ephesus (1st–2nd century CE) in *On Acute and Chronic Diseases* described the symptoms of mania and melancholia and described a range of causes for mania, which included 'continual sleeplessness, excesses of venery, anger, grief, anxiety, or superstitious fear, a shock or blow, intense straining of the senses and the mind in study, business or other pursuits' (quoted in Brown, 1997: p. 440)

The Roman encyclopaedist Celsus (*c.*25 BCE to *c.*50 CE) was a humoralist and as such favoured the use of physical treatments, to the extent that: 'If it is the mind that deceives the madman, he is best treated by torture, fetters or flogging'. However, he also advocated relieving melancholy with soft music and described the intriguing case history of a wealthy man who lived in fear of starvation. 'His attendants announced pretended legacies to him, to relieve his anxieties, until he recovered his reason' (quoted in Stone, 1998: p. 13).

Early nosologies

During the time of the Roman Empire, a distinction was drawn between illnesses that came on in adult life (e.g. mania, melancholia and paranoia), lack of normal mental functioning from birth (amentia) and loss of mental functioning (dementia). Recovery from some disorders was seen as possible, whereas recovery from amentia and dementia was not.

Similar ideas appear in a very early statute in English law, *De Praerogavita Regis*, which dates from the reign of Edward II (1307–27). It relates to the management of the property of people who, in modern terminology, lack capacity to manage their wealth. The statute makes a clear distinction between 'natural fools', who have no prospect of recovery, and 'lunatics', who may well recover. The 'lunatic', in the words of the Blackstone's 18th-century *Commentaries* (book 1, chapter 8, XVI), 'has had understanding, but by disease, grief, or other accident has lost the use of his reason'. On recovery, property would return to the control of the former 'lunatic'.

Enlightenment and later ideas about mental illness

Ideas about mental illness were refined during the Enlightenment, a period of intellectual development that saw the elaboration of the scientific method and a secular as opposed to a religious approach to mental disorder. Prominent during this period were the ideas of the English philosopher John Locke, who developed an 'associationistic' psychology, which suggested that people with a mental illness draw reasonable conclusions from false premises (a view echoed by contemporary cognitive psychology). The alternative view, that psychological diseases are diseases of the brain, became the dominant paradigm during the latter part of the 19th century (Brown, 1997). This evolved into an understanding of mental disorder as an expression of hereditary degeneracy (or in the case of general paralysis of the insane, an infective process).

These competing views of mental disorder have been greatly refined over the past 100 years. The early 20th century was dominated by 'dynamic psychiatry', under the influence of Freud and his followers (Ellenberger, 1970), although Freud's ideas had little initial impact on the care of people with severe mental illness, which remained largely institutional. The biological approach was supported by the development of effective treatments for the symptoms of mental illness during the 1950s – which saw the introduction of antipsychotic, antidepressant and anxiolytic medications. Systematic investigation of the person's social context has been added to the investigation of the causes of mental disorder (Morgan *et al*, 2008). We now know that environmental, psychological and social factors can have an effect on the expression of genes. As a result, the current dominant way of understanding the problems and needs of people with a mental illness is a biopsychosocial model, which seeks to take into account factors working at all these levels.

The care of people with mental illness

Throughout history, the primary responsibility for caring for people who were behaving abnormally has been within the family or the very local community. People of means might have access (for good or ill) to medical treatment and be looked after by attendants. Where families or local communities were unable to provide support, some care was provided haphazardly by religious institutions.

The first hospitals to be recorded as treating people with mental illness were in the major cities of the Islamic world, including Cairo, Baghdad, Basra and Aleppo (Youssef & Yousef, 1996). Similar institutions sprang up in major European cities during the Middle Ages (Bynum, 1983). In London, the Priory of St Mary of Bethlem was founded in 1247 as a focus for the collection of alms. It gradually evolved during the 1400s into a specialist institution for the confinement of the 'insane' – remaining the only one in England for over 200 years (Donnelly, 1983).

Boarding out of people with a mental illness either locally or with landlords who took residents in (for a fee) was a common practice. It was particularly associated with the small town of Geel in Belgium. Geel, site of the shrine to St Dymphna, patron saint of people who are mentally ill, attracted visitors from across Europe. (St Dymphna is said to have been killed in Geel in the 7th century by her mentally ill father, a petty Irish king.) The Church authorities encouraged local people to offer foster care.

In England there has been a system of relief for the poor and vulnerable since Tudor times. The Elizabethan Poor Law created a system that was administered by Parishes funded by the rates, a local property tax. Those who were too ill or old to work received payment and food ('outdoor relief'); in some places elderly people could reside in alms houses ('indoor relief'). Access to relief was dependent on showing a connection to the parish. Vagrants and beggars were strongly disapproved of and could be sent to a 'house of correction'. People with a mental illness might end up in a house of correction or a local gaol.

The 18th century saw the development of workhouses (the residents of which were expected to contribute by productive work). These became catch-all institutions for poor and vulnerable people. They were the central provider of support after the introduction of the New Poor Law in 1832, which drastically restricted outdoor relief. There was a parallel development of specialist institutions for people with a mental illness during the 18th century and early 19th century (Donnelly, 1983). Hospitals and asylums were opened in provincial cities as charitable foundations, along with a large number of for-profit 'madhouses'. Both would take in 'pauper lunatics' (paid for through local rates) or people of means.

Conditions in 18th-century madhouses and hospitals such as the Bethlem could be very degrading: a visit to view the lunatics at the Bethlem was seen as an enjoyable day out. However, we know that people who were sent to madhouses got better. A notable example is the poet William Cowper, who suffered from a severe recurrent affective psychosis. Cowper spent a period in 'Dr Cotton's Home for Madmen at St Albans'. While at Dr Cotton's Home Cowper was for a period bound to his bed to prevent him from killing himself. He went on to spend a productive life, living with an Evangelical Christian family, despite subsequent relapses that were managed, not without difficulty, at home (Cecil, 1933).

The magistrates visiting Ticehurst House (a purpose-built asylum catering for a wealthy clientele) noted that 'all [residents] expressed themselves well satisfied with the arrangements made for their comfort and convenience' (Scull, 1982). In 1799 the Bethlem admitted 201 patients and reported having 'cured and discharged' 179 patients and buried 20. Of the 243 residents on 31 December 1799, 130 were described as 'under cure' and 113 as 'incurable' (House of Commons, 1815: p. 388).

Moral treatment

Towards the end of the 18th century there was a movement to reform practices in asylums, exemplified by the actions of Philippe Pinel, physician successively to two large hospitals in post-revolutionary Paris, the Bicêtre and the Salpêtrière.[2] Pinel is remembered for removing the chains of inmates at the Salpêtrière and introducing a more humane approach to the treatment of the insane (*traitement moral*); in fact, similar initiatives had been taken previously, notably by Chiarugi in Florence, Daquin in Chambery and Pinel's colleague Pussin at the Bicêtre (Stone, 1998: ch. 5).

The York Retreat, moral treatment and the Tuke family

In 1791 a Quaker woman from Leeds, Hannah Mills, died some weeks after admission to the York Asylum. Investigations by her co-religionists in York, who had been asked by her family to visit her but who had been refused access, revealed very poor conditions at the Asylum. William Tuke, a tea merchant, subsequently led the foundation by subscription of an alternative asylum, initially only for Quakers. The York Retreat opened in 1796 and still exists. Although always a small institution, its design, principles and working practices, as described by Samuel Tuke, the founder's grandson, in his book *Description of The Retreat* (Tuke, 1813), were to prove highly influential. *Description of The Retreat* remains a founding text of rehabilitation psychiatry (see Chapter 17, 'Rehabilitation in hospital settings').

Samuel Tuke's book is organised in an exemplary fashion. Two introductory chapters provide a historical context, including the bureaucratic details of obtaining funding for the project. Four years elapsed between the first committee meeting and the opening of The Retreat. The third chapter describes the acquisition of the site and building work. A fourth chapter, using original notebooks Tuke had obtained, describes the approach of the first physician to The Retreat, Thomas Fowler, to medical treatment. Dr Fowler's approach was cautious and empirical and the conclusion was that

---

2. After the French Revolution, multifunctional institutions were established that contained many thousands of inmates – including people deemed 'insane' – but the Bicêtre (for men) and the Salpêtrière (for women) pre-dated these.

contemporary medical treatment was not effective, other than warm baths for women with melancholia. Tuke advocated attention to the treatment of what we would now term comorbid physical illness. A fifth and substantial chapter describes moral treatment (a term Tuke consciously appropriated from Pinel, although the practices of The Retreat evolved independently of Pinel's work). The book ends with a description of cases, some statistical material, a brief discussion of nosology and some comparative material about the ways in which particular asylums were run.

William Tuke and his committee hired a superintendent, George Jepson, and a nurse in charge of the female patients, Katherine Allen, who would have been the people most crucial to the way The Retreat worked in practice. Together they elaborated moral treatment, which was based less on theory than on practice (Samuel Tuke frequently refers to Jepson's experiences in his book). The basic tenets of moral treatment were: to strengthen and assist the power of patients to control their disorders; to be clear about the appropriate use of coercion (only when it is 'absolutely necessary'); and to promote 'the general comfort of the insane' (Tuke, 1813: p. 138). The Retreat offered a positive environment, where patients were treated with respect and encouraged to be involved in a daily routine of activity and leisure, which was specific to their previous life and interests. Patients were talked to as human beings, 'in a kind, and somewhat low tone of voice', and were encouraged to develop self-restraint. The use of chains and corporal punishment, common in the 18th-century asylum, was forbidden. Tuke discusses the limitations of punitive measures towards disturbed behaviour and value of kindness (he provides a case history). He describes how the superintendent would interact with the patient as a rational person and how the regime could foster self-esteem.

William Tuke, his son Henry and his grandson Samuel all had strong connections with The Retreat, but none was medically qualified. Samuel's book evidences a very sophisticated understanding of the care of mental illness. It is much more accessible to contemporary readers than the writings of his son, Daniel Hack Tuke, who was one of the most eminent English psychiatrists of the second half of the 19th century.

The 19th-century asylum

A complex and lightly regulated system of private madhouses and charitable hospitals and lunatic asylums had evolved in England during the 18th century. Well-publicised scandals about conditions in these institutions led to pressure for reform. A series of parliamentary investigations in the first decades of the 19th century resulted in legislation. In 1808, counties were allowed to build asylums, funded by local rates, and finally in 1845 they were required do so (Donnelly, 1983).

A Select Committee on Madhouses set up in 1815 heard evidence about abuses in asylums, madhouses and workhouses and the harm caused by traditional medical approaches to the treatment of inmates (Scull, 1982).

The Quaker Edward Wakefield provided particularly striking evidence in the case of James Norris, who was held in chains in solitary confinement at the Bethlem for over a decade. Importantly, the Committee also heard about positive practice – William Tuke gave evidence to the Committee (House of Commons, 1815: pp. 160–163). Members of the Committee had read Samuel Tuke's account of The Retreat.

Reformers in England, France and the USA were clear that what was required were purpose-built asylums organised on the therapeutic principles of moral treatment that would lead to cure and discharge. Conditions improved. Non-restraint was introduced into public asylums in England by Robert Gardiner Hill in Norwich and John Conolly at the Hanwell Asylum in Middlesex (which is now St Bernard's Hospital). Emphasis was put on engaging patients in activity. Success rates for at least some of the new therapeutically oriented asylums were initially high: over 20 years (1833–52) 71% of the patients admitted to the Worcester State Hospital, Massachusetts, who had been ill for less than a year were discharged (Bockhoven, 1954).

There was another element to the reformed asylum – the management of risk. The Criminal Lunatics Act 1800 set out a procedure for the indefinite detention of a person acquitted on the ground of insanity. Initially, such people often ended up in prison, an unsatisfactory situation that suggested the need for special provision. Following a Select Committee report in 1807, negotiation between the Home Department and the governors of the Bethlem hospital resulted in a special wing being built at its new premises (located in what is now the Imperial War Museum). This wing, the State Criminal Lunatic Asylum, opened in 1816. Its direct descendants are the three high secure hospitals in England and the ever-expanding network of forensic mental health services.

The latter half of the 19th century and the first half of the 20th century saw what has been described as the 'long sleep' of the mental hospital. Therapeutic optimism evaporated and the proportion of patients identified as curable by asylum superintendents decreased steadily (from a not very impressive 15% in 1844 to a dismal 7.7% in 1870). By 1890, more people each year were dying in the asylums than being discharged cured (Scull, 1982: ch. 6). Throughout the 19th century and in the first part of the 20th, asylums grew in size and new asylums were built, usually on the outskirts of conurbations. To contain costs, these institutions were as self-reliant as possible and depended on the labour of the better-functioning patients. These custodial asylums existed alongside an overwhelmingly organic understanding of mental disorder, which was seen as a degenerative and hereditary condition. However, even during this bleak period there was evidence of interest in supporting people who left the asylum. In 1879 the Reverend Henry Hawkins, chaplain to Colney Hatch Asylum, founded the Mental Aftercare Association (now the charity Together) 'to facilitate the readmission of the poor friendless female convalescent from Lunatic Asylums into social life'.

Rehabilitation in the 20th century

Organised rehabilitation in the UK has its beginnings in the horrors of the First World War, as attempts were made to help ex-servicemen with disabilities return to employment (Bennett, 1983). In 1919 the Ex-services Mental Welfare Society (now Combat Stress) was formed to assist shell-shocked ex-servicemen. The Society set up a convalescent home in Leatherhead and subsequently a business manufacturing electric blankets. Although this group of people had very different problems to those of patients in asylums, the Society's consultant psychiatrist, Professor Mapother, observed that a similar scheme of sheltered work would be appropriate for 'ordinary psychiatry'. It was only long after the Second World War that work rehabilitation became an integral part of the life of the mental hospital.

Asylums in the early 20th century showed no sign of awakening from their 'long sleep'. The *Journal of Mental Science* (now the *British Journal of Psychiatry*) printed a brief report on 'habit training for mental patients' (McWilliam, 1926). This was an early example of the use of occupational therapy within a mental hospital setting, which dates back to the 1900s at the Henry Phipps Clinic in Baltimore. There is no evidence that McWilliam's report had any effect on practice within the UK asylum system.

Following a Royal Commission on Lunacy and Mental Disorder, there were significant reforms to mental health law: the Mental Treatment Act of 1930 allowed, for the first time, voluntary admission to publicly funded in-patient care in what were now termed 'mental hospitals' and permitted local authorities to develop aftercare services. A study tour of mental hospitals in Holland introduced to British psychiatry the influential ideas of Dr Hermann Simon, director of the asylum in Guttersloh. Simon described 'active therapy' – which meant engaging patients in productive work to prepare them for life outside hospital.[3]

The Second World War provided a surprising stimulus to psychiatry in Britain. The army, mindful of the experience of the First World War, expected its medical officers to treat psychiatric casualties, most of whom were suffering from neurotic or stress-related conditions. Many got better; those who relapsed were reassigned to other duties or discharged back into civilian life. There were fascinating experiments in working with soldiers with a neurosis at Northfield Hospital in Birmingham and Mill Hill Hospital in London, which went on to inform group analysis and one strand of social psychiatry – the hospital as a therapeutic community (Clark, 1974). In 1944 the Disabled Persons Act set out a programme for the rehabilitation of people with both physical and mental disability. Some army doctors became psychiatrists after demobilisation and brought with

---

3. Less well known was Simon's espousal of Hitler's racist and eugenic policies, which seems at odds with the humanistic perspective that 'active therapy' implied.

them positive views on the outcome of mental illness (and quite a lot of organisational expertise).

After the war, the mental hospitals continued to accumulate patients; bed numbers reached a maximum in both the UK and the USA in 1954. However, things were changing. In the traditional mental hospital the doors to wards had been locked. Pioneering hospitals began to open these doors (T. P. Rees, medical superintendent of Warlingham Park Hospital, in Surrey, is credited as the pioneer of the 'open door movement'). From 1950, mental hospitals became more open institutions, in the sense that the numbers of both admissions and discharges increased markedly and the average length of stay decreased. This change started just before the introduction of effective pharmacological treatments for mental illness became available, the first being chlorpromazine, which was available from 1954 onwards.

Although there was increasing interest in rehabilitation, the dominant theme of mental hospital care was resettlement (Bennett, 1983). It was already apparent by the late 1950s, however, that, in the absence of adequate community care, there was a price to pay for this, in terms of the burden on families (Mills, 1962). Specific rehabilitation services initially focused on preparing people for work and mental hospitals began to offer 'industrial therapy' (Early, 1960). At one level, industrial therapy was successful (this was an era of full employment), but it became clear that other issues relating to social functioning needed to be addressed. Mental hospitals developed a gradient of increasing social expectations on patients – the ladder model of rehabilitation. The ladder was later extended to a range of supported settings out of hospital (Early, 1973).

That mental hospitals might have a bad effect on their patients had been clear since the 19th century. In 1894 the American neurologist Weir Mitchell exclaimed to the American Medico-Psychological Association, 'upon my word, I think asylum life is deadly to the insane' (quoted in Bennett, 1983). Asylum care became the focus of empirical research in the 1950s. In a seminal study the sociologist Erving Goffman (1961) described the impoverished social world of the 'inmates' of a psychiatric institution. Russell Barton (1966) viewed this effect as an illness in itself – 'institutional neurosis'. Most persuasively, Wing & Brown, in their 'Three Hospitals Study' (1970), investigated the relationship between the way that three hospitals worked and the outcome for patients with schizophrenia. They found that the quality of the social environment was associated with what we now call the negative symptoms of schizophrenia and that as the environment changed, the frequency of negative symptoms changed (in one hospital the social environment improved and negative symptoms decreased; in another it worsened and negative symptoms increased). The most important environmental factor was 'time spent doing nothing'.

The 1962 Hospital Plan envisaged the closure of 13 of the 109 large mental hospitals in England and Wales by 1975, an overall reduction in bed numbers and the opening of acute in-patient units in district general hospitals. It was not until 1986 that the first large public mental hospital (Banstead Hospital in Surrey) actually closed. Since then, almost all have closed or vastly down-sized. Most of the sites have been redeveloped for housing. The hospital closure programme in England has been the best studied in the world and has provided valuable insights about the process and outcomes of hospital closure and the impact of the social environment on people's social functioning.

The mental hospital closure programme and the TAPS study

In a relatively short period the majority of the large mental hospitals in England and Wales closed. The Team for the Assessment of Psychiatric Services (TAPS) study is the most thorough evaluation of a hospital closure programme and its aftermath that has ever been undertaken. The focus was the closure of Friern Barnet Hospital, which had opened as the second Middlesex County Asylum, or Colney Hatch, in 1851. It became the largest mental hospital in the UK, with, at its peak, some 3000 beds (and reputedly the longest hospital corridor in the world). The North East Thames Regional Health Authority resolved to close Friern and from 1985 funded a research team led by Professor Julian Leff to evaluate the closure process. The hospital closed in 1993. The site was converted to an 'exclusive residential development set within 30 acres of parkland' (according to the website marketing the properties, http://www. princessparkmanor.net) and the railings that once served to keep patients in now keep the less desirable elements out.

TAPS provided data on outcomes for patients discharged from Friern between 1985 and its closure and a cohort of patients discharged from the rather less glamorous neighbouring Claybury Hospital. TAPS also looked at the outcomes of 'difficult to place' patients from the Friern catchment area and outcomes for elderly patients with dementia. TAPs generated a huge amount of data, published in 46 named TAPS papers, a book (Leff, 1997) and a brief overview paper (Leff et al, 2000). The headline findings were that patients who were discharged to community settings (mostly offering a high level of support) gained social and domestic skills, experienced enriched social networks and had a much better living environment (Leff & Trieman, 2000). Only 10% of patients were in hospital at 5-year follow-up (Trieman et al, 1999). Many of the 'difficult to place' patients moved into newly developed specialist local services (Trieman & Leff, 2002). Challenging behaviours decreased over time and over 5 years 40% of patients moved to less supported settings.

TAPS and other studies tell us a lot about outcomes. Large mental hospitals were closed to the benefit of their residents, although local in-patient mental health services struggled for a time because of pressures following these bed reductions (Leff et al, 2000). Less well documented are the complex ideological underpinnings of the closure movement and the financial arrangements that allowed it to proceed. The earlier writings of Goffman and Barton, which suggested that the problems that long-stay hospital residents presented were largely if not entirely the result of the experience of living in an institution, were influential. Many 're-provision' services were influenced by the principles of 'normalisation'. This is a complex set of ideas first elaborated in the context of learning disability that emphasises both the right of people living with disability to occupy valued social roles and the negative impact of labelling and stigmatisation on people's ability to function (Brown & Smith, 1992).

Rehabilitation and community mental health services

It was not until 1983 that the first substantial textbook on psychiatric rehabilitation was published in the UK (Watts & Bennett, 1983). At that time, rehabilitation practice was largely limited to in-patient units (usually located within a mental hospital and focusing on people who had become long-stay patients) and day-care facilities (day hospitals and day centres). Some rehabilitation went on in hostels and group homes. Occupational therapists, whose focus is on functioning rather than illness, were already integral to mental health teams. Watts & Bennett (1983) included chapters on working with families, the importance of community support and how specific aspects of social functioning might be addressed, such as employment, daily living skills and interpersonal skills. The reality for patients leaving hospital often fell far short of the practices Watts & Bennett promoted and the deficiencies of community care became increasingly apparent (National Schizophrenia Fellowship, 1984).

Inadequacies in community support for people living with mental illness spurred the introduction of the Care Programme Approach (CPA) in 1991 (Department of Health, 1990). CPA, which is essentially a care planning mechanism for in-patient services and community mental health teams, has gone through successive subsequent refinements (Department of Health, 2008). Although the term 'rehabilitation' is not used in the policy documents, CPA is clearly rehabilitative in focus:

> Care assessment and planning views a person 'in the round' seeing and supporting them in their individual diverse roles and the needs they have, including: family; parenting; relationships; housing; employment; leisure; education; creativity; spirituality; self-management and self-nurture; with the aim of optimising mental and physical health and well-being.... Care planning is underpinned by long-term engagement, requiring trust, team work and commitment. It is the daily work of mental health services and supporting partner agencies, not just the planned occasions where people meet for reviews. (Department of Health, 2008: p. 7)

Rehabilitation into the 21st century

The National Service Framework for Mental Health was published in 1999 (Department of Health, 1999). It included a very substantial chapter on services for people with severe mental illness and specifically stated that for people discharged from in-patient care there should be 'a written after-care plan agreed on discharge which sets out the care and rehabilitation to be provided, identifies the care co-ordinator, and specifies the action to be taken in a crisis' (Department of Health, 1999: p. 41).

It is something of a historical puzzle that rehabilitation did not appear at all in the subsequent Policy Implementation Guide (Department of Health, 2001) or in the plethora of Department of Health policy documents that followed it. It is likely that policy-makers believed that the hospital closure programme had abolished the need for long-term high-support care. A review of future bed needs in England proposed that all psychiatric rehabilitation in-patient beds should close (Department of Health, 2000), although, in line with a long-term policy focus on issues of risk in mental healthcare, it did propose a massive expansion in intensive care and forensic provision.

The focus of policy in the first decade of the 21st century was on the development of functional community teams providing assertive outreach, crisis and home treatment, and early intervention in psychosis. These teams were often built from the ashes of community rehabilitation teams that had supported patients with complex needs coming out of hospital (Mountain *et al*, 2009).

It has become clear that the deinstitutionalisation promised by the hospital closure programme of the 1980s and 1990s did not in fact abolish institutional care. It was replaced by a 'virtual asylum', a complex and highly fragmented system involving public and private sector hospitals, residential and nursing home care, and various forms of supported housing (Poole *et al*, 2002). This phenomenon of transinstitutionalisation has been observed across Europe (Priebe *et al*, 2005).

Despite the lack of a clear policy lead during the past decades, both in-patient and community rehabilitation services continue to have a vital place in a comprehensive mental health system (Wolfson *et al*, 2009; Joint Commissioning Panel for Mental Health, 2012). This book seeks to put flesh on the bare bones of this statement.

References

Barton R (1966) *Institutional Neurosis* (2nd edn). John Wright.

Bennett DH (1983) The historical development of rehabilitation services. In *Theory and Practice of Psychiatric Rehabilitation* (eds FN Watts, DH Bennett): 15–42. Wiley.

Berrios GE, Freeman H (eds) (1991) *150 Years of British Psychiatry 1841–1991*. Gaskell.

Bockhoven JS (1954) Moral treatment in American psychiatry. *Journal of Nervous and Mental Diseases*, **124**: 167–94.

Brown H, Smith H (eds) (1992) *Normalisation. A Reader.* Routledge.

Brown TM (1997) Mental diseases. In *Companion Encyclopaedia of the History of Medicine* (eds WF Bynum, R Porter): 438–63. Routledge.

Bynum WF (1983) Psychiatry in its historical context. In *Handbook of Psychiatry. 1 General Psychopathology* (eds M Shepherd, OL Zangwill): 11–38. Cambridge University Press.

Cecil D (1933) *The Stricken Deer.* Constable.

Clark DH (1974) *Social Therapy in Psychiatry.* Penguin.

Department of Health (1990) *Caring for People. The Care Programme Approach for People with a Mental Illness Referred to Specialist Mental Health Services. Joint Health/Social Services Circular. C(90)23/LASSL(90)11.* Department of Health.

Department of Health (1999) *National Service Framework for Mental Health.* Department of Health.

Department of Health (2000) *Shaping the Future NHS: Long Term Planning for Hospitals and Related Services Consultation Document on the Findings of the National Beds Inquiry – Supporting Analysis.* Department of Health.

Department of Health (2001) *Mental Health Policy Implementation Guide.* Department of Health.

Department of Health (2008) *Refocusing the Care Programme Approach.* Department of Health.

Donnelly M (1983) *Managing the Mind. A Study of Medical Psychology in Early 19th Century Britain.* Tavistock.

Early DF (1960) The Industrial Therapy Organisation (Bristol). *Lancet,* ii: 754–7.

Early DF (1973) Bristol Industrial Therapy Housing Association: a contribution to domestic resettlement. *British Medical Journal,* ii: 491–4.

Ellenberger HF (1970) *The Discovery of the Unconscious.* Basic Books.

Goffman E (1961) *Asylums.* Anchor Books.

House of Commons (1815) *Report, Together with Minutes of Evidence. The Committee Appointed to Consider of Provision Being Made for the Better Regulations of Madhouses in England* (http://books.google.co.uk, accessed 22 March 2013).

Joint Commissioning Panel for Mental Health (2012) *Guidance for Commissioners of Rehabilitation Services for People with Complex Mental Health Needs* (http://www.jcpmh. info/wp-content/uploads/jcpmh-rehab-guide.pdf, accessed 27 March 2013).

Leff J (1997) *Community Care. Illusion or Reality?* Wiley.

Leff J, Trieman N (2000) Long-stay patients discharged from psychiatric hospitals. *Social and clinical outcomes after five years in the community. TAPS Project 46. British Journal of Psychiatry,* **174**: 217–23.

Leff J, Trieman N, Knapp M, *et al* (2000) The TAPS Project. A report on 13 years of research, 1985–1998. *Psychiatric Bulletin,* **24**: 165–8.

McWilliam W (1926) Habit training for mental patients. *Journal of Mental Science,* **72**: 279.

Mills E (1962) *Living with Mental Illness. A Study in East London.* Routledge and Kegan Paul.

Morgan C, McKenzie K, Fearon P (eds) (2008) *Society and Psychosis.* Cambridge University Press.

Mountain D, Killaspy H, Holloway F(2009) Mental health rehabilitation services in the UK in 2007. *Psychiatric Bulletin,* **33**: 215–18.

National Schizophrenia Fellowship (1984) Community care, the sham behind the slogan. *Psychiatric Bulletin,* **8**: 112–14.

Poole R, Ryan T, Pearsall A (2002) The NHS, the private sector, and the virtual asylum. *BMJ,* **325**: 349–50.

Priebe S, Badesconyi A, Fioritti A, *et al* (2005) Reinstitutionalisation in mental health care: comparison of data on service provision from six European countries. *BMJ,* **330**: 123–6.

Scull AT (1982) *Museums of Madness.* Penguin.

Stein G (2011) The case of King Saul: did he have recurrent unipolar depression or bipolar affective disorder? Psychiatry in the Old Testament. *British Journal of Psychiatry,* **198**: 212.

Stone MH (1998) *Healing the Mind. A History of Psychiatry from Antiquity to the Present.* Pimlico.

Trieman N, Leff J (2002) Long-term outcome of long-stay inpatients considered unsuitable to live in the community. TAPS Project 44. *British Journal of Psychiatry*, **181**: 428–432.

Trieman N, Leff J, Glover G (1999) Outcome of long stay psychiatric patients resettled in the community: prospective cohort study. *BMJ*, **319**: 13–16.

Tuke S (1813) *Description of The Retreat, An Institution Near York For Insane Persons of the Society of Friends*. W Alexander (http://books.google.co.uk, accessed 22 March 2013).

Watts FN, Bennett DH (eds) (1983) *Theory and Practice of Psychiatric Rehabilitation*. Wiley.

Wing JK, Brown GW (1970) *Institutionalism and Schizophrenia*. Cambridge University Press.

Wolfson P, Holloway F, Killaspy H (2009) *Enabling Recovery for People with Complex Mental Health Needs. A Template for Rehabilitation Services*. Faculty Report FR/RS/1. Faculty of Rehabilitation and Social Psychiatry, Royal College of Psychiatrists.

Yapijakis C (2009) Hippocrates of Kos, the father of clinical medicine, and Asclepiades of Bithynia, the father of molecular medicine. *In Vivo*, **23**: 507–14.

Youssef HA, Youssef FA (1996) Evidence for the existence of schizophrenia in medieval Islamic society. *History of Psychiatry*, **7**: 55–62.

CHAPTER 2

What is psychiatric rehabilitation?

Tom Craig and Helen Killaspy

Introduction

Rehabilitation is defined by the World Health Organization (1980) as the application of measures aimed at reducing the impact of disabling and handicapping conditions and enabling people with a disability to achieve social integration. Implicit in this definition are two components: first, an active process through which a person adapts or acquires the skills needed to mitigate the constraints of disease; and second, an acknowledgement that there may also need to be changes in the environment, including the attitudes of people without a disability, if optimal social integration is to be achieved.

For William Anthony, product champion of psychiatric rehabilitation in the USA, rehabilitation involves 'improving the psychiatrically disturbed person's capabilities and competence' by bringing about 'behavioural improvement in their environment of need' (Anthony *et al*, 1984: 140). In subtle contrast, Douglas Bennett (1978), whose views strongly influenced UK practice, emphasised helping individuals adapt to their deficits in personal skills by 'making best use of [their] residual abilities in order to function in as normal environment as possible'.

Psychiatric rehabilitation is frequently defined as the activity of a set of specialist services. An alternative formulation would be in terms of the needs or characteristics of people who would benefit from rehabilitation inputs. Wykes & Holloway (2000) defined the potential client group as people with severe and long-term mental illnesses who have both active symptomatology and impaired social functioning as a consequence of their mental illness. From this definition they argued that rehabilitation services should have the joint aims of minimising the symptoms of illness and promoting the social inclusion of clients.

Recent years have seen a growing focus on mental health rehabilitation in the UK. Killaspy *et al* (2005) collated responses from rehabilitation practitioners into a contemporary definition:

> A whole systems approach to recovery from mental illness that maximises an individual's quality of life and social inclusion by encouraging their skills,

promoting independence and autonomy in order to give them hope for the future and leads to successful community living through appropriate support (p. 163).

Although rehabilitation services were marginalised during the period of investment in specialist community teams described in the *National Service Framework for Mental Health* (Department of Health, 1999), there has been a resurgence of interest in mental health rehabilitation over the past decade, as it has become increasingly clear that the new teams (providing assertive outreach, early intervention and crisis resolution) were not able to offer a viable alternative for people with the most complex mental health problems. There is now an acceptance of the ongoing need for specialist rehabilitation services that provide assessment, treatment and longer-term support to individuals whose needs cannot be met by general adult mental health services.

Around 10% of people entering mental health services will have particularly complex needs that require rehabilitation and intensive support over many years (Craig *et al*, 2004a). The majority have a diagnosis of psychosis complicated by prominent 'negative' symptoms that impair their motivation and organisational skills to manage everyday activities and that place them at risk of self-neglect (Wykes & Dunn, 1992; Wykes *et al*, 1992; Green, 1996). Many also have 'positive' symptoms (delusions and hallucinations) that have not responded fully to medication and can make communication and engagement difficult (Holloway, 2005). It is estimated that around a third of people with a diagnosis of schizophrenia do not respond adequately to antipsychotic medication (Meltzer *et al*, 1997).

Many also have coexisting problems that further complicate their recovery, including other mental health issues (such as depression and anxiety), long-term physical health conditions (such as chronic obstructive pulmonary disease and cardiovascular disease), pre-existing disorders (such as intellectual disability and developmental disorders, including those on the autistic spectrum) and substance misuse. Most have considerable disability and impaired mental capacity to make everyday decisions, which may lead to vulnerability to exploitation and abuse by others and may require safeguarding. They may present with challenging behaviours, including aggression to others. All these complex problems may result in lengthy hospital stays (Holloway, 2005).

Typically, the contemporary pathway to a rehabilitation service involves many years of illness and disability (see Case example 2.1, which relates Simon's story). A recent survey of in-patient mental health rehabilitation services found that service users had experienced mental health problems for an average of 13 years and had been recurrently admitted to hospital before referral for rehabilitation (Killaspy *et al*, 2013). By this time the patient, the family and the supporting services will have, at best, low expectations or, at worst, may have lost hope altogether.

Case example 2.1 Simon's journey into a rehabilitation service

Simon is in his early 40s. He has had a diagnosis of schizophrenia for 15 years. He has been hospitalised five times, being compulsorily detained three times. A prominent feature of his illness is his unshakeable conviction that he is under constant surveillance by a government organisation. He believes he is followed wherever he goes and frequently sees people who he believes are these agents, on the street and in local shops. Partly through fearfulness and partly through apathy, he spends most of his time alone in his flat. He takes no interest in his appearance or hygiene. He has problems managing the upkeep of his flat and owes a considerable amount of unpaid rent. He has not worked for many years. The view of some clinicians is that his is a pretty hopeless case. In the course of the long illness, he has received all the usual (and some not so usual) pharmacological and psychosocial interventions, but to apparently little effect.

Simon's view is just as bleak, if not more so. In the past 10 years he has had two consultant psychiatrists, who he has seen mostly during his spells in hospital, and a string of trainee psychiatrists, seen fleetingly in an out-patient clinic. His main contact had been with a community psychiatric nurse but she moved away just as he was beginning to believe someone might have had his interests at heart. Conversations with mental health staff have mainly concerned medication or been disapproving of his lifestyle. He has picked up the air of hopelessness that surrounds his case, noticing that the enthusiastic promises of new treatments and new referrals (in which he had little faith anyway) have long since dropped away. Having been out of employment for many years, he does not believe he is employable or indeed able to work, and cannot see the point of attending a day centre to mingle with strangers or to work without reward. He feels quite powerless to do anything himself and has come to the view that there is little anyone else can do either.

Despite this background of hopelessness and mistrust, it is the common experience of every professional with an interest in rehabilitation that such apparently intractable situations can be turned around to a surprising degree. The ingredients for this success are: (1) the development of a culture of empowerment, healing and hope; (2) the provision of interventions to limit the impact of disability; and (3) making adjustments to the environment that ease the burden of handicap.

Rehabilitation services adopt a 'recovery' approach that values service users as partners in a collaborative relationship with staff to identify and work towards personalised goals. The concept of recovery encompasses the values of hope, agency, opportunity and inclusion, themes that resonate well with the aims of mental health rehabilitation.

Mental health rehabilitation services aim to enable people with complex mental health problems to acquire or regain the skills and confidence to live successfully in the community. They focus on addressing and minimising the symptoms and functional impairment associated with complex and longer-term severe mental health problems while enabling individuals to achieve as much autonomy and independence as possible. This includes optimal management of symptoms, promotion of activities of daily living and meaningful occupation, screening for physical health problems and promoting healthy living, as well as providing support and evidence-based interventions to support carers.

In order to deliver these interventions, rehabilitation services operate as a whole system that includes a range of in-patient and community services, supported accommodation and vocational services provided by statutory, independent and voluntary sector organisations.

This chapter provides a brief and critical outline of how the key ingredients of rehabilitation can be provided. Specific elements of the rehabilitation process are described in much more detail elsewhere in this book. The 'What is psychiatric rehabilitation?' of the chapter title is clarified by answering the question 'How can we best carry out psychiatric rehabilitation?' Throughout the chapter, the focus is on rehabilitation services. It is important to emphasise that the task of rehabilitation can, of course, be undertaken in a wide range of alternative services and settings, or indeed in no particular setting at all. To an important extent, rehabilitation is as much an approach or attitude of mind as it is a treatment technology. At the same time, the rehabilitation care pathway is key in ensuring that the necessary components of treatment, care and support are available to enable individuals in their recovery. Rehabilitation is therefore not one specific intervention or even one complex intervention; it does not take place in one particular ward, unit or supported accommodation facility. It is a process that needs to be tailored to each individual's particular and changing needs over the longer term.

Promoting a culture of healing and instilling hope

Rediscovering recovery

Long before the discovery of effective medical and psychological treatments for psychosis, it was known that better outcomes could be obtained where people were treated with respect and dignity and in settings that emphasised collaboration between staff and patients. This understanding was seen in the moral treatment provided in the best early 19th-century asylums and in the social psychiatry revolution of the 1950s (see Chapter 1, 'Rehabilitation in a historical context').

These earlier insights have re-emerged in the 'recovery' paradigm, which has its origins in the consumer/ex-patient empowerment movement (see Chapter 3, 'Rehabilitation as a values-led practice'). In this latest formulation, a distinction is drawn between the technologies of rehabilitation and the process of recovery, the latter being defined as: 'the lived or real life experience of persons as they accept and overcome the challenge of the disability' (Deegan, 1988: p. 11). This recovery process is understood to be unique to the individual. In large part it is the discovery of a purpose and meaning to life. It calls for an active daily life, the assumption of personal responsibility, the exercise of choice and a degree of risk-taking. The individual may find purpose and meaning through work, in personal relationships, or even through political action or advocacy on behalf of others. Importantly, there is no assumption of 'cure' in the sense of entirely escaping symptoms or impairments; instead, the emphasis is on achieving a fulfilling existence despite enduring disability.

These ideas emphasise the critical importance of collaboration in therapy, of choice rather than coercion, positive reinforcement of success rather than punishment for failure and a shared involvement with professionals in how the service is provided. For practitioners, this is the difference between viewing a patient as a person who happens to suffer from schizophrenia and labelling him or her 'a schizophrenic'. This is a subtle but important distinction, as it opens the door for conversations about what might be attempted or achieved despite the diagnosis or such and such symptom or experience. This focus and emphasis on the possibility of success rather than of failure, looking forward rather than backward and making much of small steps to instil hope and fuel self-esteem and self-respect.

Empowerment

In addition to instilling hope, a core task of rehabilitation is empowerment. Empowerment is both something provided externally by the way services are structured and an internal psychological state of self-worth, self-confidence and courage to take calculated risks and to take responsibility for them. In terms of how services are structured, empowerment is facilitated both by ensuring that therapeutic interventions are collaborative, negotiated and their purpose transparent and by encouraging patients to take more personal responsibility for setting goals, working to achieve them and making decisions.

Much of what is involved in recovery is the business of picking up lost social roles – as tenant, employee, friend and so forth. In this respect, 'dependency' is not an entirely bad word. Recognising a state of dependency is typically the starting point of a recovery, although it is not without risks, in terms both of being let down by those on whom one depends and of sapping initiative and self-directed action. In the recovery approach, the aim is to move from dependency towards progressively more personal responsibility for choices and goals and their associated risks.

Principles into practice

For people entering a typical rehabilitation service (Case example 2.1), changes in their experiences might begin the moment they are admitted to the unit. Instead of a frantic acute ward, here is a relaxed, even-paced setting with a clear purpose to the day. Staff are interested in them as people, their views are taken seriously and therapeutic arrangements occur when they are scheduled. They are expected to contribute to the life of the unit and it is clear that their contributions are valued and matter. Although they may not be entirely convinced that treatment is likely to be helpful, they may be pleased nonetheless that its purpose is explained and that it is delivered at a pace they can manage. During the course of their stay their experiences are listened to seriously and as much, if not more, attention is paid to the successes in life as to the consequences of their illness. It is within this context that technical interventions that have failed in the past may succeed.

Limiting disability: processes and services

Impairment, disability and handicap

The recovery paradigm within mental health services is fashionable. Much less fashionable is an analysis of the complex effects of mental illness on the sufferer. It is helpful in understanding these effects to make distinctions between *impairment, disability* and *handicap:*

- In the context of severe mental illness, *impairments* comprise the positive and negative, affective and cognitive symptoms of the illness (e.g. distressing auditory hallucinations, social withdrawal, depression and impaired concentration, all commonly experienced by someone with schizophrenia)
- *Disabilities* are the difficulties someone experiences in performing everyday tasks (e.g. shopping, cooking, functioning at work) as a result of impairment.
- *Handicap* is the disadvantage and exclusion from social roles consequent on impairments and disabilities, but also on external factors such as stigma, alienation from friends and family, unemployment, homelessness and poverty. (People with severe mental illness have also commonly experienced significant social disadvantage *before* becoming ill.)

An additional and important issue is the *personal reaction* to the impairments, disabilities and social disadvantage they experience as a result of an episode of illness. People often experience depression and despair or, conversely, deny that there are problems that need to be addressed. Adverse personal reactions can compound and amplify the effects of illness on an individual.

Simon (Case example 2.1), for instance, suffers severe disabilities in terms of self-care, occupational functioning and social skills as a consequence of the symptomatic and cognitive impairments of his illness. Even if the severity of the symptomatic impairments could be reduced, there would remain much work to do in order to rebuild Simon's self-esteem, confidence and day-to-day coping skills. Handicaps from the illness have already arisen – debt, unemployment and alienation of friends and family. Thus it should come as little surprise that managing symptoms alone is not enough. The stigma, shabby accommodation and poverty Simon has experienced will serve to erode self-esteem, destroy confidence and promote disability: instilling hope becomes a central requirement for Simon's chances of recovery from his illness.

Vulnerability, stress, coping and competence

Another useful way of conceptualising the focus of psychiatric rehabilitation is to consider the *vulnerability–stress–coping–competence* model (Anthony & Liberman, 1986). In this model, biological vulnerabilities predispose people to illness when they are exposed to environmental stress (e.g. interpersonal tensions or life events). Even if the biological vulnerability is impervious to intervention, the triggering and maintaining stressors can be mitigated by medication or by interventions that teach skills to cope with arousal or that provide buffering support. Rehabilitation can aim to reduce exposure to stress, to optimise protective factors and to develop living and coping skills.

Organising rehabilitation services

The ideal rehabilitation service provides a comprehensive, continuous, coordinated, collaborative and patient-oriented approach. Interventions are linked to individualised needs assessments and to the personal goals of patients, each step negotiated and aiming at end-points that are personally meaningful and desired. The rehabilitation care pathway provides a continuum of treatment and support settings that facilitate this graduated, step-by-step approach (see Fig. 2.1).

A key aspect of effective rehabilitation is the recognition that people's behaviour varies substantially from one situation to another. In general, task performance is more stable than social behaviour and simple skills are more transferable than complex ones. Many of the improvements seen in a narrow rehabilitation setting are transient responses to the particular characteristic of that environment and do not readily transfer or generalise to more complex settings and situations. Therefore, rehabilitation assessment should focus more on an individual's capacities than on fixed behaviours, and should ideally be carried out across a wide spectrum of settings and conditions in an attempt to work out what may be achieved under optimal conditions and what problems are likely in suboptimal conditions. People should be prepared for the environments in which they will be expected to function and, in general, it is better to rehabilitate *in vivo* than in the contrived setting of the hospital clinic.

Transitions between different settings along the rehabilitation care pathway can be destabilising in an individual's recovery. It is not uncommon for people to have to make more than one attempt at a transition from a more highly supported to a less supported setting. Being willing to adapt

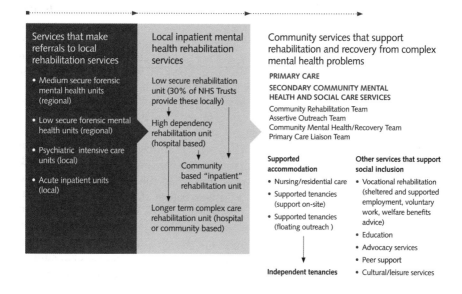

Fig. 2.1 Components of a 'whole system' rehabilitation care pathway (from Joint Commissioning Panel for Mental Health, 2012, reproduced with permission)

and reset goals to facilitate a successful move even after many previous failed attempts is one example of how rehabilitation practitioners can hold and work with therapeutic optimism for an individual. Conversely, transitions can sometimes prove surprisingly empowering in promoting people's abilities that they had had little motivation to use in a more supported setting.

It is also worth distinguishing long-term targets from short-term goals. The former are often couched in fairly broad terms, while the latter are the stepping stones to take the person to where he or she wants to go. Short-term goals need to be 'SMART' (Specific, Measurable, Achievable, Realistic and Time-limited) and set in collaboration with the patient, relatives and other relevant people. Specific interventions can then be devised with these short-term goals in mind that aim to produce a series of consistent, if modest achievements, backed up by frequent praise, encouragement and support.

Some 30 years ago Watts & Bennett (1983: p. 12) drew attention to the need to avoid setting goals that are unrealistically high or demoralisingly low. It is important to emphasise the individual's positive capacities and achievements, not only for the good this does to self-esteem but also as 'the most effective antidote to the paternalistic attitudes that develop when psychiatric services try merely to care for long term patients'.

Minimising impairment and disability

Pharmacological management

The past decade has seen advances in the pharmacological treatment of severe mental illness. Currently, the vogue is the newer 'atypical' antipsychotics. These drugs are as effective, at least in the short term, as traditional treatments, while having fewer troublesome extrapyramidal side-effects (Davis *et al*, 2003). (The exception is clozapine, which is undoubtedly more effective than other antipsychotics.) The initial enthusiasm with which 'atypicals' were greeted by many rehabilitation psychiatrists has waned somewhat now that the majority of patients have already received these 'new' drugs before their first contact with rehabilitation services.

We have also seen the emergence of longer-term side-effects of atypical antipsychotics with protracted use. Of these, weight gain is probably the feature of most concern to patients. It is difficult to predict for the individual but the risk factors include a younger age and good clinical response to treatment (Jones *et al*, 2001). The prevalence of diabetes in people with schizophrenia is almost twice that in the general population and may be further increased with some antipsychotic treatment (Baptista *et al*, 2002). These caveats aside, there is clearly an important role for the expert management of psychotropic medication in severe and enduring mental illness, not only for the control of symptoms but also for the management of co-occurring depression and cognitive impairment.

The challenge for medication management in rehabilitation is seldom a matter of finding an effective cocktail to address a range of comorbidities and more often a matter of a systematic appraisal of the diagnosis and of what treatments have been tried before, for how long and with what effect, sometimes returning to an earlier approach but for a longer or modified trial. Occasionally this throws up a gem – a previous failure to have considered clozapine or a missed mood component to the illness – but more typically it is a matter of adopting a different, more collaborative approach to choosing and administering medication, tackling practical difficulties and attending to and minimising side-effects. Decisions should always be framed in the context of individual responsibility for patients' self-management of their condition. Chapter 14, 'Management of medication when treatment is failing', offers authoritative advice on this difficult topic.

Cognitive–behavioural interventions

Cognitive–behavioural interventions have wide applicability for enduring mental illness (see Chapter 9, 'Cognitive approaches'). For schizophrenia, for example, the main aim is to reduce distress and disability, and to help the individual develop an understanding of his or her illness (Fowler *et al*, 1995). Patients are encouraged to re-evaluate their beliefs through a gradual process of reviewing the evidence and constructing alternative explanations and to identify and manipulate factors that contribute to symptom maintenance. The therapist works collaboratively, taking an active, enquiring stance towards the patient's account of the experiences. Direct confrontation of delusions is avoided, as this has been shown to be counterproductive. Moderately severe thought disorder can be tackled by disentangling the most emotionally relevant themes and helping the patient focus on these themes using thought linkage techniques. Patients are encouraged to develop and use a variety of coping strategies, including anxiety management, activity scheduling and attention control to reduce the occurrence and duration of hallucinations and of distressing experiences of anxiety or suspiciousness (Tarrier, 1992). An impressive number of randomised controlled trials have now been carried out, from which it appears that cognitive–behavioural therapy for psychosis (CBTp) is beneficial in terms of reduction of positive symptoms and distress (Pilling, *et al*, 2002a; Wykes *et al*, 2008; NICE, 2009).

As with most treatments in medicine, early enthusiasm is often tempered by experience of larger, more rigorously controlled clinical trials and the same can be said for CBTp. The original claims for efficacy in terms of reducing relapse have been questioned by a failure to replicate earlier observations (Garety *et al*, 2008), but even the most rigorous meta-analyses support the assertion that the intervention is helpful for reducing the experience of positive symptoms and distress, with reported effect sizes of 0.2–0.4 (Wykes *et al*, 2008). This compares favourably with a recent meta-analysis of placebo-controlled randomised trials of second-generation antipsychotic medication that showed a pooled effect size of 0.51, with that for positive symptoms of 0.48 (Leucht *et al*, 2009), or with the introduction of clozapine in treatment-resistant cases (Conley *et al*, 2009).

While CBTp may be effective and has been around for more than two decades, it is still not widely available. Surveys suggest that as few as 10% of eligible patients get access to CBTp if a rigorous definition of an adequate dose of therapy is adopted (Prytys *et al*, 2011). A way of achieving a step change in service capacity is needed. A distinction between 'low-intensity' and 'high-intensity' therapy has been made for psychological therapy in other guidelines from the National Institute for Health and Clinical Excellence (NICE) and has now formed the basis of the national Improving Access to Psychological Therapies (IAPT) programme for implementing the NICE guidelines on anxiety and depression. There is some evidence to support the use of these low-intensity methods such as graded exposure and behavioural activation with people with schizophrenia (e.g. Turkington *et al*, 2002; Mairs *et al*, 2011; Waller *et al*, 2013). Furthermore, non-specialist staff can deliver these interventions effectively after brief training (e.g. Ekers *et al*, 2011, Waller *et al*, 2013).

Family interventions

In the UK, there has been a long-standing interest in the effect of the family environment on major mental illness. This led to the development of family interventions that include education about the nature of the illness, emotional support and training in how to cope with illness-related symptoms and behaviours. Family interventions have been shown in repeated clinical trials to be effective in preventing relapse and rehospitalisation, possibly partly through increased adherence to pharmacological treatment (Pilling *et al*, 2002*a*; NICE, 2009; Pharoah *et al*, 2010). By and large, as is the case for CBTp, later studies have produced somewhat less positive results than the earliest investigations, possibly because the early studies were led by charismatic enthusiasts (Mari & Streiner, 1994) or because later ones used less-potent family group methods (Pilling *et al*, 2002*a*).

The NICE guideline for schizophrenia (2009) in the UK and the Schizophrenia Patient Outcomes Research Team (PORT; Lehman *et al*, 2004) in the USA recommend that family interventions be routinely available for the families of people with schizophrenia. A recent meta-analysis of 53 randomised controlled trials concluded that family interventions reduced relapse and rehospitalisation (with number needed to treat of around 6), encouraged compliance with prescribed medication, and improved general social function and levels of expressed emotion (Pharoah *et al*, 2010).

As is the case for CBTp, it remains a challenge to put this research into routine clinical practice (see Chapter 10, 'Family interventions').

Skills training

Interventions aimed at correcting deficits in daily living skills such as poor personal hygiene, problems managing the home or dealing with finances are ubiquitous in rehabilitation practice; indeed, they form the basis for the daily work of nurses and occupational therapists in most if not all services. Many of these interventions involve simple advice, coaching and modelling. The more elaborate schemes draw upon operant conditioning theory. In the most elaborate (but now largely defunct) approach, programmes were developed based on patients collecting tangible rewards ('tokens') for performing desired behaviours. These were hugely complex programmes that were very difficult to implement and have proven untenable outside of very specialised settings. The skills acquired in the hospital or clinic setting often failed to generalise to daily life, which had far more complexity than could be managed by a simple contingency-based reward system.

One skills training approach with a well-developed research base is the modular programme developed by Liberman and his colleagues at the UCLA Clinical Research Center for Schizophrenia and Psychiatric Rehabilitation. This behavioural programme teaches a range of skills, including medication self-management, basic conversational skills, grooming and self-care, job-finding and interpersonal problem-solving. A broad range of interventions are employed, including videotape demonstrations, role-play, *in vivo* exercises and homework practice (Wallace *et al*, 1985).

There have been numerous clinical trials showing benefits over standard care in terms of improved conversational skills, assertiveness and medication management (Heinssen *et al*, 2000). These methods have been successfully employed with acute in-patients, patients with residual symptoms and patients with severe and persistent illness. Not surprisingly, given the focus on specific social behaviours, social skills training has only a modest impact on symptoms, relapse and hospitalisation. Some studies have found no significant advantage over more traditional occupational therapy or group-based supportive psychotherapy. Evidence on the extent to which new skills learnt in specific programmes generalise across settings or fade with time is sparse, though what there is points to a severe problem in generalisation from the classroom to real life. There is some evidence for the benefit of including 'top-up' sessions and for carrying out some training away from the initial treatment setting (Eckman *et al*, 1992).

These formal programmes have proven much less popular in Europe than in the USA. A meta-analysis of randomised controlled trials of skills training found no consistent evidence for any benefit on relapse rate, global adjustment, social functioning or quality of life (Pilling *et al*, 2002*b*). There is, however, little reason to expect that an intervention aimed at improving self-care should have any impact on relapse or rehospitalisation. Perhaps the prevailing view in the UK reflects a wider shift towards the cognitive end of the cognitive–behavioural spectrum of psychological interventions in recent years. Whatever the reason, it is striking that the interventions that comprise so much of nursing, occupational therapy and psychological practice in rehabilitation settings is so under-researched in the UK.

Cognitive remediation

Cognitive impairment in schizophrenia predicts poor rehabilitation outcomes. So it is an appealing thought that remediation of the impairments of memory and executive function commonly seen in people with severe mental illness might facilitate skills training and contribute to improved social functioning (see Chapter 9, 'Cognitive approaches'). Cognitive remediation seeks to retrain and improve memory, attention and speed of information processing using a variety of 'exercise' programmes that were originally developed for neurological rehabilitation (e.g. after head injury or stroke).

Wykes *et al* (2007) randomised 85 patients to 40 sessions of cognitive remediation or to 'treatment as usual'. Patients receiving the intensive remediation attended at least three times weekly until 40 sessions were completed. The cognitive remediation focused on deficits in executive functioning (cognitive flexibility, working memory and planning). Cognitive remediation led to durable improvements in working memory as well as improvement in cognitive flexibility. Furthermore, memory improvement predicted improvement in social functioning.

A meta-analysis of randomised trials (Wykes *et al*, 2011) found that cognitive remediation has an enduring impact on global cognition and functioning. It was more effective when the patient's condition was stable and where it was provided as part of a wider rehabilitation programme. The effect sizes are similar to that found for CBTp, although of course focused on cognitive rather than symptomatic outcomes.

As we have seen for CBTp and family interventions, such benefits achieved in research settings do not necessarily transfer easily to routine care. In one attempt to introduce cognitive remediation as a routine intervention, a total of 23 rehabilitation staff received training but of these 13 subsequently moved to new jobs, where it is unlikely their new skills were utilised. Of the 16 clients who had been identified as suitable for cognitive remediation, only five were willing and able to participate and only two completed the course, one of whom was thought to have benefited substantially (Cupitt *et al*, 2004).

Addressing handicap

A home of one's own?

Throughout the 1970s and early 1980s, rehabilitation came to be regarded as synonymous with resettlement of the long-stay hospital population. This narrow view was rightly criticised at the time, not least because of the danger that, once the patient had been resettled, the job of rehabilitation might be seen to be over. A range of accommodation options, from highly staffed residential homes through to independent flats with visiting support forms an essential ingredient of any modern psychiatric service (see Chapter 19, 'Housing'). However, there is surprisingly little research into the relative benefits of different configurations of housing and support.

Perhaps the best-known British research was carried out into the closure and re-provision of Friern Barnet Hospital in north London (see Leff, 1997, for a summary of the main findings). The majority of re-provision was into group homes with shared facilities. These settings were less regimented and restrictive than the hospital and were preferred by patients to the hospital ward. Living in the community had some advantages, such as low rehospitalisation rates and, for some, the opportunity to develop friendships with ordinary members of the public. While individual patients showed large fluctuations in symptoms over the follow-up, there was no overall change in psychiatric state for the whole sample and behavioural problems also remained stable. There was little difference in cost between hospital and community care once account was taken of the few patients with particularly challenging behaviours who could not be immediately discharged to the community.

Comparable outcomes of hospital closure programmes have been reported both elsewhere in the UK and internationally (for a comprehensive review see Fakhoury & Priebe, 2002). The number of residents living in such shared accommodation has risen substantially in the past decade, in line with Europe-wide trends in psychiatric care (Priebe *et al*, 2005).

In the UK, investment in new specialist community teams promoted by the *National Service Framework for Mental Health* (Department of Health, 1999) led to a disinvestment in mental health rehabilitation services (Mountain *et al*, 2009). This was followed by a rapid and uncontrolled rise in the provision of 'out-of-area placements' in hospital, nursing homes and residential care homes in the independent sector for people with longer-term and complex mental health problems who could not be discharged from acute admission wards (Davies *et al*, 2005; Department of Health, 2011). This phenomenon has been referred to as the 'virtual asylum', since, until recently, there was little attention paid to the ongoing review of these individuals' needs and their potential for recovery and progress to more independent living (Poole *et al*, 2002). Concerns have been raised about the social dislocation caused when service users are placed many miles from their homes and criticisms have been made of the quality of care and lack of rehabilitative ethos in some out-of-area facilities (Ryan *et al*, 2004). It is also the case that out-of-area placements cost, on average, around 65% more than similar local services (Killaspy & Meier, 2010) and there are often inadequate systems for monitoring the quality of care and the ongoing need for the level of support provided (Ryan *et al*, 2007). Thus, the 'virtual asylum' at best replaces the asylum ward with more 'homely' environments but at worst substitutes one order of neglect with another (Geller, 2000).

An alternative model relies more on a partnership between the providers of ordinary public housing and mental health services, the latter coordinating and providing a range of training and treatment. Such models are preferred by patients and carers (Carling, 1993). But this is not to say that such an approach guarantees a better outcome. The default approach is not to provide continuing monitoring and care through a specialist rehabilitation service, but rather to leave the case management to already overstretched generic community teams or to inexperienced housing support workers who may have little appreciation of the complexity of severe mental illness. Without close attention, there are real risks of neglect, abuse and institutionalisation in these settings (Carling, 1995). Chapter 18, 'Community-based rehabilitation and recovery', discusses the importance of specialist community rehabilitation teams.

No substantial evaluations of the 'mobile support' model have been carried out in the UK. Limited evidence is available from the USA. In one thought-provoking study, Susser *et al* (1997) randomised 96 homeless men with mental illness who were being rehoused to receive either 9 months of a 'critical time' service (comprising intensive case management, including tenancy support) or care as usual. At 18-month follow-up, the average number of homeless nights was 30 for the 'critical time' group and 91 for the group receiving usual services. Overall costs of care were similar in the two groups (Jones *et al*, 2003).

Attempts have also been made to implement and evaluate city-wide programmes. One such effort was sponsored by the Robert Wood Johnson Foundation and the US Department of Housing and Urban Development. This brought together housing and health authorities in nine cities to provide and evaluate a comprehensive system of housing subsidy and mobile support for people suffering from severe mental illness. The success of this programme varied widely from city to city, with some benefits in terms of quality of life but no substantial effect on clinical outcomes or rehospitalisation (Goldman *et al*, 1994). Social isolation and the lack of recreational opportunities were frequently cited problems in these programmes, any expansion in social contacts often being confined to health professionals and fellow residents (Friedrich *et al*, 1999).

A job to do

The importance of meaningful occupation and employment to recovery has been recognised since the dawn of 'moral treatment' (see Chapter 20, 'Work and employment'). Shockingly, employment rates for people with severe mental illness are far lower now than in the 1950s (Marwaha & Johnson, 2004). There are many reasons for this, not least profound changes in the nature of available work and the demands for performance made on employees and employers in the 21st-century economy. There may be a tendency for mental health professionals to overestimate the negative impact of the stress of employment on mental health and to underestimate their clients' capacity for work (Secker *et al*, 2001). Negative symptoms of schizophrenia, poor social skills and neuropsychological impairments have all been shown to impair performance at work. Medication side-effects can also be problematic, particularly sedation: this will be less of an issue in contemporary practice, where high-dose regimes are avoided.

The earliest models in the post-asylum era involved the transfer of hospital-based industrial therapy units and work crews into smaller community-based offices on the high street, where part-time, low or unpaid occupation was provided. Movement from these settings to competitive employment in the open labour market is rare and the model has fallen out of favour, though the risks of dependency and institutionalisation can be minimised by an emphasis on market orientation, employee involvement and regularly reviewed action plans.

These early occupational models took it for granted that patients with severe mental illness required extensive training in work habits before they could attempt to find employment in open society. This belief has been challenged with the emergence of new models of supported employment that adopt a 'place then train' approach, with an emphasis instead on rapid job search and the provision of support once in the job. The approach now has a solid evidence base in terms of achieving off-welfare open employment in the USA (where it originated), in Australia and in some countries in Europe. Employment rates as high as 60% are quoted, compared with

20% or less in traditional vocational rehabilitation (Bond, 2004; Burns *et al*, 2007; Bond *et al*, 2008). The approach achieves high rates of competitive employment without increasing hospitalisation, but, on the down side, job turnover is high, the majority of placements are in rather low-paid, unskilled occupations and a continuing high level of support is essential to job retention (McHugo *et al*, 1998). There are now a few long-term follow-up studies that suggest that people do move on to periods of longer job tenure (Salyers *et al*, 2004; Becker *et al*, 2007).

Another development worth mentioning is the 'Clubhouse' model (Beard *et al*, 1982), which provides a sheltered and supported employment programme. This emerged in the USA in the 1950s as a setting for support and preparation for employment. Clubhouse is particularly interesting as it has many characteristics reminiscent of therapeutic communities. People attending clubhouse are members, not patients or clients, and are expected to participate in all aspects of the organisation, sharing responsibility with staff for maintaining the building, preparing meals, working in the office and greeting visitors. Staff and members work side by side and there are no member-only or staff-only areas. Members are involved at every level of the organisation, including on the clubhouse board. Two models of employment support are provided. In the more sheltered approach, work placements are arranged in a variety of temporary jobs with mainstream employers, the employment contract being held by the clubhouse and placements capable of being shared on a part-time basis between members. But clubhouse also provides a supported employment service for those who express readiness for work. The model has been compared favourably to other supported employment schemes and, if anything, achieves somewhat better tenure in higher-quality jobs (Macias *et al*, 2006; Schonebaum *et al*, 2006). Clubhouse members are members for life and have open access to support as and when needed. In this way, clubhouse is rather better than other community services in providing the open-ended support that is advocated by the supported employment model. There are now over 300 clubhouses worldwide, mostly in the USA and Europe.

In Europe, many of the sheltered workshops have evolved or been trans-formed into 'social firms' – small market-oriented business ventures that are run by and/or employ significant numbers of people with various disabilities. There is some evidence for their commercial viability, high user satisfaction and reduced use of mental health services (Grove & Drurie, 1999).

There have been several successful programmes in which patients have been employed in front-line caring roles, typically in peer-support roles, in both the USA (Mowbray *et al*, 1998; Solomon & Draine, 1998) and the UK (Craig *et al*, 2004*b*). Peer-support programmes have great potential, providing service users with a community of people who have a shared experience of mental ill-health and of psychiatric services. Benefits accrue to both service users and the peer providers themselves (Salzer & Shear, 2002). But most services have a poor record in recruiting people who have suffered from mental health problems and there must be every precaution to guard against employing service users as a cheaper alternative to statutory care (see Chapter 21, 'Peer support in mental health services').

The evaluation of these different models of employment is methodologically difficult, as they often involve small schemes with different local circumstances, patient populations and programme details. With this caveat in mind, there is now a fair amount of data available on what works, and practice guidelines are beginning to emerge. These essentially boil down to managing the tension between individual rehabilitation needs on the one hand and the market-oriented demands of the job on the other. For example, coping strategies such as taking frequent short breaks that may be helpful to maintain concentration or minimise intrusive hallucinations can be problematic in the workplace and viewed poorly by employers (Cook & Razzano, 2000). Also, while a comprehensive assessment of an individual's suitability for a particular post may take several weeks, many employers demand maximum productivity from the outset. Finally, no one model is likely to be sufficient for all rehabilitation needs. Each approach is likely to be helpful to different people at different times in their recovery (O'Flynn & Craig, 2001).

Many younger people in rehabilitation services will have had their education interrupted by the onset of their illness and for them a return to complete or supplement education may be an appropriate choice. There is far less research on how best to manage such a return to education. It seems logical to presume that similar considerations to those for returning to employment should apply here – with an emphasis on using ordinary education settings, on-site support and individualised programmes.

Conclusions

Although the thrust of this chapter has concerned people with chronic and persistent mental illness, the principles and ingredients of rehabilitation are also applicable to the early stages of illness, where they may play an important role in preventing disability. The 2 or 3 years following the first onset of severe mental illness have been identified as a critical period for intervention (Birchwood *et al*, 1998). It is during these early years that much damage is done to self-esteem and social networks, and when education and employment opportunities may be lost, never to come again.

Depression and anxiety are major causes of disability worldwide. The specific interventions for the management of severe neuroses and personality disorder are likely to be rather different from those described in this book, which largely concerns services for people with psychotic illnesses. However, the guiding principles of rehabilitation – *in vivo* delivery of goal-directed therapy managed in partnership and provided in a culture of empowerment and optimism – remain the cornerstone of all branches of mental healthcare. These rehabilitation principles are therefore not solely applicable to services with a designated 'rehabilitation' label, but are applicable to all mental health services operating at any stage in an individual's career of contact with the mental health system.

References

Anthony WA, Liberman RP (1986) The practice of psychiatric rehabilitation: historical, conceptual and research base. *Schizophrenia Bulletin*, **12**: 542–59.

Anthony WA, Cohen MR, Cohen BF (1984) Psychiatric rehabilitation. In *The Chronic Mental Patient. Five Years Later* (ed JA Talbott): 135–57. Grune & Stratton.

Baptista T, Kin N, Beaulieu S, *et al* (2002) Obesity and related metabolic abnormalities during antipsychotic drug administration: mechanisms, management and research perspectives. *Pharmacopsychiatry*, **35**: 205–19.

Beard JH, Propst RN, Malamud TJ (1982) The Fountain House model of rehabilitation. *Psychosocial Rehabilitation Journal*, **5**: 47–53.

Becker D, Whitley R, Bailey E, *et al* (2007) A long-term follow-up of adults with psychiatric disabilities who receive supported employment. *Psychiatric Services*, **58**: 922–8.

Bennett DH (1978) Community psychiatry, *British Journal of Psychiatry*, **132**: 209–20.

Birchwood M, Jackson C, Todd P (1998) The critical period hypothesis. *International Clinical Psychopharmacology*, **12**: 27–38.

Bond GR (2004) Supported employment: evidence for an evidence-based practice. *Psychiatric Rehabilitation Journal*, **27**: 345–59.

Bond GR, Drake RE, Becker DR (2008) An update on randomized controlled trials of evidence-based supported employment. *Psychiatric Rehabilitation Journal*, **31**: 280–90.

Burns T, Catty J, Becker T, *et al* (2007) The effectiveness of supported employment for people with severe mental illness: a randomised controlled trial. *Lancet*, **370**: 1146–52.

Carling PJ (1993) Housing and supports for persons with mental illness: emerging approaches to research and practice. *Hospital and Community Psychiatry*, **44**: 439–49.

Carling PJ (1995) *Returning to Community, Building Support Systems for People with Psychiatric Disabilities*. Guilford Press.

Conley R, Tamminga C, Kelly D, *et al* (2009) Treatment resistant schizophrenic patients respond to clozapine after olanzapine non-response. *Biological Psychiatry*, **43**: 76–7.

Cook JA, Razzano L (2000) Vocational rehabilitation for persons with schizophrenia: recent research and implications for practice. *Schizophrenia Bulletin*, **26**: 87–103.

Craig T, Garety P, Power P, *et al* (2004*a*) The Lambeth Early Onset (LEO) Team: randomised controlled trial of the effectiveness of specialised care for early psychosis. *BMJ*, **329**: 1067–71.

Craig T, Doherty I, Jamieson-Craig R, *et al* (2004*b*) The consumer-employee as a member of a mental health assertive outreach team. 1. Clinical and social outcomes. *Journal of Mental Health*, **13**: 59–69.

Cupitt C, Byrne L, Tompson N (2004) Delivering cognitive remediation therapy in a clinical setting. *Clinical Psychology*, **37**: 10–14.

Davies S, Mitchell S, Mountain D, *et al* (2005) *Out of Area Treatments for Working Age Adults with Complex and Severe Psychiatric Disorders: Review of Current Situation and Recommendations for Good Practice* (Faculty of Rehabilitation and Social Psychiatry Working Group Report). Royal College of Psychiatrists (http://www.rcpsych.ac.uk/workinpsychiatry/faculties/rehabilitationandsocial/resources.aspx).

Davis JM, Chen N, Glick ID (2003) A meta-analysis of the efficacy of second-generation antipsychotics. *Archives of General Psychiatry*, **60**: 553–64.

Deegan PE (1988) Recovery: the lived experience of rehabilitation. *Psychosocial Rehabilitation Journal*, **11**: 11–19.

Department of Health (1999) *National Service Framework for Mental Health*. TSO (The Stationery Office).

Department of Health (2011) In sight and in mind: A toolkit to reduce the use of out of area mental health services (www.rcpsych.ac.uk/pdf/insightandinmind.pdf).

Eckman TA, Wirshing WC, Marder SR, *et al* (1992) Technique for training schizophrenic patients in illness self-management: a controlled trial. *American Journal of Psychiatry*, **149**: 1549–55.

Ekers D, Richards D, McMillan D, *et al* (2011) Behavioural activation delivered by the non-specialist: phase II randomised controlled trial. *British Journal of Psychiatry*, **198**: 66–72.

Fakhoury W, Priebe S (2002) The process of deinstitutionalisation: an international review. *Current Opinion in Psychiatry*, **15**: 187–92.

Fowler D, Garety P, Kuipers E (1995) *Cognitive Behaviour Therapy for People with Psychosis*. John Wiley and Sons.

Friedrich RM, Hollingsworth B, Hradek E, *et al* (1999) Family and client perspectives on alternative residential settings for persons with severe mental illness. *Psychiatric Services*, **50**: 509–14.

Garety PA, Fowler DG, Freeman D, *et al* (2008) Cognitive behaviour therapy and family intervention for relapse prevention and symptom reduction in psychosis: randomised controlled trial. *British Journal of Psychiatry*, **192**: 412–23.

Geller JL (2000) The last half century of psychiatric services as reflected in 'Psychiatric Services'. *Psychiatric Services*, **51**: 41–67.

Goldman HH, Morrissey JP, Ridgely MS (1994) Evaluating the Robert Wood Johnson Foundation program on chronic mental illness. *Milbank Quarterly*, **72**: 37–47.

Green MF (1996) What are the functional consequences of neurocognitive deficits in schizophrenia? *American Journal of Psychiatry*, **153**: 321–30.

Grove B, Drurie S (1999) *Social Firms – An Instrument for Economic Empowerment and Inclusion*. Social Firms UK.

Heinssen RK, Liberman RP, Kopelowicz A (2000) Psychosocial skills training for schizophrenia: lessons from the laboratory. *Schizophrenia Bulletin*, **26**: 21–46.

Holloway F (2005) *The Forgotten Need for Rehabilitation in Contemporary Mental Health Services: A Position Statement from the Executive Committee of the Faculty of Rehabilitation and Social Psychiatry*. Royal College of Psychiatrists (http://www.rcpsych.ac.uk/pdf/frankholloway_oct05.pdf, accessed December 2014).

Joint Commissioning Panel for Mental Health (2012) *Guidance for Commissioners of Rehabilitation Services for People with Complex Mental Health Needs*. Royal College of Psychiatrists.

Jones B, Basson BR, Walker DJ, *et al* (2001) Weight change and atypical antipsychotic treatment in patients with schizophrenia. *Journal of Clinical Psychiatry*, **62** (suppl 2): 41–4.

Jones K, Colson PW, Holter MC, *et al* (2003) Cost-effectiveness of critical time intervention to reduce homelessness among persons with mental illness. *Psychiatric Services*, **54**: 884–90.

Killaspy H, Meier R (2010) A fair deal for mental health rehabilitation services. *The Psychiatrist*, **34**: 265–7.

Killaspy H, Harden C, Holloway F, *et al* (2005) What do mental health rehabilitation services do and what are they for? A national survey in England. *Journal of Mental Health* **14**: 157–66.

Killaspy H, Marston L, Omar R, *et al* (2013) Service quality and clinical outcomes: an example from mental health rehabilitation services in England (2013). *British Journal of Psychiatry*, **202**: 28–34.

Leff J (ed) (1997) *Care in the Community – Illusion or Reality?* Wiley.

Lehman AF, Kreyenbuhl J, Buchanan RW, *et al* (2004) The Schizophrenia Patient Outcomes Research Team (PORT): updated treatment recommendations. *Schizophrenia Bulletin*, **30**: 193–217.

Leucht S, Arbter D, Engel RR, *et al* (2009) How effective are second-generation antipsychotic drugs? A meta-analysis of placebo controlled trials. *Molecular Psychiatry*, **14**: 429–47.

Macias C, Rodican CF, Hargreaves WA, *et al* (2006) Supported employment outcomes of a randomized controlled trial of ACT and clubhouse models. *Psychiatric Services*, **57**: 1406–15.

Mairs H, Lovell K, Campbell M, *et al* (2011) Development and pilot investigation of behavioural activation for negative symptoms. *Behavior Modification*, **35**: 486–506.

Mari DJ, Streiner D (1994) An overview of family interventions and relapse on schizophrenia: meta-analysis of research findings. *Psychological Medicine*, **24**: 565–78.

Marwaha S, Johnson S (2004) Schizophrenia and employment: a review. *Social Psychiatry and Psychiatric Epidemiology*, **39**: 337–49.

McHugo GJ, Drake RE, Becker DR (1998) The durability of supported employment effects. *Psychiatric Rehabilitation Journal*, **22**: 55–61.

Meltzer HY, Rabinowitz J, Lee MA, *et al* (1997) Age of onset and gender of schizophrenic patients in relation to neuroleptic resistance. *American Journal of Psychiatry*, **154**: 475–82.

Mountain D, Killaspy H, Holloway F (2009) Mental health rehabilitation services in the UK in 2007. *Psychiatric Bulletin*, **33**: 215–18.

Mowbray CT, Moxley DP, Collins ME (1998) Consumers as mental health providers: first-person accounts of benefits and limitations. *Journal of Behavioural Health Services and Research*, **25**: 397–411.

National Institute for Health and Clinical Excellence (NICE) (2009) *Core Interventions in the Treatment and Management of Schizophrenia in Primary and Secondary Care (Update)*. NICE.

O'Flynn D, Craig T (2001) Which way to work? Occupations, vocations and opportunities for mental health service users. *Journal of Mental Health*, **10**: 1–4.

Pharoah F, Mari J, Rathbone J, *et al* (2010) Family intervention for schizophrenia. *Cochrane Database Systematic Reviews*, **8**: CD000088.

Pilling S, Bebbington P, Kuipers E, *et al* (2002a) Psychological treatments in schizophrenia I: Meta-analyses of family intervention and cognitive behaviour therapy. *Psychological Medicine*, **32**: 763–82.

Pilling S, Bebbington P, Kuipers E, *et al* (2002b) Psychological treatments in schizophrenia: II. Meta analyses of randomized controlled trials of social skills training and cognitive remediation. *Psychological Medicine*, **32**: 783–91.

Poole R, Ryan T, Pearsall A (2002) The NHS, the private sector, and the virtual asylum. *BMJ*, **325**: 349–50.3

Priebe S, Badesconyi A, Fioritti A, *et al* (2005) Reinstitutionalisation in mental health care: comparison of data on service provision from six European countries. *BMJ*, **330**: 123–6.

Prytys M, Garety P, Jolly S, *et al* (2011) Implementing the NICE guideline for schizophrenia recommendations for psychological therapies: a qualitative analysis of the attitudes of CMHT staff. *Clinical Psychology and Psychotherapy*, **18**: 48–59.

Ryan T, Pearsall A, Hatfield B, *et al* (2004) Long term care for serious mental illness outside the NHS: a study of out of area placements. *Journal of Mental Health*, **13**: 425–9.

Ryan T, Hatfield B, Sharma I, *et al* (2007) A census study of independent mental health sector usage across seven strategic health authorities. *Journal of Mental Health*, **16**: 243–53.

Salyers MP, Becker DR, Drake RE, *et al* (2004) A ten-year follow-up of a supported employment program. *Psychiatric Services*, **55**: 302–8.

Salzer M, Shear L (2002) Identifying comsumer–provider benefits in evaluations of consumer-delivered services. *Psychiatric Rehabilitation Journal*, **25**: 281–8.

Schonebaum AD, Boyd JK, Dudek KJ (2006) A comparison of competitive employment outcomes for the clubhouse and PACT models. *Psychiatric Services*, **57**: 1416–20.

Secker J, Grove B, Seebohm P (2001) Challenging barriers to employment, training and education for mental health service users: the service users perspective. *Journal of Mental Health*, **10**: 395–404.

Solomon P, Draine J (1998) Consumers as providers in psychiatric rehabilitation. *New Directions for Mental Health Services*, **79**: 65–77.

Susser E, Valencia E, Conover S, *et al* (1997) Preventing recurrent homelessness among mentally ill men: a 'critical time' intervention after discharge from a shelter. *American Journal of Public Health*, **87**: 256–62.

Tarrier N (1992) Management and modification of residual positive psychotic symptoms. In *Innovations in the Psychological Management of Schizophrenia* (eds M Birchwood, N Tarrier): 147–69. John Wiley and Sons.

Turkington D, Kingdon D, Turner T, *et al* (2002) Effectiveness of a brief cognitive behavioural therapy intervention in the treatment of schizophrenia. *British Journal of Psychiatry*, **180**: 523–7.

Wallace CJ, Boone SE, Donahoe CP, *et al* (1985) The chronic mentally disabled: independent living skills training. In *Clinical Handbook of Psychological Disorders: A Step-by-Step Treatment Manual* (ed D Barlow): 147–68. Guilford Press.

Waller H, Garety PA, Jolley S, *et al* (2013) Low intensity cognitive behavioural therapy for psychosis: a pilot study. *Journal of Behavior Therapy and Experimental Psychiatatry*, **44**: 98–104.

Watts F, Bennett D (1983) The concept of rehabilitation. In *Theory and Practice of Psychiatric Rehabilitation* (eds FN Watts, DH Bennett): 3–14. John Wiley & Sons.

World Health Organization (1980) *International Classification of Impairment, Disabilities and Handicaps: A Manual of Classification Relating to the Consequences of Disease*. WHO.

Wykes T, Dunn G (1992) Cognitive deficit and the prediction of rehabilitation success in a chronic psychiatric group. *Psychological Medicine*, **22**: 389–398.

Wykes T, Holloway F (2000) Community rehabilitation: past failures and future prospects. *International Review of Psychiatry*, **12**: 197–205.

Wykes T, Katz R, Sturt E, *et al* (1992) Abnormalities of response processing in a chronic psychiatric group. A possible predictor of failure in rehabilitation programmes? *British Journal of Psychiatry*, **160**: 244–52.

Wykes T, Reeder C, Landau S, *et al* (2007) Cognitive remediation therapy in schizophrenia: randomised controlled trial. *British Journal of Psychiatry*, **190**: 421–7.

Wykes T, Steel C, Everitt B, *et al* (2008) Cognitive Behaviour Therapy for schizophrenia: Effect sizes, clinical models and methodological rigor. *Schizophrenia Bulletin*, **134**: 523–37.

Wykes T, Huddy V, Cellard C, *et al* (2011) A meta-analysis of cognitive remediation for schizophrenia: methodology and effect sizes. *American Journal of Psychiatry*, **168**: 472–85.

CHAPTER 3

Rehabilitation as a values-led practice: the contribution of recovery, social inclusion and personalisation

Glenn Roberts, Jed Boardman and Kevin Lewis

Introduction

Developments in rehabilitation practice and services have arisen in reaction to prevailing social attitudes and norms, scandals and crises in care, and in pursuit of improvements for the life experience of people with severe and complex mental health conditions. The language and concepts given to these initiatives have changed over the years, keeping pace with shifting therapeutic philosophies and social policy. Current approaches are built upon the legacy of innovations, which include: moral treatment, deinstitutionalisation, social role valorisation, strengths-based approaches, normalisation and community care. Each in its day arose from a struggle to reconcile humanitarian ideals with the care and treatment of people with disabling mental illness. Each was a reaction to well-documented limitations and failings in the quality of services, and each pushed for progress and flourished for a while before losing popularity and momentum, and, like waves upon a beach, receding in impact and influence until overtaken by a successor. Few, if any, of their advocates would be fully satisfied with what they achieved or would have regarded these 'movements' as having fulfilled their potential. But the wider impression, albeit with setbacks and less favourable periods, is that the tide has been steadily coming in and there has been an increasing ethical impetus towards social justice, respect, inclusion, integration and acceptance for people with severe and complex mental health problems, in open society, as fellow citizens.

A notable recent contribution has been publication of the Francis report into the failed care, excess suffering and death of vulnerable, mostly elderly, people in physical healthcare in mid-Staffordshire, which has given further momentum to (and renewed public concern about) the need for compassion, kindness and person-centred approaches to healthcare (Francis, 2013).

In among the complex details of service evaluation, the emerging standard is, 'Would you regard the service you work in as good enough for your own friends and family'? There are undoubtedly services that do exemplify good practice, but recurrent inquiries by regulators, user-led reports (MIND, 2011) and independent commissions (Rethink, 2012) have noted that this remains patchy and that there continue to be concerns over the quality of many services and the outcomes experienced by the people they serve.

In their recommendations, these reviews have correspondingly offered clarification of what people do want and value, and it is not technically complex or inherently unattainable. As a broad generalisation, people want a service that is both kind and effective, in which they are treated as people by people with humanity and compassion. They want helpers (staff) to know not just about the technicalities of symptoms, diagnoses and evidence-based treatments but also what it is like to face such challenges and how to find a way through them so as to be able to get back into life. They want to be able to choose from a range of interventions offered and to be supported in working out what works best for them, based on their personal perspective of the relative merits and difficulties of treatments as they experience them. They want people to offer and express hope for their futures and have confidence that they will recover a pattern of living in society that they value, even if their condition cannot be cured.

These are not unreasonable expectations but meeting them has not been a cultural hallmark of mental health services for people with severe mental health problems. Such aspirations have, though, informed what have emerged as the major values-led drivers of rehabilitation practice in the past 20 years. Indeed, few of these drivers, if any, have arisen primarily from clinicians or professional concerns so much as from the testimony and advocacy of people with personal experience. These have drawn attention to the disabling consequences of social exclusion, impersonal or depersonalised service contacts and lack of a hopeful and ambitious focus on recovery for people with severe mental health problems. There can be few practitioners in rehabilitation unfamiliar with the corresponding emphasis on recovery, social inclusion and personalisation, but perhaps equally few who work in service settings where the full implications and potential of these principles have been realised in practice.

This chapter offers a succinct conceptual clarification of these key principles but also invites readers to engage with these as valued supports for improving their practice and the experience and outcomes of those they work with. Each principle holds considerable potential to support the development of services towards those that are genuinely person-centred, valued and appreciated by those who use them and about which we would have little doubt that they are good enough for our families.

Recovery: a common purpose

The past decade has seen a gathering interest and sharpening focus on recovery as the guiding purpose of mental health and social care services (Repper & Perkins, 2003; Care Services Improvement Partnership *et al*, 2007; Roberts & Hollins, 2007). There has been increasing recognition that what has become the dominant approach of traditional services – focusing on getting *better from* symptoms, problems, difficulties and disorders (i.e. clinical recovery) does not necessarily enable people to get *forwards into* a satisfactory pattern of life and living, with or without ongoing problems (i.e. personal recovery) (Slade, 2009). Hence, alongside continuing to value guidance on evidence-based treatment, there has been a growing emphasis on the importance of choice, opportunity, hope, self-determination, social inclusion and personalisation as overarching mediators of well-being.

Clarification of concepts: defining and redefining recovery

'Recovery' is an ordinary word in common usage that has come to be used in several ways, all relevant to mental health services and practice (Box 3.1).

As a 'natural healing process' it reminds us of the role of resilience in health, but if equated to 'cure' or a return to how things were before the injury occurred or illness began, it points to the limits of achieving this when applied to people with long-term conditions (Whitwell, 2005). When

---

Box 3.1 Understanding recovery: one word, three meanings, five usages

- *Recovery* is commonly regarded as a natural healing process and an approximation to cure – most people get better from most things, most of the time
- *Clinical recovery* – recovery from symptoms and difficulties in response to effective care and treatment, as described in most evidence-based guidelines (e.g. those produced by the National Institute for Health and Care Excellence)
- *Personal recovery* – recovery of a valued pattern of life and living, with or without ongoing symptoms and difficulties, linked to an active personal commitment to working on recovery
- *Recovery-oriented approaches and services* – the overall pattern of care, support and professional practice based on learning 'what works' from people in recovery, conducted by staff with appropriate qualities and skills in recovery-supportive relationships
- *The recovery movement* – a values-led collaborative endeavour of people in recovery, practitioners and many others, working to develop and transform mental healthcare and treatment. This recognises the concurrent value of diverse expertise developed though personal experience, research and training, and the benefit of working together in partnership to co-construct and co-produce learning, teaching and change

---

used to define a social movement, it highlights the key importance of social justice and civil rights to the lives of people with mental health problems (Davidson *et al*, 2010*a*).

Personal recovery has at its heart a reconceptualisation of recovery as a personal process of learning how to live and how to live well, with or without enduring symptoms or vulnerabilities. It is concerned with gaining hope, meaning, purpose and control over patterns of living, as valued and chosen by the person himself or herself (Slade, 2009). There appears to be broad acceptance of the validity of distinguishing between clinical and personal recovery and how people can progress in each, independent of the other. This shift of perspective has enabled people to redefine themselves from being 'chronically ill' to 'in recovery' and realise that it is possible to have an illness or ongoing symptoms and difficulties but nonetheless to take actions to discover how to become more well and to develop a more satisfactory life experience.

Mental health policy has developed over more than a decade (Department of Health, 2001) using Anthony's (1993) internationally accepted definition of personal recovery to underpin its strategic aim that 'More people will recover' (Department of Health, 2011: p. 16). This goal is described practically as occurring when people who develop mental health problems increasingly experience 'a good quality of life, greater ability to manage their own lives, stronger social relationships, a greater sense of purpose, improved chances in education, better employment rates and a suitable and stable place to live'. These are clearly ambitions close to the heart of what psychiatric rehabilitation seeks to achieve. Learning how to support people in achieving these goals is what 'recovery-oriented practice' is described as focusing upon, which similarly overlaps with good practice in rehabilitation.

International understanding and policy

The recovery approach in UK services is a product of international collaboration and an open exchange of ideas and innovations from a broad and growing network of recovery researchers and development leads. This has resulted in a consensus which has seen the concept of recovery explicitly adopted in national policy across England (2001/11), Ireland (2005) and Scotland (2006), as well as in other Anglophone countries, including New Zealand (1998), the USA (2003), Australia, (2003) and Canada (2009). There has also been a close engagement with the concept in Italy (Davidson *et al*, 2010*b*) and northern Europe (Amering & Schmolke, 2009; Amering *et al*, 2012). There are some cultural differences and initial explorations in some Asian (Ahmed *et al*, 2012; Thara, 2012) and African countries (Katontoka, 2012; Parker, 2012) have illustrated variations in non-Western concepts of recovery which tend to emphasise spirituality and a collective, rather than an individual, identity (Slade *et al*, 2012).

Recovery and the Royal College of Psychiatrists

The College's Joint Position Statement advocating for recovery as a 'common purpose' in future mental health services (Care Services Improvement Partnership *et al*, 2007) was reaffirmed in its 'Fair Deal' campaign. The College's membership of the Future Vision Coalition led to it being a co-signatory of a 'vision statement' that prioritised recovery as a key driver for future services and endorsed the ambition that, in future: 'Workforce training and continuing professional development for mental health workers is built around recovery principles as a matter of course' (Future Vision Coalition, 2009: p. 5).

The influence of this lobbying group was clear in subsequent mental health policy under both Labour (Department of Health, 2010) and Coalition (Department of Health, 2011) governments. The latter adopted recovery as one of its six overall aims, with an associated commitment to 'test the key features of organisational practice to support the recovery of those using mental health services' (Department of Health, 2011: p. 22). This became the programme 'Implementing Recovery through Organisational Change' (ImROC), established by the Centre for Mental Health & NHS Confederation (2012).

Psychiatrists in the UK work almost invariably in multiprofessional teams and it is therefore significant that each of the core mental health professions has also made some form of statement similar to that of the British Psychological Society (BPS) (Kinderman & Tai, 2009) that 'mental health services should fully embrace the recovery approach'. Endorsement of recovery has also formed a basis for inter-agency collaboration, for example that between the Royal College of Psychiatrists and the Association of Directors of Adult Social Services (2013), which state a shared belief that:

> the purpose of mental health services should be to support each person's recovery journey and the achievement of goals that matter to that individual, rather than to focus exclusively on clinical recovery. This means a shift in the relationship between professionals and individuals to one with a greater emphasis on partnership. (Royal College of Psychiatrists & Association of Directors of Adult Social Services, 2013: p. 4)

And also that:

> Personalisation and recovery are part of a common agenda for mental health system transformation. At their core, both are rooted in self-determination and reclaiming the rights of full citizenship for people with a lived experience of mental health problems. (Royal College of Psychiatrists & Association of Directors of Adult Social Services, 2013: p. 4)

When considering how to achieve this, they place an emphasis on the expertise of lived experience and the need for significant changes in the culture, practice and organisation of mental health services.

As with the above, much of the discussion about recovery emphasises the need for change, development and transformation. Not all are in favour of this or even see the need for it, and there are those who are confident that we are 'doing it already' and that to assert a need for a development agenda around 'recovery' is misguided or a form of shallow rebranding of what may otherwise be simply called 'good practice' (Roberts & Boardman, 2014a). A key confusion is that much of what is described as needing to change *is* described in existing policy, but that this remains largely unimplemented or at best inconsistently so. The broad consensus on policy is, though, leading to reasonable international agreement on an emerging curriculum to guide implementation of these principles in practice and to equip practitioners to be more supportive of personal recovery (Box 3.2), some of which constitutes a re-emphasis of existing guidance, but other elements represent innovations (see Roberts & Boardman, 2014a,b, for a full description).

Rehabilitation and recovery

The present volume is titled *Enabling Recovery* and connections between the recovery movement and rehabilitation psychiatry are obvious and plentiful. Virtually all the professional leads in recovery have come from rehabilitation backgrounds (e.g. Bill Antony, Larry Davidson, Mike Slade, Geoff Shepherd, Julie Repper and Rachel Perkins). Similarly, the founding stories of personal recovery were almost entirely from people with long-standing psychosis and often unrewarding or damaging experiences of care and treatment, which overlapped with the focus of rehabilitation psychiatry, on which they were often critical commentators (e.g. Pat Deegan, Mary O'Hagan, Ron Colman and Rufus May).

This close association has led to many teams and services being relabelled 'rehabilitation and recovery' or simply 'recovery'. Initially this seemed a positive and invigorating shift, as rehabilitation practice became the test bed of many recovery innovations, but more recently it is clear there is both a cost and a risk. For although a core emphasis on enabling recovery remains pivotal to rehabilitation, the recovery movement did not arise from and does not belong to the mental health professions so much as to people in recovery themselves (Social Perspectives Network, 2007). Casual co-option of the word to relabel rehabilitation risks a backlash from service users, who may suspect 'colonisation' or 'tokenism', to the point where, ironically, they may wish to dissociate themselves from (professionalised) 'recovery' as a damaged concept before it has even been properly engaged with.

The other risk in conflating recovery and rehabilitation is that it carries an implication that, from a clinical point of view, it is only rehabilitation services that 'do recovery'. The Joint Commissioning Panel for Mental Health (2012), in its 'Ten Key Messages for Commissioners', clearly states that rehabilitation services always aim to work in partnership with service users and carers, adopting a recovery orientation that places collaboration at the centre of all activities, and describes professionals' role and purpose

Box 3.2 An outline curriculum for training in recovery-oriented practice

Understanding for all practitioners
- Understanding the origins and guiding principles of recovery
- Personal reflections on recovery: learning from your own experience
- Reflections on personal recovery: learning from recovery narratives
- Personal approaches to distress: culturally appropriate and trauma-informed care
- The importance of language that enables and supports recovery
- Concerns and challenges: problems raised with the recovery approach

Skills for all practitioners
- Creating a hospitable and welcoming environment
- Supporting self-management: use of tools and frameworks
- Building on strengths and working towards personal goals
- Enabling self-direction and control: personalisation and personal budgets
- Working with peer support
- Educational supports for personal recovery
- Bringing it all together: recovery-oriented care planning
- Developing natural supports and promoting community participation

Specific issues in relation to medical responsibilities
- Engaging with knowledge and skills for all recovery-oriented practitioners

Additional understanding
- Recovery and realism: is it 'open to all'?

Additional skills
- Promoting recovery for people detained under the Mental Health Act
- Reconsidering risk assessment and safety planning
- Medication management and supported decision-making
- Practitioners in context: participating in organisational change
- Practitioners in context: participating in societal and cultural change
- Tracking progress: evaluation and outcome measures
- Continuing professional development: supports and resources

Abridged from Roberts & Boardman (2014a,b)

as providing 'specialist assessment, treatment, interventions and support to enable the recovery of people whose complex needs cannot be met by general adult mental health services' (1.2). However, it also states that 'Rehabilitation services are not the same as recovery services' because 'A recovery orientation should be at the centre of all health and social care service provision to people with mental health problems and is not limited to rehabilitation services'. Hence, 'Rehabilitation services adopt a "recovery" approach that values service users as partners in a collaborative relationship with staff to identify and work towards personalised goals'.

This key description of what rehabilitation services are and do, and who provides them, goes on to say that 'The concept of recovery encompasses the values of hope, agency, opportunity and inclusion, themes that resonate well with the aims of mental health rehabilitation'. This clearly underlines the breadth of application of recovery as 'a common purpose' (Care Services Improvement Partnership *et al*, 2007) and a new vision (Future Vision Coalition, 2009) which is 'Open to all' (Roberts & Wolfson, 2004; South London and Maudsley NHS Foundation Trust & South West London and St George's Mental Health NHS Trust, 2010) and which offers a revising philosophy for practice (Roberts & Boardman 2014*a,b*) and services (Centre for Mental Health *et al*, 2012). Rehabilitation should therefore be seen as one, perhaps a leading one, of a wide range of recovery-oriented services, but care is needed not to lose what is distinctive about rehabilitation, which is its role in enabling recovery for people with particular profiles of need.

The challenge to rehabilitation from the recovery movement

Although one of the experience-based founders of the recovery movement wrote of rehabilitation as 'The lived experience of recovery' (Deegan, 1988), it is unclear to what degree the current endorsement of recovery principles has yet converted to enhancement of the kind of outcomes valued by people themselves (Killaspy *et al*, 2012).

Part of the difficulty is, as the Mental Health Implementation Framework observes, that 'there are key aspects of mental health, such as recovery, for which agreed outcome measures are not yet available' (Centre for Mental Health *et al*, 2012: 15). A recent ImROC briefing paper (Shepherd *et al*, 2014) has summarised quality indicators and outcome measures including personal measures of personal progress, personal measures of service experience and more objective assessments of gains in valued social achievements such as secure housing, sufficient finances, suitable work and satisfactory relationships, to which could be added service evaluation of being up to standard (e.g. Scottish Recovery Indicator, www.sri2.net). However, there is not yet any wide experience of using such measures in practice and some previously promoted recovery measures, such as the Recovery Star, are better regarded as engagement or coaching tools than outcome measures (Killaspy *et al*, 2012).

The recovery movement is fundamentally informed and led by experience-based expertise, whose viewpoint offers additional challenges to current rehabilitation practice. These include: an ambition to eliminate coercion, seclusion and restraint and a progressive reduction in compulsory measures (Ashcraft & Anthony, 2008); workforce changes that increasingly value 'lived experience' and engagement with peer-support workers as colleagues (see Chapter 21, 'Peer support in mental health services'); the shift from an emphasis on giving treatment towards offering co-produced education experiences that enable people to learn how to make progress in their own recovery (Perkins *et al*, 2012); developing more substantial opportunities for people to exercise informed choice over treatments (Roberts *et al*, 2008; Baker *et al*, 2013); and reaching beyond traditional service boundaries to increase routes to participation and inclusion though working not just in the community but with the community and as practitioners taking on some aspects of social activism (Slade, 2010). These progressive ideas recur as we move on to consider the overlapping contributions of social inclusion and personalisation.

Social inclusion

Understanding exclusion and enabling participation

Historically, we have recognised that people with mental health problems are disadvantaged in many ways, not only because of the incapacities and impairments that arise from their disorders, but also from social and institutional barriers. Over recent years the term 'social exclusion' has been used to describe and analyse the disadvantages faced by many groups of people in society, including those with mental health problems (Boardman *et al*, 2010).

The term 'social exclusion' belongs to the social policy literature and originated in France during the 1970s, referring to *Les Exclus*, people who slip though the social security net and thus become administratively excluded by the state (Burchardt *et al*, 2002a; Morgan *et al*, 2007). This concept of social exclusion was influential in European social policy and policies adopted by the UK government from 1997 to 2010.

Some definitions of social exclusion are presented in Box 3.3. A common thread linking these definitions is *social participation*: the extent to which individuals are able to participate in key areas of the economic, social and cultural life of society. This lack of participation is seen to arise owing to constraint, rather than individual choice.

Traditionally, the literature on disadvantage has focused on material deprivation (poverty, hardship, destitution). While poverty remains an important factor limiting participation, the concept of social exclusion directs our attention to the range of phenomena that influence participation, for example discrimination, long-term illness, social isolation, culture and ethnicity, which in turn highlights possible causes and solutions.

Social exclusion and mental health problems

There are several key areas in which people can be excluded from participation (Boardman *et al*, 2010). These domains include:

- *consumption* – exclusion from material resources and the capacity to purchase goods and services (income poverty)
- *production* – exclusion from (socially valued) productive activity, such as participation in economically or socially valuable activities (employment, education, etc.)

Box 3.3 Definitions of social exclusion

A shorthand term for what can happen when people or areas suffer from a combination of linked problems such as unemployment, poor skills, low incomes, poor housing, high crime environments, bad health and family breakdown. (Social Exclusion Unit, 2001: p. 11)

An individual is socially excluded if (a) he or she is geographically resident in a society, (b) he or she cannot participate in the normal activities of citizens in that society, and (c) he or she would like to so participate, but is prevented from doing so by factors beyond his or her control. (Centre for Analysis of Social Exclusion (CASE) – Burchardt *et al*, 1999: p. 228)

An individual is socially excluded if he or she does not participate in key activities of the society in which he or she lives. (Centre for Analysis of Social Exclusion (CASE) – Burchardt *et al*, 2002*b*: p. 30)

Social exclusion is a process over time that deprives individuals and families, groups and neighbourhoods of the resources required for participation in the social, economic, and political activity of society as a whole. This process is primarily a consequence of poverty and low income, but other factors such as discrimination, low educational attainment and depleted environments also underpin it. Through this process people are cut off for a significant period in their lives from institutions and services, social networks and developmental opportunities that the great majority of a society enjoys. (Pierson, 2010: p. 12)

- *social interaction* – exclusion from social relations and neighbourhoods, from interaction with family, friends, community (isolated networks)
- *political engagement* – exclusion from civic participation and involvement in local or national decision-making (having a voice, choice and control)
- *services* – including utility services, public services, private services, health services.

We can readily recognise that people with mental health problems are often excluded in all of these domains. Some examples are outlined in Box 3.4. For a more complete account see Boardman *et al* (2010).

Overall, people with mental health problems and people with intellectual disabilities are at greater risk of risk of exclusion than the general population. Nevertheless, people with mental health problems are not a homogeneous group and have a range of incapacities and have varying risks and experiences of exclusion. Notwithstanding individual differences, it is generally clear that some groups face a higher risk of exclusion, particularly those who experience psychoses and those whose problems fall into multiple diagnostic categories. In addition, people with mental health problems will face differential levels of exclusion related to their

Box 3.4 Exclusion of people with mental health problems

Consumption – exclusion from material resources
- Low incomes among people with severe mental health problems (Foster *et al*, 1996; Jenkins *et al*, 2008)
- High rates of people receiving welfare benefits (Meltzer *et al*, 1995; Jenkins *et al*, 2008)
- High proportions of people in debt (Fitch *et al*, 2007; Jenkins *et al*, 2008)
- Lack of basic necessities (Payne, 2006)
- High proportions living in deprived neighbourhoods and poor housing (Boardman *et al*, 1997; Meltzer *et al*, 2002; Payne, 2006)
- Poor access to transport (Thornicroft, 2006)

Production – exclusion from (socially valued) productive activity
- Low levels of educational attainment (Melzer *et al*, 2003)
- Early termination of education (Fergusson & Woodward, 2001)
- Low levels of employment (Boardman, 2003; Marwaha & Johnson, 2004)

Social interaction – exclusion from social relations and neighbourhoods
- Low rates of marriage and high proportions living alone (Foster *et al*, 1996; Meltzer *et al*, 2002)
- Small social networks (Meltzer *et al*, 1995)
- Small primary support groups (Foster *et al*, 1996)
- Restricted participation in social and leisure pursuits (Trauer *et al*, 1998; Mayers, 2000)

Political engagement – exclusion from civic participation
- There is a lack of research in this area – but the Poverty and Social Exclusion Survey (Pantazis *et al*, 2006) suggests that civic participation is limited among people with mental health problems. There is evidence of a curtailment of citizenship and of political and human rights for people with mental health problems (Sayce, 2000; Thornicroft, 2006)

Exclusion in relation to health, and health services in particular
- Selective exclusion of certain diagnostic groups from mental health services (people with dual diagnoses, personality disorders, intellectual disabilities and substance misuse) (Department of Health, 2002; National Institute for Mental Health in England, 2003; Alcohol Needs Assessment Research Report Project, 2004; Cooper *et al*, 2004)
- Increased risk of premature death (Harris & Barraclough, 1998; Hippisley-Cox, 2006*a,b*)
- Reduced access to primary care services (Disability Rights Commission, 2006; Samele *et al*, 2006)

membership of different social identity groups (e.g. Black and minority ethnic groups, women, sexual orientation groups), or because they are excluded owing to the nature of their situation, for example prisoners, those who are homeless and refugees and asylum seekers.

Value of the concept of social exclusion to people with mental health problems

Several concepts related to social exclusion are of value in identifying the position of people with mental health problems in society and in directing national social policies and the future organisation and delivery of mental health services.

Agency and process

Social exclusion can be seen as a dynamic process that places an emphasis on agency. It implies that someone or something (e.g. political, economic and social institutions) is doing the exclusion. This points to the value of adopting a 'social model' of disability for understanding the obstacles faced by people with mental health problems. This model stresses the role of social and environmental factors in producing disability (Oliver, 1996) and, while this acknowledges the reality of people's impairments and the pain and distress associated with them, it separates the experience of impairments from those of disability. This provides a helpful framework for describing the experiences of people with mental health problems and the social barriers they face, including those of stigma – ignorance, prejudice and discrimination (Thornicroft, 2006).

Citizenship and social justice

There is little doubt that people with mental health problems face prejudice and discrimination in their daily lives (Sayce, 2000; Thornicroft, 2006). This draws our attention to the areas of citizenship, social justice, equality and human rights. Entitlement to human rights is based on one's humanity and citizenship implies that people are active agents. Both apply to people with mental health problems. This leads us to a consideration of choice (the power to make decisions) and access as a means of facilitating engagement and participation.

Causation: a life-course and a longitudinal perspective

The relationship between mental health problems and social exclusion is complex and multifactorial. A life-course and longitudinal perspective is helpful in understanding the effects of early-life factors that determine the pathways to exclusion and of intergenerational and intragenerational aspects of the transmission of exclusion (Centre for Longitudinal Studies, 2008).

Pointers to action

Understanding the factors associated with social exclusion provides indicators for action to promote the inclusion of people with mental health problems. This will require broad social and economic policies to create sustainable social justice (Coote & Franklin, 2009; New Economics Foundation, 2009). These may be linked to policies for health and social

Box 3.5 Proposed principles for socially inclusive mental health services

- Place people at the forefront of services – aiming to build meaningful and satisfying lives
- Adopt the organisational aim of supporting personal recovery
- Embed recovery principles (hope, agency, opportunity) at all levels of the organisation and services
- Use the best available knowledge in service and treatment developments to improve clinical and social outcomes
- Give primacy to outcomes valued by service users
- Emphasise prevention, promotion and early intervention
- Place increased emphasis on educational and training opportunities for service users within mental health services
- Place an emphasis on co-production, developing partnerships with service users and partnerships between all provider and commissioning agencies
- Increase employment opportunities for people with mental health problems, including development of peer roles in mental health services
- Focus on inclusion in the community, not just integration
- Fight discrimination and champion respect, rights and equality for people with mental health problems
- Challenge and dismantle barriers to recovery and inclusion

Adapted from Boardman *et al* (2010: p. 371)

services, education and training, poverty and social welfare, housing, transport, leisure, civil and human rights, stigma and discrimination, family support and community participation (Office of the Deputy Prime Minister, 2004; Thornicroft, 2006; Mental Health Europe, 2008; Duffy, 2011). The challenge for mental health services is how to make them recovery-oriented and in turn promote social inclusion for people with mental health problems (Repper & Perkins, 2003; Sainsbury Centre for Mental Health, 2009; Shepherd *et al*, 2010). Some principles for socially inclusive practice are shown in Box 3.5.

Social inclusion and recovery

'Recovery' is not usually included in the literature on social exclusion, but there is a clear overlap between the ideas of recovery and the concepts of social exclusion. Social exclusion belongs in the social policy literature and describes the position of people in relation to society, whereas the ideas of recovery have largely emerged from the accounts of people who have experienced mental ill-health and may have used mental health services. Social exclusion emphasises the social and political processes that determine participation, whereas recovery focuses on the individual's personal experience and the importance of hope, agency (control) and opportunity in fostering better health (Repper & Perkins, 2003). However, recovery and social inclusion may be linked by agency and opportunity: the opportunity to participate in one's community and gain a sense of control. In addition, many of the outcomes associated with recovery are also markers of social inclusion, such as working, studying, living independently, having good family relationships, having a social life, being part of the community. One way in which mental health services can contribute to the social inclusion of people with mental health problems is to develop practices and services that are 'recovery oriented' (see Box 3.5) (Shepherd *et al*, 2008; Sainsbury Centre for Mental Health, 2009).

Personalisation: restoring authority through choice and control

A Google search on the term 'personalisation' will elicit more than 5.5 million results; there's a lot of it about. Two definitions are particularly informative: 'Personalisation means starting with the individual as a person with strengths and preferences who may have a network of support and resources' (*Personalisation: A Rough Guide*; Social Care Institute for Excellence, 2008); and 'efforts to make public services more people-centred, i.e. more tailored to their needs, more controlled by them, and more "co-produced" by them' (*Making It Personal*; ACEVO, 2009). These two definitions capture the way in which personalisation starts with the individual but, scaled up, can reform whole systems.

Personalisation is more than the mechanisms for the purchase of services, with which it is sometimes confused. However, personalisation is often enabled by transferring control of the budget to the individual. At present in the National Health Service, this can be done in the following ways:

- A *personal budget* (PB) involves 'being clear with the person at the start how much money is available to meet their needs, then allowing them maximum choice over how the money is spent'. This is subject to means testing through the Fair Access to Care Services (FACS) system.
- A *personal health budget* (PHB) 'is an amount of money to support your individual healthcare and wellbeing needs, planned and agreed between you or your representative and your local NHS team' (Department of Health, 2012).
- A *direct payment* is the receipt of cash to buy the services the individual and doctor or care manager decide are needed.

Personal budgets and personal health budgets can be held by the citizen or a third party, or can be a notional budget only, that is, identified as a sum dedicated to the individual, but held by a commissioning body. The concern that people may be unable to manage a budget owing to the illness can be accommodated through these mechanisms and robust advance planning.

Personalisation is an essentially simple concept (put the citizen at the centre of all discussion, and planning and building a solution to suit them, with them) yet it is often elusive when it comes to the delivery of services. To deliver personalised services, professionals have to cede some power to the individual and rethink the nature of engagement: it is about choice and control, but it is about more than that.

In our effort to understand personalisation, it can be illuminating to think about our experience of public services that are depersonalised. A mundane example: public transport fails. You are now going to be late. All of that talk of 'valued customers' sounds hollow. There is no information, no engaging with you to meet your needs. You are left feeling powerless and angry. Or consider a devastating example: the neglect of vulnerable and elderly people who have been treated without humanity in hospitals and care homes in recent times. Both cases are the antithesis of a personalised approach.

Where has an emphasis on personalisation come from?

Personalisation began with physical disability lobby groups in the USA during the 1970s and the 'independent living' movement. Tired of their lives being limited because they were defined by their disability, often being condemned to lifelong institutional care, activists sought to realise their constitutional rights. In the UK, policy evolved informed by these developments. The moves to close long-stay hospitals and to introduce inclusive education in the 1980s and 1990s can be seen as direct products of the paradigm shift: people were more than their diagnostic label and could participate in defining their world.

Emerging political consensus about personalisation

It is important to consider personalisation in the context not just of mental health. In fact, there is a broad political consensus that the citizen should be placed at the heart of the provision of most public services. The focus on the individual is implicit in Conservative thinking. In 2004, Charles Leadbeater wrote a seminal paper, 'Personalisation through participation: a new script for public services' (DEMOS). This paper, very influential with the Blair government, argued that both the individual and the state could benefit from a new approach whereby each citizen is actively involved in designing and delivering any care or support needed. Giving the individual control of the funds to achieve that was the next logical step. This broad political support is important in that it signals that personalisation is not a short-term issue but rather a new underpinning policy that all will have to embrace. Duffy (2010) proposes 'that the real choice, underlying these debates, is whether the welfare state wishes to move from a paternalistic model of service delivery towards a model which treats people as citizens, and not as service users'.

Benefits of personalisation

Historically, many people have complained that their condition – 'the appendix in bed two', 'the schizophrenic in the side room' – too frequently defines them. This is both demeaning and unhelpful. In mental health services there is increasing evidence that the active engagement of the individual seeking help is pivotal to successful management of the condition and to recovery. We know from personal experience that when we are engaged in something, it is likely to succeed; when we are half-hearted or antagonistic, failure is likely. We also know that we are more than the sum of our labels and we see ourselves as multifaceted. Working with the individual and, where appropriate, the family, clinicians are able to bring into play the whole person. The mental health issue is considered juxtaposed with the whole personal story. Support is provided in the context of formal inputs but there are natural supports too: family, friends and colleagues. Housing, work and something meaningful to do all contribute to the management of illness.

Personalisation and recovery

Personalisation and recovery have grown in parallel in mental health. Alakeson & Perkins (2012) observe in *Recovery, Personalisation and Personal Budgets*:

> There are two strands of thinking currently shaping mental health policy and practice in the UK and internationally: recovery and personalisation. Both have emerged independently but in similar ways, both challenge the current predominance of professional, clinical knowledge over the expertise of lived experience in the mental health system. Both require significant changes in the culture, practice and organisation of mental health services encompassing both the NHS and social care.

Both are central tenets of the strategy 'No health without mental health' (Department of Health, 2011).

The challenge of personalisation to clinicians

When surveyed, the majority (56%) of clinicians say they already offer adequate patient choice (NHS Confederation, 2011: p. 10). Conversely, when people who use services are asked about being included in decision-making, the majority said they are not: 'A common theme in both the survey and focus groups was that people felt neither managers nor professionals were listening to their views' (NHS Confederation, 2011: p. 12). Both groups can't be right, and this apparent contradiction goes to the heart of the difficulty in shifting the balance of power. Personalisation is not anti-psychiatry, nor anti-professional. However, it does demand a reframing of our assumptions and practice to include the unique expertise of each patient who seeks help. The clinician brings academic knowledge, melded by years of experience. Patients bring their own unique experiences of illness, and their unique understanding and circumstances. Engaging in a different kind of dialogue and establishing a different relationship – one of equals – can and does achieve more satisfactory outcomes.

The equalities agenda

Personalisation is a means of addressing the equalities agenda. Historically, the NHS has provided a range of services into which the individual has to fit. This has led to complaints that services are often not sensitive and appropriate to gender, sexuality, faith or culture. Given the need for any service to be congruent with the experience of the individual, personalisation offers a simple, cheap, effective way forwards.

By meeting all patients on their own terms, listening to them and building a package of care and support together, all facets of their life can be attended to. There are frequently complaints that the patient is non-compliant, or does not engage. By providing a response sensitive to the whole individual, satisfaction and compliance increase, and, with that, we may expect better outcomes (Personal Social Services Research Unit, 2012).

The impact of personal budgets on services

Giving citizens control of the purse strings confers ultimate power on them as consumers of services. Often for the first time, they are able to tailor the help they require to suit their unique needs and wishes. Historically, private medicine offered the same thing; its USP ('unique selling proposition') was the way in which it ceded choice and control to the patient, establishing a fundamentally different relationship where payment was not a given, but had to be earned. Over time, successive governments have sought to mirror that shift by increasing the information available about services, and offering some choice, but this has had less impact in mental health than in other areas of medicine, until now.

The offer of a personal health budget (PHB) will, potentially, change service responsiveness rapidly. Provider organisations will have to attend to the real wishes of potential customers. For example, in the PHB pilot programme, one primary care trust offered a PHB to 20 people who had been waiting (up to 9 months) for cognitive–behavioural therapy (CBT) from the local foundation trust. Three found, through their broker, other ways of dealing with their sense of isolation, while the other 17 chose to stick with CBT but on their own terms. From a list of accredited practitioners, they chose on the basis of gender, location and time. Only one of the group returned to the general practitioner for more assistance. The others got the support they wanted in timely fashion. The foundation trust lost business.

Although many people develop support packages with their clinician that include things not traditionally associated with psychiatric practice (going to the gym, taking classes), many also want to use traditional services but on their own terms – as we all do in most domains of our lives. The PHB pilots demonstrate that few people reject conventional services out of hand, but they do want to be engaged actively in understanding how best to meet their needs. Having agreed a plan, they then expect to have some choice about its delivery. Given that abuse is so prevalent in the history of many people with a mental illness, it is not surprising that they wish to choose the gender of their clinician: services have too often been insensitive to this. So, patients seeking to buy a community psychiatric nurse's time via a PHB because they want to choose their clinician are not rejecting traditional services, merely the arrogance of an organisation saying 'you'll have what we offer'. A patient who bought support out of hours (when he was most likely to self-harm) did so because NHS services did not offer support when he needed it. The days of 'Hobson's choice' in the provision of public services are numbered.

Why is personalisation so difficult to achieve?

Clinicians and other professionals are accustomed to being competent and in control, and to holding a professional distance. It is difficult to empathise with a patient who feels utterly lost, powerless and frightened: it can become just another assessment for the clinician, but is perhaps a life-defining moment for the patient. We know that staff in stressful clinical settings hide behind task and process to contain possibly overwhelming anxiety (Menzies Lyth, 1959). Through personalisation, clinicians engage with each individual as a fellow citizen with equal import, and in doing so drop some of the defences all professionals build, making themselves more vulnerable, but more effective too. So one of the most fundamental challenges of personalisation is to engage more deeply but without being overwhelmed by the distress of others.

The benefit of working through the lens of personalisation is that a different, more equal and more dynamic relationship can be established between patient and clinician, with both benefiting, both taking responsibility for moving forward.

Looking ahead: valuing the values

Recovery, social inclusion and personalisation are all supported by national work programmes, and all three uphold ambitious aspirations for changing the relationships people have with supports and services, their carers and fellow citizens. In terms of implementation, all are 'work in progress'. These overlapping, companionable and mutually supportive approaches embody some of the core values that underpin rehabilitation practice in its aspiration to enable people with severe mental illness live well, as judged by themselves.

Rehabilitation practitioners live with the mixed fortunes of a professional inheritance based on support for such person-centred approaches but also the shame of being party to periods dominated by dehumanising institutionalisation, abuse and neglect. There continues to be a necessary agenda for quality improvement and transformation and there is still much to do in relation to teaching, training, mentoring, continued professional development and provision of collegial support. But these values-led considerations also encourage professionals to take opportunities to go beyond the usual emphasis on progressive acquisition of knowledge and skills and give time and thought to cultivating qualities too. Each of these domains invites professionals to do that in the company of those they serve as they look ahead to co-design, co-produce and co-evaluate progressive change. In doing so they have more chance of upholding their guiding values and rise to the challenge of working out how best to implement them in practice.

References

ACEVO (2009) *Commission on Personalisation. Making It Personal: A Social Market Revolution.* ACEVO.

Ahmed A, Buckley P, Mabe P (2012) International efforts at implementing and advancing the recovery model. *International Psychiatry,* **9**: 4–6.

Alakeson V, Perkins R (2012) *Recovery, Personalisation and Personal Budgets.* Centre for Mental Health.

Alcohol Needs Assessment Research Project (ANARP) (2004) *The 2004 National Alcohol Needs Assessment for England.* Department of Health.

Amering M, Schmolke M (2009) *Recovery in Mental Health: Reshaping Scientific and Clinical Responsibilities.* Wiley–Blackwell/World Psychiatric Association.

Amering M, Mikus M, Steffen S (2012) Recovery in Austria: mental health trialogue. *International Review of Psychiatry,* **24**: 11–18.

Anthony W (1993) Recovery from mental illness: the guiding vision of the mental health service system in the 1990s. *Psychosocial Rehabilitation Journal,* **16**: 11–23.

Ashcraft L, Anthony W (2008) Eliminating seclusion and restraint in recovery-oriented crisis services. *Psychiatric Services,* **59**: 1198–202.

Baker E, Fee J, Bovingdon L, *et al* (2013) From taking to using medication: steps towards a recovery-focused approach to prescribing and medicines management. *Advances in Psychiatric Treatment,* **19**: 2–10.

Boardman AP, Hodgson R, Lewis M, *et al* (1997) Social indicators and the prediction of psychiatric admissions in different diagnostic groups. *British Journal of Psychiatry,* **171**: 457–62.

Boardman J (2003) Work, employment and psychiatric disability. *Advances in Psychiatric Treatment,* **9**: 599–603.

Boardman J, Currie A, Killaspy H, *et al* (2010) *Social Inclusion and Mental Health.* Royal College of Psychiatrists.

Burchardt T, LeGrand J, Piachaud D (1999) Social exclusion in Britain 1991–1995. *Social Policy and Administration,* **33**: 227–44.

Burchardt T, LeGrand J, Piachaud D (2002a) Introduction. In *Understanding Social Exclusion* (eds J Hills, J LeGrand, D Piachaud): 1–12. Oxford University Press.

Burchardt T, LeGrand J, Piachaud D (2002b) Degrees of exclusion: developing a dynamic, multidimensional measure. In *Understanding Social Exclusion* (eds J Hills, J LeGrand, D Piachaud): 30–43. Oxford University Press.

Care Services Improvement Partnership, Royal College of Psychiatrists, Social Care Institute for Excellence (2007) *A Common Purpose: Recovery in Future Mental Health Services*. Social Care Institute for Excellence.

Centre for Longitudinal Studies (2008) *Now We Are 50. Key Findings from the National Child Development Study*. Centre for Longitudinal Studies.

Centre for Mental Health & NHS Confederation (2012) *Implementing Recovery Through Organisational Change: Continuing the Journey*. Centre for Mental Health.

Centre for Mental Health, Department of Health, MIND, *et al* (2012) *No Health Without Mental Health: Implementation Framework*. TSO (The Stationery Office).

Cooper SA, Melville C, Morrison J (2004) People with intellectual disabilities. *BMJ*, **329**: 414–15.

Coote A, Franklin J (2009) *Green Well Fair. Three Economies for Social Justice*. New Economics Foundation.

Davidson L, Rakfeldt J, Strauss J (2010a) *The Roots of the Recovery Movement in Psychiatry: Lessons Learned*. Wiley–Blackwell.

Davidson L, Mezzina R, Rowe M, *et al* (2010b) 'A life in the community': Italian mental health reform and recovery. *Journal of Mental Health*, **19**: 436–43.

Deegan P (1988) Recovery: the lived experience of rehabilitation. *Psychosocial Rehabilitation Journal*, **11**: 11–19.

Department of Health (2001) *The Journey to Recovery*. Department of Health.

Department of Health (2002) *Mental Health Policy Implementation Guide: Dual Diagnosis Good Practice Guide*. Department of Health.

Department of Health (2010) *New Horizons: A Shared Vision for Mental Health*. Department of Health.

Department of Health (2011) *No Health Without Mental Health: A Cross-Government Mental Health Outcomes Strategy For People Of All Ages*. Department of Health.

Department of Health (2012) *Evaluation of the Personal Health Budgets Pilot Programme*. Department of Health.

Disability Rights Commission (2006) *Equal Treatment: Closing the Gap. A Formal Investigation into Physical Health Inequalities Experienced by People with Learning Disabilities and/or Mental Health Problems*. Disability Rights Commission.

Duffy S (2010) *The Future of Personalisation: Implications for Welfare Reform*. Centre for Welfare Reform.

Duffy S (2011) *A Fair Income. Tax-Benefit Reform in an Era of Personalization*. Centre for Welfare Reform.

Fergusson DM, Woodward LJ (2001) Mental health, educational and social role outcomes of adolescents with depression. *Archives of General Psychiatry*, **59**: 225–31.

Fitch C, Chaplin R, Trend C, *et al* (2007) Debt and mental health: the role of psychiatrists. *Advances in Psychiatric Treatment*, **13**: 194–202.

Foster K, Meltzer H, Gill B, *et al* (1996) *Economic Activity and Social Functioning of Adults with Psychiatric Disorders* (OPCS Surveys of Psychiatric Morbidity in Great Britain. Report No. 8. OPCS, Social Survey Division). TSO (The Stationery Office).

Francis R (2013) *Report of the Mid Staffordshire NHS Foundation Trust Public Inquiry*. TSO (The Stationery Office).

Future Vision Coalition (2009) *A Future Vision for Mental Health*. Future Vision Coalition.

Harris EC, Barraclough B (1998) Excess mortality of mental disorder. *British Journal of Psychiatry*, **173**: 11–53.

Hippisley-Cox C, Vinogradova Y, Coupland C, *et al* (2006a) *Study One: A Comparison of Survival Rates for People with Mental Health Problems and the Remaining Population with Specific Conditions*. Disability Rights Commission.

Hippisley-Cox C, Parker C, Coupland C, *et al* (2006*b*) *Study Two: Use of Statins in Coronary Heart Disease Patients With and Without Mental Health Problems*. Disability Rights Commission.

Jenkins R, Bhugra D, Bebbington P, *et al* (2008) Debt, income and mental disorder in the general population. *Psychological Medicine*, **38**: 1485–93.

Joint Commissioning Panel for Mental Health (2012) *Guidance for Commissioners of Rehabilitation Services for People with Complex Mental Health Needs*. Royal College of Psychiatrists.

Katontoka S (2012) Consumer recovery: a call for partnership between researchers and consumers. *World Psychiatry*, **11**: 170–1.

Killaspy H, White S, Taylor T, *et al* (2012) Psychometric properties of the Mental Health Recovery Star. *British Journal of Psychiatry*, **201**: 65–70.

Kinderman P, Tai, S. (2009) *Psychological Health and Well-Being: A New Ethos for Mental Health*. British Psychological Society.

Leadbeater C (2004) Personalisation through participation: a new script for public services. DEMOS.

Marwaha S, Johnson S (2004) Schizophrenia and employment. *Social Psychiatry and Psychiatric Epidemiology*, **39**: 337–49.

Mayers CA (2000) Quality of life: priorities for people with enduring mental health problems. *British Journal of Occupational Therapy*, **63**: 591–7.

Meltzer H, Gill B, Petticrew M, *et al* (1995) *Economic Activity and Social Functioning of Adults with Psychiatric Disorders* (OPCS Surveys of Psychiatric Morbidity in Great Britain. Report No. 3. OPCS, Social Survey Division). HMSO.

Meltzer H, Singleton N, Lee A, *et al* (2002) *The Social and Economic Consequences of Adults with Mental Disorders*. TSO (The Stationery Office).

Melzer D, Fryers T, Jenkins R (2003) *Social Inequalities and the Distribution of the Common Mental Disorders* (Maudsley Monograph 44). Psychology Press.

Mental Health Europe (2008) *From Exclusion to Inclusion – The Way Forward to Promoting Social Inclusion of People with Mental Health Problems in Europe*. Mental Health Europe.

Menzies Lyth, I. (1959) *Containing Anxiety in Institutions (Selected Essays, Volume 1)*. Free Association Books.

MIND (2011) *Listening to Experience: An Independent Inquiry into Acute and Crisis Mental Healthcare*. MIND.

Morgan C, Burns T, Fitzpatrick R, *et al* (2007) Social exclusion and mental health. Conceptual and methodological review. *British Journal of Psychiatry*, **191**: 477–83.

National Institute for Mental Health in England (2003) *Personality Disorder. No Longer a Diagnosis of Exclusion: Policy Implementation Guidance for the Development of Services for People with Personality Disorder*. Department of Health.

New Economics Foundation (2009) *National Accounts of Well-Being: Bringing Real Wealth onto the Balance Sheet*. New Economics Foundation.

NHS Confederation (2011) *Facing Up to the Challenge of Personal Health Budgets*. NHS Confederation.

Office of the Deputy Prime Minister (2004) *Mental Health and Social Exclusion*. Office of the Deputy Prime Minister.

Oliver M (1996) *Understanding Disability. From Theory to Practice*. Palgrave.

Pantazis C, Gordon D, Levitas R (2006) *Poverty and Social Exclusion in Britain. The Millennium Study*. Policy Press.

Parker JS (2012) Developing the philosophy of recovery in South African mental health services. *African Journal of Psychiatry*, **15**: 417–20.

Payne S (2006) Mental health, poverty and social exclusion. In *Poverty and Social Exclusion in Britain* (eds C Pantazis, D Gordon, R Levitas): 285–311. Policy Press.

Perkins R, Repper R, Rinaldi M, *et al* (2012) *Recovery Colleges: Implementing Recovery Organisational Change* (ImROC Briefing Paper 1). NHS Confederation/Centre for Mental Health.

Personal Social Services Research Unit (2012) *Evaluation of Personal Health Budget Pilot Programme*. PSSRU.

Pierson J (2010) *Tackling Social Exclusion* (2nd edn). London: Routledge.

Repper J, Perkins R (2003) *Social Inclusion and Recovery*. Baillière Tindall.

Rethink (2012) *The Abandoned Illness: A Report by the Schizophrenia Commission*. Rethink.

Roberts G, Boardman J (2014a) Understanding recovery. *Advances in Psychiatric Treatment*, **19**: 400–9.

Roberts G, Boardman J (2014b) Becoming a recovery-oriented practitioner. *Advances in Psychiatric Treatment*, **20**: 37–47.

Roberts G, Hollins S (2007) Recovery: our common purpose? Editorial. *Advances in Psychiatric Treatment*, **13**: 397–9.

Roberts G, Wolfson P (2004) The rediscovery of recovery: open to all. *Advances in Psychiatric Treatment*, **10**: 37–48.

Roberts G, Dorkins E, Wooldridge J, *et al* (2008) Detained: what's my choice. A discussion paper. *Advances in Psychiatric Treatment*, **14**: 172–80.

Royal College of Psychiatrists & Association of Directors of Adult Social Services (2013) *The Integration of Personal Budgets in Social Care and Personal Budgets in the NHS* (Joint Position Statement PS01/2013). Royal College of Psychiatrists.

Sainsbury Centre for Mental Health (2009) *Implementing Recovery. A New Framework for Organisational Change* (Position Paper). Sainsbury Centre for Mental Health.

Samele C, Seymour L, Morris B, *et al* (2006) *A Formal Investigation into Health Inequalities Experienced by People with Learning Difficulties and People with Mental Health Problems – Area Studies Report*. Disability Rights Commission

Sayce L (2000) *From Psychiatric Patient to Citizen. Overcoming Discrimination and Social Exclusion*. Macmillan.

Shepherd G, Boardman J, Slade M (2008) *Making Recovery a Reality*. Sainsbury Centre for Mental Health.

Shepherd G, Boardman J, Burns M (2010) *Implementing Recovery. A Methodology for Organisational Change*. Sainsbury Centre for Mental Health.

Shepherd G, Boardman J, Rinaldi M, *et al* (2014) *Supporting Recovery in Mental Health Services: Quality and Outcomes* (ImROC Briefing Paper 8). NHS Confederation/Centre for Mental Health.

Slade M (2009) *Personal Recovery and Mental Illness*. Cambridge University Press.

Slade M (2010) Mental illness and well-being: the central importance of positive psychology and recovery approaches. *BCM Health Services Research*, **10**: 26 (http://www.biomedcentral.com/1472-6963/10/26, accessed December 2014).

Slade M, Leamy M, Bacon F, *et al* (2012) International differences in understanding recovery: systematic review. *Epidemiology and Psychiatric Sciences*, **21**: 353–64.

Social Care Institute for Excellence (2008) *Personalisation: A Rough Guide*. SCIE.

Social Exclusion Unit (2001) *Preventing Social Exclusion*. TSO (The Stationery Office).

Social Perspectives Network (2007) *Whose Recovery Is It Anyway?* Social Perspective Network.

South London and Maudsley NHS Foundation Trust & South West London and St George's Mental Health NHS Trust (2010) *Recovery Is For All. Hope, Agency and Opportunity in Psychiatry. A Position Statement by Consultant Psychiatrists*. SLAM/SWLSTG.

Thara R (2012) Consumer perceptions of recovery: an Indian perspective. *World Psychiatry*, **11**: 169–70.

Thornicroft G (2006) *Shunned: Discrimination Against People with Mental Illness*. Oxford University Press.

Trauer T, Duckmanton RA, Chiu E (1998) A study of the quality of life of the severely mentally ill. *International Journal of Social Psychiatry*, **44**: 79–91.

Whitwell D (2005) *Recovery Beyond Psychiatry*. Free Association Books.

CHAPTER 4

A comprehensive approach to assessment in rehabilitation settings

Alan Meaden and Sridevi Kalidindi

Introduction

People requiring rehabilitative interventions are first and foremost individuals, who are likely to have had difficult experiences in their lives, both before and since the emergence of their mental health condition(s). They are likely to have been in contact with services for some years. By the time of referral for rehabilitation they may feel a loss of hope, having seen several clinicians and having received many interventions, none of which have been adequately effective.

The guideline on schizophrenia produced by the National Institute for Health and Care Excellence (NICE) begins with a statement about optimism:

> Work in partnership with people with schizophrenia and their carers. Offer help, treatment and care in an atmosphere of hope and optimism. Take time to build supportive and empathic relationships as an essential part of care. (NICE, 2014)

These sentiments are central to our approach to working with service users, work that starts during the assessment process.

It is important to recognise that clinicians hold a position of relative power when they meet with an often disempowered person, sometimes unwilling and often anxious, to consider the current position, how it has been arrived at and to propose a way forward. Starting at the first meeting, an empathic effort is crucial to understand clients and their story, to engage with them as people who have, or can be supported to have, goals, aspirations, strengths and resources. Alongside this, it is important to assess the complex mix of mental health conditions, comorbidities and behavioural needs that they experience, taking a truly biopsychosocial approach.

There is a clear role for personal self-assessment, to ascertain what the service users make of their condition and situation and how and what they would envisage as being of use to them from clinicians and services more generally. Different frameworks can be adopted: service users at the South London and Maudsley NHS Foundation Trust are encouraged to use the

Recovery and Support Plan, which is discussed in more detail in Chapter 8, 'Rehabilitation at the coalface'. This approach resonates with Copeland's Wellness Recovery Action Plan (Copeland, 2002). Telling one's own story as a narrative in written form is also to be encouraged, as it can be validating and a way of making sense of one's illness. This process takes a collaborative approach between clinician and service user, to consider and negotiate options and opportunities. The aim must be for service users to become self-managing of their conditions and to live as independently as possible and as they wish. Many people who come to rehabilitation services will not be in a position to engage fully in the process at the outset, but with persistence and consistency, across the whole multidisciplinary team, some degree of collaborative working alliance should be possible.

In this chapter we provide a guide to the process of assessment, set out the areas to consider and describe some useful tools. Most importantly we suggest how findings from this assessment process can be drawn together and used to devise a formulation (a basis for care planning and treatment) that can be shared and agreed as much as possible with service users themselves and all those involved in their care.

The process of assessment

A responsive and flexible approach is key when assessing people who come to a rehabilitation service. Some people are unable to tolerate a more formal approach. Assessment in the person's own home is often preferable, if he or she does not find this too intrusive, although if admission to an in-patient unit is planned, a visit to the unit is helpful with engagement. The assessment should be person-centred if it is to be effective and ideally experienced as a collaboration between the clinician, the service user and carers. This ensures that needs are properly identified and addressed, including comorbid conditions. Unidentified or unmet needs can result in recurrent hospital admissions, further decline in function and further loss of hope.

A good starting point for each new person referred is to conduct a thorough case-note review. A pictorial method such as a life chart or timeline can be invaluable to clarify which factors (adopting a biopsychosocial framework) have contributed to periods of relative stability and wellness, as well as those that correlate with periods of illness. Ensuring a good corroborative history from multiple sources, including staff members who know the person and family members, is imperative to give a rounded view of the individual's needs, risks, general level of functioning, strengths and goals. Such assessment also provides the opportunity to highlight any interpersonal or relationship issues, including social isolation or possible abuse or exploitation.

Initial meetings can be lengthy; even so, multiple meetings will often be necessary for an adequate assessment. The process needs to take account of cognitive problems, negative symptoms, suspicion and hostility as well anxiety levels. Some may benefit from a series of shorter meetings. Those who are socially withdrawn may require a slower pace and greater time to reply. It is especially important to use open questions with people who are suggestible and may passively conform to leading questions. People with social anxieties may prefer the involvement of fewer professionals and a less directive approach. When, as is often the case, engagement is an issue, practical support and social activities may provide an appropriate forum for assessment.

Rehabilitation can be a slow process and assessment needs to be ongoing. Longitudinal assessments are preferred, although repeated snapshots may suffice, with the interval determined by the nature and frequency of the problems. A truly multidisciplinary team approach is invaluable in understanding the needs and story of the individual and this context can ensure good, collaborative and SMART (Specific, Measurable, Attainable, Realistic and Timely) goal setting and care planning. Occupational therapy and psychology assessments, alongside the psychiatric assessment, assist in forming a particularly rounded view of the individual. The more informal relationship that people develop with support time and recovery workers (STaR workers) or peer-support workers along with the relatively greater face-to-face time spent with them can also provide very valuable insights of the service user.

Subsequently, an initial assessment conference, with presentations to the wider team, should reach a consensus on some key issues (e.g. fulfilment of service criteria, risk, interests, strengths, goals and initial treatment options) and indicate lines of further assessment and investigation needed to reach a shared formulation. Rating scales may contribute to this process, alongside interviews and accurate observations. Rating scales can be particularly useful as an objective measure of the current levels of symptoms and disability, and as a means of evaluating the impact of interventions and the care plan.

An initial formulation should, where practicable, be shared with the service user and areas of agreement and dissent noted. When issues of lack of capacity arise, then a clear assessment of this and use of the Mental Capacity Act 2005 in the UK, or similar legal frameworks in other countries, should come into play. Family, carers and friends also have a role in the initial assessment and beyond, when the service user wishes their inclusion.

Although, broadly, the principles will be the same, there are different considerations for ongoing assessment to guide the course of rehabilitative care. Clinicians will need to be aware of milestones marking transitions (e.g. for leave if someone is detained) and for preparation for leaving in-patient care or transfer from a specialist to generic community teams.

Unmet or unrecognised needs are common among people requiring a rehabilitation approach. This can result in increased risk, slow progress and a greater probability of relapse, alongside long-term disability, social exclusion and stigma. Some will have received a comprehensive range of therapeutic interventions and the reasons for their success or failure need to be carefully examined. Others may have proved hard to reach or have received a limited range of treatments and experienced an impoverished social or care environment that has had low expectations of them. Finding a way to support people with complex needs, while working from a 'strengths and opportunities' perspective, can be challenging. However, the potential to change the outlook to a more hopeful one, with improved service user engagement and ownership and progress towards recovery, is to be highly prized.

Care planning

A formal process of review should monitor the effectiveness and acceptability of treatment as well as provide an opportunity for further information-gathering and dialogue. Assessment findings and formulations are all too often not reflected in care plans. A process for ensuring that findings are routinely translated into care plans is key to making the best use of assessment and formulation.

What should we assess?

In its schizophrenia guideline, NICE (2014) identifies a number of assessment domains over and above the symptoms of the illness: accommodation; culture and ethnicity; economic status; occupation and education (including employment and functional activity); prescribed and non-prescribed drug history; quality of life; responsibility for children; risk of harm to self and others; sexual health; and social networks. These form a vital background to care planning.

Box 4.1 suggests how to prepare for an assessment after someone is referred. Box 4.2 provides a comprehensive list of the areas that a good rehabilitation assessment covers. This importantly includes a thorough assessment of the person's physical health needs, which is relevant because

---

Box 4.1 Preparations on receiving a referral

- Share and discuss the information with the multidisciplinary team (MDT).
- Come to an initial preliminary view of the main issues and plan the way forward.
- Think who in the MDT will be best placed to assess the person, the location and who else needs to be present (e.g. family, carers, care home staff).
- Consider whether any further information is necessary prior to organising the first meeting

Box 4.2 Initial assessment for rehabilitation

- *Personal self-assessment, engagement and recovery factors:* the person's understanding of his or her condition and situation, as well as of services and treatment (including adherence); the person's hopes and aspirations, valued roles and goals, personal strengths and preferences of options and hopes of support; the person's understanding of difficulties, insight and attitude to illness; motivation for self-management
- *History and pattern of illness:* a life chart/timeline can be useful; detailed history of previous treatments and treatment response – medication, psychological and social interventions; premorbid functioning; duration of untreated psychosis; personal and developmental history
- *Current mental state:* type of symptoms (include depressive and negative symptoms); severity of symptoms; impact on mood and behaviour; change in symptoms, mood, behaviour; non-psychotic symptoms; secondary difficulties (e.g. social anxiety)
- *Risk assessment* – as part of initial, extended and ongoing assessments: deliberate self-harm, violence to others (including sexual violence) and property (including arson), self-neglect, vulnerability to abuse, victimisation and exploitation; specialised risk assessment for those presenting with significant risk behaviours to support a structured professional judgement approach (e.g. HCR-20)
- *Medication:* efficacy in reducing symptoms and distress; efficacy in improving functional level; assessment of side-effects, including questionnaires and physical health investigations – see below
- *Early warning signs:* observed and self-reported, of relapse and risk
- *Substance use:* type, amount, frequency and dependency; impact on self and others, finances, employment and accommodation
- *Coping:* personal coping and coping style; attempts to cope with difficulties
- *Current physical health:* weight; general physical symptoms; mobility; sensory impairment; sexual functioning; monitoring and assessment of the potential side-effects of medication (electrocardiography, metabolic syndrome; drug plasma levels; medication dependant tests); pre-existing physical health conditions and whether they are being adequately managed
- *Social functioning:* longitudinal picture of family and social networks (including family dynamics); quality of life; lifestyle assessment; support systems
- *Cultural, spiritual, gender and sexual issues*
- *Finances*, including the need for benefit advice and support, budgeting skills
- *Accommodation needs* (whether accommodation is safe and supportive)
- *Employment and education (history, attainment and needs)*
- *Carers' assessment:* impact of care and quality of life; psychiatric/psychological symptoms; unmet needs; family members (genogram); clarification of confidentiality/information-sharing issues between services, service user, friends and family; identification of a key point of contact for significant others (whom to contact in a crisis)

of the excess mortality and consequent shortened lifespan associated with a diagnosis of severe mental illness (Vreeland, 2007). The assessment of physical health needs is discussed in detail in Chapter 15, 'Physical healthcare'.

Assessments should be meaningful, be sensitive to the person's stage of illness and recovery, and have a clear purpose. They should be targeted towards the task at hand and be no more detailed or systematic than the circumstances require. They should wherever possible have a recovery focus, incorporating personal goals, hopes, aspirations and motivation for self-management. Additionally, assessment measures should reflect the aims of the service. If a team's rehabilitation approach is based on social recovery and quality of life, then their assessments should reflect this. In the case of assertive outreach teams, it may be useful to assess engagement on an ongoing basis. In residential care, the focus may be to determine the level of independence required for the service user to move on from the service (with account being taken of the types of housing or supported accommodation available).

One vital component of the assessment process is a consideration of the individual's functional skills. Often referred to as 'activities of daily living', these are basic life skills such as shopping, cooking, cleaning, budgeting and interacting with others. Assessment of functional skills is best undertaken in the environment where the person is most likely to use them: one that allows (and expects) the person to use these skills. Assessment for and provision of aids and adaptations may be required to improve and restore function in personal and daily activities of living.

Once treatment has been optimised, symptoms are less significant than function in planning for a person's future care needs, although some specific behavioural problems have been shown to have a marked impact on placement options (Cowan *et al*, 2012). If not adequately assessed and planned for, these may result in the breakdown of placements and repeated acute in-patient admissions.

The growth in psychological interventions has helped to refine the level at which assessments may be targeted. Assessment as described by Haddock & Tarrier (1998) may be carried out at a symptom or syndrome level (e.g. eliciting whether a person is hearing voices), at the level of dimensions of experience (e.g. frequency and severity of voices), or used to inform therapy (e.g. assessing the antecedents and consequences of hearing voices).

The value of diagnostic assessments

Accurate diagnosis guides evidence-based pharmacological and psychological treatments and can support the person's own research and link her or him to other individuals and organisations. Some people find a formal diagnosis such as schizophrenia stigmatising. Historically, important comorbidity has been obscured by the label of 'psychosis'. Problems and distress related to depression, anxiety, obsessional symptoms, substance misuse, personality disorder, intellectual disability, acquired brain injury and autistic spectrum disorder will certainly colour the clinical picture and may require specific therapeutic intervention. Where such difficulties go unrecognised, well-intentioned rehabilitation efforts may fail, which will be frustrating for all concerned and may lead to reduced empathy among staff and subsequent 'heart sink.'

Substance misuse

Individuals diagnosed with schizophrenia present with an increased risk of substance misuse, which in turn is associated with an increased risk of relapse, medication non-compliance, aggression, depression, suicide, unstable housing and family burden (Drake & Mueser, 2001; NICE, 2011). Chapter 12, 'Working with coexisting substance misuse', provides an up-to-the-minute and practical account of the assessment and treatment of substance misuse.Detection and screening are important in any assessment.

Autism spectrum disorder

Impairments in social interaction and communication in autism, which occurs in approximately 1% of adults, may be misinterpreted as evidence of both positive and negative symptoms of schizophrenia spectrum disorders. Chapter 25, 'Autism spectrum disorder', provides a detailed account of both assessment and the therapeutic options that are available.

Some people in this group require high levels of support, whereas others live independently but may be significantly disadvantaged in social terms (Brugha *et al*, 2011). The increased recognition that those with autism can go unrecognised, with unmet needs, has resulted in national clinical guidance (NICE, 2012, 2013) and UK legislation (Autism Act 2009). The overvalued ideas, often with persecutory content, and the way in which experiences are explained, thought to be in keeping with theory-of-mind deficits, can be incorrectly labelled by psychiatrists as psychosis. Autism may coexist with a psychotic disorder and there is some evidence to suggest the prevalence of schizophrenia is increased in people with autism (Stahlberg *et al*, 2004; Rapoport *et al*, 2009) and indeed some evidence that suggests shared genetic factors (Carroll & Owen, 2009).

Obtaining a good developmental history and assessing as far as possible social interaction and communication difficulties are essential. Where both disorders are present, people may fall between services, partly owing to lack of staff training and confidence in how to manage autism and partly to commissioning structures in some countries.

Personality difficulties and personality disorder

Persons presenting with personality difficulties often engender a degree of hostility from staff. Personality characteristics influence the way in which people engage with treatment. However, for some this influence may be more marked and may significantly impair the rehabilitation process. Certain personality disorders are more closely associated with schizophrenia than others. Those with paranoid, schizoid or schizotypal personality disorder often present with psychotic-like symptoms (Derksen, 1995), and these personality disorders are implicated as vulnerability factors in the development of schizophrenia (Nuechterlein & Subotnik, 1998). Psychotic-like symptoms may also emerge in borderline personality disorder. It is important therefore to give consideration to premorbid functioning, and the persistence of psychotic symptoms when conducting an assessment. The development of a 'shared formulation', described later in this chapter, may be particularly relevant when working with people with comorbid personality disorder.

The value of structured assessments

Formal measures provide a valuable guide and structure to asking the most relevant questions. A rating system is often used. This supports the prioritising of needs and helps to capture any change. In an era that demands the routine evaluation of care, structured tools can provide valuable feedback and evidence to clinicians, carers and most importantly the client that progress is being made and that the often careful, undramatic and persistent efforts of a rehabilitation process are of benefit. 'Goal attainment scaling', developed by Kiresuk *et al* (1994), can be particularly helpful in this respect. This process helps to define progress, measured in terms of specific short-term achievable goals that are concrete and clear and relevant to enabling recovery. If well selected to match service aims, measures can provide outcomes to commissioners and also support research into the unfashionable area of rehabilitation, developing its evidence base.

Assessment tools in rehabilitation practice

Assessment tools have been developed that aim to standardise direct observations or interviews. Interviews can be structured, such as the Present State Examination (Wing *et al*, 1974) or systematic, in the form of a rating scale, such as the Brief Psychiatric Rating Scale (Lukoff *et al*, 1986) or the Health of the Nation Outcome Scales (HoNOS; Wing *et al*, 1996). Structured interviews are mainly used in research, while rating scales are more widely used in clinical practice. The assessment process and tools should together be used to provide as comprehensive a view as possible.

Box 4.3 lists some basic assessment tools that are used successfully in rehabilitation services. These look at need, social functioning, symptoms, side-effects of medication and the service user's perspective. There are particular difficulties in capturing the service user's perspective on rehabilitation needs. The Recovery and Support Plan is in routine use within South London & Maudsley NHS Foundation Trust. Another tool, the Recovery Star, is popular in rehabilitation settings. It is perceived as providing a personal and self-rated perspective on an individual's priorities

Box 4.3 Basic assessment tools for assessment in psychiatric rehabilitation

- Camberwell Assessment of Need Short Assessment Schedule (Slade *et al*, 1999)
- Social Functioning Questionnaire (Clifford & Morris, 1983)
- Life Skills Profile (Rosen *et al*, 1989)
- Health of the Nation Outcome Scales (Wing *et al*, 1996)
- Model Of Human Occupation Screening Tool (MOHOST; Baron *et al*, 1998)
- Liverpool University Neuroleptic Side-Effect Scale (LUNSERS; Day *et al*, 1995)
- Recovery and Support Plan (South London & Maudsley NHS Foundation Trust, unpublished)

and quality of life. It can be used to monitor progress in reaching personal goals or recovery as defined by the individual. Although there are concerns with its psychometric properties, as an outcome measure the Recovery Star can undoubtedly facilitate discussions between service user, clinicians and family/carers to feed into collaborative care and support planning (Killaspy *et al*, 2012).

These tools can be supplemented as necessary to provide a more extended assessment relevant to the planning and monitoring of occupational therapy and psychological interventions. For the assessment and monitoring of psychological interventions we routinely use: the Beliefs About Voices Questionnaire–Revised (Chadwick *et al*, 2000); the schedule for the Cognitive Assessment of Voices (Chadwick & Birchwood, 1995); and the Beliefs and Convictions Scale (Brett-Jones *et al*, 1987); as well as psychotic symptom rating scales such as: the Postive and Negative Syndrome Scale (Kay, 1991); the Calgary Depression Scale (Addington *et al*, 1993), and the Beck Anxiety Inventory (Beck *et al*, 1988). The Early Signs Scale (Birchwood *et al*, 1989) is useful for developing relapse plans and monitoring early signs of relapse. The Personal Beliefs About Illness Questionnaire (Birchwood *et al*, 1993), Attitude to Relapse Interview and Scale (Smith, 2003), Recovery Style Questionnaire (Drayton *et al*, 1998) and Hall Engagement Scale (Hall *et al*, 2001) are useful for assessing attitude to relapse, recovery style and service engagement, respectively. The Model of Human Occupation Screening Tool (MOHOST; Baron *et al*, 1998) is valuable in assessing functional abilities, supplemented as necessary by other scales to measure activities of daily living and interests. We add to this a good quality-of-life measure such as the Manchester Short Assessment of Quality of Life (Priebe *et al*, 1999).

There may be a need for supplementary specialist assessments to ensure that there is a full profile of the difficulties and needs. It may be necessary to use tools for the diagnosis of comorbid disorders such as autism, personality disorder, substance misuse and physical health conditions. For some people, more specialist forensic or other risk assessments are required, such as the HCR-20 (Douglas *et al*, 2013). Assessment of cognitive deficits is discussed below.

Structured assessment tools may be helpful in the decision-making process surrounding transitions within and between settings. If assessment tools are, as we recommend, to be used routinely, the team will need training so that, ideally, all members feel confident to carry out such assessments. Training is as important as experience and administering these tools, and analysing and interpreting the results are complex skills.

Assessment of cognitive impairment

There is evidence that approximately 70% of people with schizophrenia show specific cognitive deficits in the context of generalised cognitive impairment (Harvey & Sharma, 2002; Sharma & Antonova, 2003; Leeson *et al*, 2009). These affect quality of life (Maat *et al*, 2012). Cognitive impairments show a greater relationship to negative symptoms than to positive symptoms but do not appear to be caused by them and may persist even when negative symptoms improve (Leff *et al*, 1994).

Cognitive impairments are a significant predictor of outcome in terms of social and occupational functioning and independent living (Green *et al*, 2000; Sharma & Antonova, 2003) and predict success in acquiring daily living skills and in work rehabilitation (Bell & Bryson, 2001). Knowledge of cognitive impairment is therefore important when planning rehabilitation interventions. Box 4.4 outlines the specific cognitive deficits commonly experienced by people with a diagnosis of schizophrenia.

Assessing cognitive difficulties is a specialist task best undertaken by a clinical psychologist who has, ideally, undertaken further specialist training in neuropsychology. Occupational therapists will also be able

---

Box 4.4 Areas in which people with a diagnosis of schizophrenia commonly have cognitive deficits

- Learning new verbal information
- Sustained attention or vigilance and distractibility
- Executive functions (a range of higher-level cognitive functions, including attentional inhibition and attentional switching, initiation of action, planning and error monitoring)
- Verbal fluency
- Working memory (the ability to hold information in mind for a short time and mentally manipulate that information to perform a task)
- Recall of information
- Visuo-motor skills

From Harvey & Sharma (2002)

to assess cognition, with an emphasis on functional abilities. Functional assessment, using tools such as MOHOST is helpful in monitoring progress and assessing the functional impact of cognitive impairment, and should be part of a comprehensive multidisciplinary assessment.

A vast number of tools for cognitive assessment are available. The Wechsler Adult Intelligence Scale (4th edition) (WAIS-IV; Wechsler, 2008) provides a useful measure of current intellectual functioning and problem-solving ability; the Wechsler Memory Scale (4th edition) (WMS-IV; Wechsler, 2009) provides a useful and detailed measure of memory function. Tools for assessing executive functions include the Delis Kaplan Executive Functions System (DKEFS; Delis & Kaplan, 2001), the Hayling and Brixton (Burgess & Shallice, 1997) and the Behavioural Assessment of Dysexecutive Syndrome (BADS; Wilson *et al*, 1996). Assessing premorbid intelligence (taking into account educational opportunities) using the Test of Premorbid Functioning (Wechsler, 2011) will give an estimation of any decline from pre-illness abilities.

It is essential that clinicians consider the validity of the test results obtained, by assessing the degree to which the individual has applied him- or herself to the test situation. A number of tools exist for this purpose but the Test of Memory Malingering (TOMM; Tombaugh, 1996) has been shown to be relatively insensitive to the symptoms of schizophrenia and so is valid for use in this population as a symptom validity test (Duncan, 2005).

Given the increasing recognition of cognitive impairment in schizophrenia, together with the general failure of conventional drug treatment to treat this impairment, there is currently much interest from the pharmaceutical industry in developing drugs that target negative symptoms. Several recent studies have evaluated the potential for cognitive rehabilitation in schizophrenia and this topic is covered in detail in Chapter 9, 'Cognitive approaches'.

Risk assessment

Risk assessment is a core element of psychiatric practice. In reality, assessment of risk is of no value unless it is associated with the development of plans to manage the risk. It is also necessary to emphasise at the outset that positive therapeutic risk-taking is of key importance in enabling people to learn and move on from an apparently 'stuck' situation. Chapter 26, 'Risk management in rehabilitation practice', provides a detailed account of the issues surrounding the topic.

Estimates for risk behaviour vary, depending on the type of behaviour chosen and the specific population studied (Meaden & Hacker, 2011). The assessment and management of risk are both continuous and iterative processes. Reassessment is necessary at key points in a service user's transition between different levels of service, as the same risks may have to be managed very differently and new risks may come to the fore, for example if the service user moves from an in-patient ward to a community setting.

People with mental health problems present with a wide range of risk behaviours, including: physical (non-sexual) violence or aggression (hitting others, use of weapons); verbal aggression (shouting, insults, threats to harm); suicide (overdose, hanging, jumping, cutting wrists, carbon monoxide poisoning); self-harm (cutting, stubbing out cigarettes on oneself, ingesting noxious substances); self-neglect; vulnerability to exploitation or assault; self-denial of personal possessions or food; and poor road safety skills. Less common are arson and sexual violence (rape, indecent assault, child molestation, exposure, stalking).

Methods of risk assessment

Risk assessment can take a variety of forms: unstructured clinical judgement; structured professional judgement, as recommended by the Department of Health (2007), which draws on both clinical experience and the evidence base; actuarial assessment, involving scoring individuals on tools that cover known risk factors predictive of particular future risks (e.g. the Violence Risk Appraisal Guide; Harris *et al*, 1993), which supports a structured professional judgement approach; and anamnestic assessment, based on what the person has done before and the circumstances involved.

Unstructured judgements are no better than chance at estimating risk (Monahan, 1981). A useful framework for conceptualising risk and how best to manage it is to consider the following about individuals:

- What will they do?
- What have they done before? The best predictor of future behaviour is past behaviour.
- Under what circumstances did the behaviour occur? Why does this risk behaviour occur and what factors drive it?
- Are those circumstances present now? Answering this question facilitates positive risk-taking.
- Will the circumstances emerge if the context changes (e.g. on discharge from hospital)?
- Can the factors driving the behaviour be changed? Are these factors treatable?
- How is the risk best managed? Can the individual be monitored and supervised?

The risk of violent behaviour is linked to: a history of violence (Bonta *et al*, 1998; Andrews *et al*, 2006); the use of alcohol and other drugs (Swanson *et al*, 1990; Monahan *et al*, 2001); personality disorder, especially if antisocial attitudes are evident (Monahan *et al*, 2001); poor involvement in treatment and medication non-compliance (Swartz *et al*, 1998; Monahan *et al*, 2001); the presence of paranoid delusions, particularly when 'threat-control override' symptoms are present (Swanson *et al*, 1996; Appelbaum *et al*, 2000); and the presence of command hallucinations that command violence (Birchwood *et al*, 2011).

The forensic literature delineates three types of risk factor (Beech & Ward, 2004; Douglas & Skeem, 2005): *static, dynamic stable* and *dynamic acute*. These may usefully be combined into a risk formulation framework to guide treatment and supervision.

Static (including historical) factors cannot, by definition, change over time. They are based on factors known to predict specific types of risk behaviour (e.g. age, age at first offence, gender, number of previous offences) as well as what the person has done previously. Identifying static factors helps to answer the question 'How likely is this person, compared with others who have committed an offence, to engage in this behaviour again (within a specified time period)?'

Dynamic stable factors are enduring factors linked to the likelihood of risk behaviours occurring. These are considered dynamic since they may change spontaneously or with treatment, but change may be slow. Assessment of dynamic stable factors involves attempts to understand what factors were involved in previous risk behaviours and how they might be linked to risk. Such an assessment helps to define treatment targets (e.g. command hallucinations or substance use), with the aim of reducing risk and promoting positive risk-taking.

Dynamic acute factors are more rapidly changing and their presence increases the likelihood of the risk behaviour imminently: increased substance use; non-compliance with medication; isolation; distress; increased preoccupation with delusions. These factors relate most closely to the immediate management of risk.

Team processes

In order to carry out a comprehensive assessment, a great deal of information needs to be elicited, recorded, shared and made useful. This requires a clear structure, which should be developed locally and fit in with current guidance and national policies. Findings from various assessment tools can then be organised into this structure (described below) and the relevant interventions planned. Team skills need to include an understanding of benefit and accommodation issues, ability to assess capacity and guardianship, knowledge of the mental health legislation, vulnerability legislation (including adult and child protection), familiarity with carer needs, skills to assess occupational, work and education problems, psychological needs and management of treatment resistance.

Assessment should not be seen as comprising a static 'tick box' exercise but as an ongoing collaborative process. If undertaken sensitively and carried out collaboratively, assessment can be an engaging and therapeutic process in itself. Clinicians may usefully begin by asking whether the person needs a specialist rehabilitation service (community or in-patient), whether the person's needs can be met in more generic services, or whether advice and support for the existing care team may suffice. An evaluation of risk may indicate the need for urgency or the need for an alternative care setting. Emerging goals of the care plan should be clear, realistic, relevant to enabling recovery and measurable.

Drawing it all together: the formulation

In order to make assessment findings meaningful, they should be collated and shared as part of a process that facilitates care planning and problem-solving. Formulation is a useful method for drawing together assessment findings. Formulation may best be described as 'a map of a person's presenting problems that describes the territory of the problems and explains the processes that caused and maintain the problems' (Bieling & Kuyken, 2003: p. 53). Various formats exist, including the '5 Ps': Presenting problems and Precipitating, Perpetuating, Predisposing and Protective factors (Johnstone & Dallos, 2006). A sixth P (Plan) may be usefully added. However, this is a broad level of formulation and specific formulations may be needed to address specific clinical issues and problems, such as risk (Meaden & Hacker, 2011).

Formulation should not involve simply completing a template. As Westermeyer (2003) has noted, the process of formulation is equally important, if not more so, as the end product itself. Indeed, mixed results have been reported when completed templates are presented to patients. The formulation process should therefore provide a collaborative problem-solving framework and promote a shared view and consistent approach. Meaden & Hacker (2011) have argued that an overarching framework is required that incorporates the person's own unique personal goals, hopes and values as well as environmental, social and person-based barriers to participation in ordinary community living. Fig. 4.1 provides an example of a formulation.

As Chapter 2, 'What is psychiatric rehabilitation?', describes, the biopsychosocial perspective is now a widely accepted way of conceptualising the difficulties presented by those who experience psychosis. This perspective is usually framed within a stress–vulnerability model and recognises how biological, psychological and social factors combine and interact in the onset and maintenance of psychotic symptoms and their associated difficulties. The model provides a valuable perspective when developing a formulation. All too often formulations are not reflected in the client's care plan, which is often centred on broad goals that are non-specific and therefore unlikely to lead to any meaningful change in the delivery of care. Formulation elements may usefully be adopted as SMART goals and goal attainment scaling (described earlier in this chapter, under 'The value of structured assessments') may be used to gauge progress in meeting specific goals.

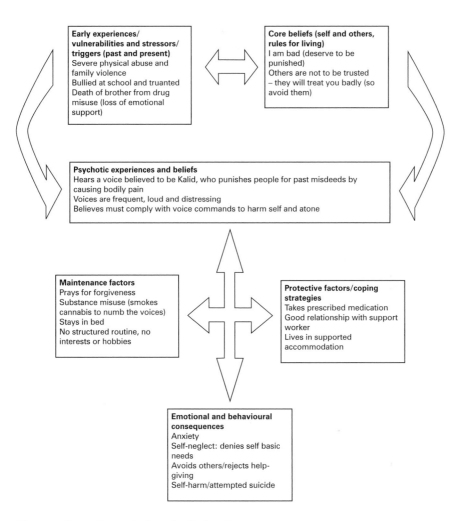

Fig. 4.1 Shared formulation of a fictional case

Conclusions

Assessment is a crucial element in the provision of good mental healthcare and service user rehabilitation and recovery. In this chapter we have outlined a comprehensive process of assessment and highlighted the importance of promoting meaningful, collaborative and relevant outcomes for service users, carers and clinical staff. Appropriate training for staff and ongoing support for staff and service users to engage more actively in this process are vitally important.

References

Addington D, Addington J, Maticka-Tyndale E (1993) Assessing depression in schizophrenia: The Calgary Depression Scale. *British Journal of Psychiatry*, **163** (suppl. 22): 39–44.

Andrews D, Bonta J, Wormith S (2006) The recent past and near future of risk and/or need assessment. *Crime and Delinquency*, **52**: 7–27.

Appelbaum PS, Robbind PC, Monahan J (2000) Violence and delusions: data from the MacArthur Violence Risk Assessment Study. *American Journal of Psychiatry*, **157**: 566–72.

Baron K, Kielhofner G, Iynger A, *et al* (1998) *The Occupational Self Assessment (OSA) Version 2.2*. Model of Human Occupation Clearinghouse, University of Illinois of Chicago.

Beck AT, Epstein N, Brown G, *et al* (1988) An inventory for measuring clinical anxiety: psychometric properties.*Journal of Consulting and Clinical Psychology*, **56**: 893–7.

Beech AR, Ward T (2004) The integration of aetiology and risk in sex offenders: A theoretical model. *Aggression and Violent Behaviour*, **10**: 31–63.

Bell MD, Bryson G (2001) Work rehabilitation in schizophrenia: does cognitive impairment limit improvement? *Schizophrenia Bulletin*, **27**: 269–79.

Bieling P, Kuyken W (2003) Is cognitive case formulation science or science fiction? *Clinical Psychology: Science and Practice*, **10**: 52–69.

Birchwood M, Smith J, MacMillan F, *et al* (1989) Predicting relapse in schizophrenia: The development and implementation of an early signs monitoring system using patients and families as observers, a preliminary investigation. *Psychological Medicine*, **19**: 649–56.

Birchwood M, Mason R, Macmillan F, *et al* (1993) Depression, demoralization and control over psychotic illness: a comparison of depressed and non-depressed patients with a chronic psychosis. *Psychological Medicine*, **23**: 387–95.

Birchwood M, Peters E, Tarrier N, *et al* (2011) A multi-centre, randomised controlled trial of cognitive therapy to prevent harmful compliance with command hallucinations. *BMC Psychiatry*, **11**: 155.

Bonta J, Hanson K, Law M (1998) The prediction of criminal and violent recidivism among mentally disordered offenders: a meta-analysis. *Psychological Bulletin*, **123**: 123–42.

Brett-Jones J, Garety P, Hemsley D (1987) Measuring delusional experiences: A method and its application. *British Journal of Clinical Psychology*, **26**: 257–65.

Brugha TS, McManus S, Bankart J, *et al* (2011) Epidemiology of autism spectrum disorders in adults in the community in England. *Archives of General Psychiatry*, **68**: 59–65.

Burgess P, Shallice T (1997) *The Hayling and Brixton Tests. Test Manual*. Thames Valley Test Company.

Carroll LS, Owen MJ (2009) Genetic overlap between autism, schizophrenia and bipolar disorder. *Genome Medicine*, **1**: 102.

Chadwick P, Birchwood M (1995)The omnipotence of voices II: The Beliefs About Voices Questionnaire. *British Journal of Psychiatry*, **166**: 773–6.

Chadwick P, Lees S, Birchwood M (2000) The revised Beliefs About Voices Questionnaire (BAVQ-R). *British Journal of Psychiatry*, **177**: 229–32.

Clifford P, Morris I (1983) *The Social Functioning Questionnaire*. Research and Development for Psychiatry.

Copeland M (2002) *Wellness Recovery Action Plan*. Peach Press.

Cowan C, Meaden A, Commander M, *et al* (2012) In-patient psychiatric rehabilitation services: Survey of service users in three metropolitan boroughs. *Psychiatric Bulletin*, **36**: 85–9.

Day JC, Wood G, Dewey M and Bentall RP (1995) A self-rating scale for measuring neuroleptic side-effects. Validation in a group of schizophrenic patients. *British Journal of Psychiatry*, **166**: 650–3.

Delis DC, Kaplan E (2001) *Delis-Kaplan Executive Function System: Examiner's Manual*. Psychological Corporation.

Department of Health (2007) *Best Practice in Managing Risk*. Department of Health.

Derksen J (1995) *Personality Disorders: Clinical and Social Perspectives.* Wiley.

Douglas KS, Skeem JL (2005) Violence risk assessment: Getting specific about being dynamic. *Psychology, Public Policy and Law,* **11**: 347–83.

Douglas KS, Hart SD, Webster CD, *et al* (2013) *HCR-20 V3: Assessing Risk of Violence – User Guide.* Mental Health, Law, and Policy Institute, Simon Fraser University.

Drake RE, Mueser KT (2001) Substance abuse comorbidity. In *Comprehensive Care of Schizophrenia: A Textbook of Clinical Management* (eds JA Lieberman, RM Murray), 243–55. Taylor and Francis.

Drayton M, Birchwood M, Trower P (1998) Early attachment experience and recovery from psychosis. *British Journal of Clinical Psychology,* **37**: 269–84.

Duncan A (2005) The impact of cognitive and psychiatric impairment of psychotic disorders on the test of memory malingering (TOMM). *Assessment,* **12**: 123–9.

Green MF, Kern RS, Braff DL, *et al* (2000) Neurocognitive deficits and functional outcome in schizophrenia: are we measuring the 'right stuff'? *Schizophrenia Bulletin,* **26**: 119–36.

Haddock G, Tarrier N (1998) Assessment and formulation in the cognitive behavioural treatment of psychosis. In *Treating Complex Cases: The Cognitive Behavioural Therapy Approach* (eds N Tarrier, A Wells): 155–75. Wiley.

Hall M, Meaden A, Smith J, *et al* (2001) Brief report: The development and psychometric properties of an observer-rated measure of engagement with mental health services. *Journal of Mental Health,* **10**: 457–65.

Harris GT, Rice ME, Quinsey VL (1993) Violent recidivism of mentally disordered offenders: the development of a statistical prediction instrument. *Criminal Justice and Behaviour,* **20**: 315–35.

Harvey PD, Sharma T (2002) *Understanding and Treating Cognition in Schizophrenia: A Clinician's Handbook.* Martin Dunitz.

Johnstone L, Dallos R (2006) *Formulation in Psychology and Psychotherapy.* Routledge.

Kay SR (1991) *Positive and Negative Syndromes in Schizophrenia: Assessment and Research.* Brunner/Mazel.

Killaspy H, White S, Taylor TL, *et al* (2012) Psychometric properties of the Mental Health Recovery Star. *British Journal of Psychiatry,* **201**: 65–70.

Kiresuk TJ, Smith A, Cardillo JE (1994) *Goal Attainment Scaling: Applications, Theory and Measurement.* Lawrence Erlbaum Associates.

Leeson V, Robbins T, Matheson E, *et al* (2009) Discrimination learning, reversal, and set-shifting in first episode schizophrenia: stability over six years and specific associations with medication type and disorganization syndrome. *Biological Psychiatry,* **66**: 586–93.

Leff J, Thornicroft G, Coxhead N, et al (1994) The TAPS project: A five-year follow-up of long-stay psychiatric patients discharged to the community. *British Journal of Psychiatry,* **165** (suppl. 25): 13–17.

Lukoff D, Nuchterlein K, Ventura J (1986) Manual for Expanded Brief Psychiatric Rating Scale (BPRS). *Schizophrenia Bulletin,* **4**: 594–602.

Maat A, Fett AK, Derks E, *et al* (2012) Social cognition and quality of life in schizophrenia. *Schizophrenia Research,* **137**: 212–18.

Meaden A, Hacker D (2011) *Problematic and Risk Behaviours in Psychosis: A Shared Formulation Approach.* Routledge.

Monahan J (1981) *The Clinical Prediction of Violent Behavior.* Government Printing House.

Monahan J, Steadman HJ, Silver E, *et al* (2001) *Rethinking Risk Assessment: The Macarthur Study of Mental Disorder and Violence.* Oxford University Press.

National Institute for Health and Care Excellence (2014) *Psychosis and Schizophrenia in Adults: Treatment and Management* (NICE Clinical Guidance 178). NICE.

National Institute for Health and Clinical Excellence (2011) *Psychosis with Coexisting Substance Misuse* (NICE Clinical Guideline 120, Full Guideline). British Psychological Society and Royal College of Psychiatrists.

National Institute for Health and Clinical Excellence (2012) *Autism: Recognition, Referral, Diagnosis and Management of Adults on the Autism Spectrum* (NICE Clinical Guidance 142). NICE.

National Institute for Health and Clinical Excellence (2013) *Autism – Management of Autism in Children and Young People* (NICE Clinical Guidance 170). NICE.

Nuechterlein KH, Subotnik KL (1998) The cognitive origins of schizophrenia and prospects for intervention. In *Outcome and Innovation in Psychological Treatment of Schizophrenia* (eds T Wykes, N Tarrier, S Lewis): 17–43. Wiley.

Priebe S, Huxley P, Knight S, *et al* (1999) Application and results of the Manchester Short Assessment of Quality of Life (MANSA). *International Journal of Social Psychiatry*, **45**: 7–12.

Rapoport J, Chavez A, Greenstein D, *et al* (2009) Autism spectrum disorders and childhood-onset schizophrenia: clinical and biological contributions to a relation revisited. *Journal of the American Academy of Child and Adolescent Psychiatry*, **48**: 10–18.

Rosen A, Hadzi-Pavlovic D, Parker G (1989) The Life Skills Profile: a measure assessing function and disability in schizophrenia. *Schizophrenia Bulletin*, **15**: 325–37.

Sharma T, Antonova L (2003) Cognitive function in schizophrenia. Deficits, functional consequences, and future treatment. *Psychiatric Clinics of North America*, **26**: 25–40.

Slade M, Thornicroft G, Loftus L, *et al* (1999) *CAN: Camberwell Assessment of Need*. Gaskell.

Smith J (2003) *Early Warning Signs: A Self-Management Training Manual for Individuals with Psychosis*. Worcester Community and Mental Health Trust.

Stahlberg O, Soderstrom H, Rastam M, *et al* (2004) Bipolar disorder, schizophrenia, and other psychotic disorders in adults with childhood onset AD/HD and/or autism spectrum disorders. *Journal of Neural Transmission*, **111**: 891–902.

Swanson JW, Holzer CE, III, Ganju VK, *et al* (1990) Violence and psychiatric disorder in the community: evidence from the Epidemiologic Catchment Area surveys. *Hospital and Community Psychiatry*, **41**: 761–70.

Swanson JW, Borum R, Swartz MS (1996) Psychotic symptoms and disorders and the risk of violent behaviour in the community. *Criminal Behaviour and Mental Health*, **6**: 309–29.

Swarz MS, Swanson JW, Hiday VA, *et al* (1998) Violence and severe mental illness: the effects of substance abuse and nonadherence to medication. *American Journal of Psychiatry*, **155**: 226–31.

Tombaugh TN (1996) *TOMM: Test of Memory Malingering (Test Manual)*. Multi-Health Systems Inc.

Vreeland B (2007) Treatment decisions in major mental illness: weighing the outcomes. *Journal of Clinical Psychiatry*, **68** (suppl. 12): 5–11.

Wechsler D (2008) *Wechsler Adult Intelligence Scale, Fourth Edition*. Pearson.

Wechsler D (2009) *Wechsler Memory Scale, Fourth Edition*. Pearson.

Wechsler D (2011) *Test of Premorbid Functioning*. Pearson.

Westermeyer H (2003) On the structure of case formulations. *European Journal of Psychological Assessment*, **19**: 210–16.

Wilson BA, Alderman N, Burgess PW, *et al* (1996) *Behavioural Assessment of the Dysexecutive Syndrome (BADS)*. Thames Valley Test Company.

Wing JK, Cooper JE, Sartorius N (1974) *Measurement and Classification of Psychiatric Symptoms*. Cambridge University Press.

Wing JK, Cooper JE, Beevor A (1996) *The Health of the Nation Outcome Scales*. Royal College of Psychiatrists.

CHAPTER 5

Understanding madness: a psychosocial perspective

Elina Baker and Glenn Roberts

Much madness is divinest sense to a discerning eye.
Emily Dickinson, 1890

Introduction

Understanding madness may at first seem a futile prospect, for psychosis, madness, has historically been defined as 'un-understandable' and can appear bizarre, confusing or completely unintelligible to those encountering it from the outside. We disagree, and we are not alone, for there is historical precedent and current interest in reconsidering how to understand both the occurrence of psychosis and the link between psychotic symptoms and people's life experiences.

There has been a historical division of understanding between the now dominant biomedical approach, which understands madness as an illness with essentially meaningless symptoms, and psychosocial perspectives, which understand madness, in both form and content, as a personal reaction, meaningfully related to life experience. In the equivalent chapter in the first edition of this book, one of us (G.R.) offered a potential bridge across this divide, through suggesting that the contents of many symptoms of madness may arise from people's attempts to ascribe meaning to a confusing psycho-physiological process. In revisiting the chapter together, we have agreed to offer a psychosocial perspective, reviewing some of the related theory and evidence that have become available since the first edition was published in 2006. Our different backgrounds and training have led to us wanting to give greater or lesser emphasis to the possible causal role of life events and we will reflect on how our understanding of causes has implications for the relationships we establish in therapeutic settings and the nature of and rationale for our treatments. Nonetheless, we share the previous conclusion: that a collaborative search for meaning can be 'antipsychotic', by fostering trusting, compassionate and thus healing relationships with people to whom it could otherwise be difficult to relate. Our argument constitutes a balancing rather than balanced contribution; it aims for an expectation and appreciation of meaningfulness in our work as a foundation for helpful relationships with people travelling through this profound experience, in support of their recovery.

Our shared premise is thus that, whatever the origins of psychosis, in common with Emily Dickinson's observation above, it may be possible to find meaning in experiences that at first glance appear purely nonsensical. We believe that there are good reasons to be interested in the sense that people make of their psychotic experience and particularly the connections that can be made between the context of their lives and the nature of their experiences. In this chapter we will review these reasons, by looking at what is known about personal recovery processes and by discussing possible links between childhood adversity and psychosis. We will also describe how these understandings can be translated into practice, in ways that support collaborative and creative working and break down barriers. As part of this, we will discuss what it takes to develop a 'discerning eye', in ourselves, the teams with which we work and in the people we are seeking to support, identifying ways in which such an approach can contribute to moving forward from the confusion, helplessness and alienation that so often characterises madness.

Why try to make sense of madness?

The recovery and service user movements (see Chapter 3, 'Rehabilitation as a values-led practice') have documented a strong interest among many people with lived experience of mental health difficulties in identifying connections between their experiences and the context of their lives. They have both emphasised the need for people exploring this to be supported by mental health services. This has translated into good practice guidance, with the guideline for schizophrenia from the National Institute for Health and Clinical Excellence (2009) recommending that 'service users should be offered help to better understand the period of illness, and given the opportunity to write their account in their notes'. Despite the pivotal status of guidance from the Institute, in our experience personal narratives are rarely recorded alongside professional accounts of a person's difficulties in this way. There is an ongoing call from service user organisations, such as the Hearing Voices Network, for professionals to have a greater focus on the links between psychosis and life events and to be more concerned with 'what has happened to this person?' rather than 'what is wrong with this person?' (Dillon, 2013).

Systematic analysis of people's accounts of living successfully with psychotic experience has identified that finding a way to understand and accept the experience that makes sense to the person (and not necessarily one that reflects a traditional definition of 'insight') is important. This has been described as 'developing a coherent account of experience' (May, 2004), which is similar to Slade's (2009: p. 85) identification, as one of his four key tasks in personal recovery, of 'developing a personally satisfactory meaning to frame the experience which professionals would understand as mental illness'. This suggests that it may be useful to incorporate into rehabilitation practice the search for a personally acceptable framework of meaning that accounts for the experience of psychosis.

Slade (2009) suggests that having a way of making sense of the experience may support recovery by allowing the person to see the possibility of moving beyond it and to sustain an identity separate from 'illness'. We have also found it to be a useful starting point for rehabilitation, as it may point towards new strategies for managing the experience. Many people will come to use rehabilitation services because their condition is resistant to treatment: there is emerging evidence that antipsychotic medication may have more limited effectiveness than previously thought (Morrison *et al*, 2012), suggesting a pressing need to develop alternative or adjunctive approaches. Resistance to treatment often also takes the form of treatment refusal, possibly reflecting this evidence of limited therapeutic benefits, as well as its adverse effects. Drawing on the person's preferred framework for understanding creates the possibility of collaborative problem-solving and may lead to the identification of strategies that are acceptable to and valued by the person. We will discuss a range of potential approaches in more depth below.

Just as having a personally satisfactory understanding of their condition may enable people to overcome the self-stigma that results from the experience of mental health difficulties, viewing madness as meaningful may mitigate the associated stigma from others, resulting in more compassionate and productive engagement with mental health workers, families and the wider community. Making psychosis understandable supports efforts to see beyond it, to a person's wider identity and the range of qualities, strengths and priorities that good rehabilitation practice seeks to identify and amplify. Positive relationships and valued social roles have also been identified as key to the recovery process (Slade, 2009) and enabling understanding may powerfully counteract processes of 'othering' (Tew, 2005). We will also discuss ways in which greater understanding between people with mental health problems and their social networks can be fostered.

Is madness a meaningful reaction to life events?

It has not always been the case that madness has been predominantly understood as the meaningless consequence of a biological process. At the inception of the schizophrenia concept, and based upon an unusually close relationship with his patients, we find Bleuler (1950: p. 403) observing that 'At first all this may appear sheer nonsense', but that 'on closer scrutiny we find understandable connections in every one of these cases ... the delusions of the paranoiac form a logical structure with only a few false premises and inferences in its foundation, or among its building stones; the delusions of the schizophrenic are not as systematic, yet they are not the chance heap of unruly chaos which they seem on superficial observation'. Jung, working alongside Bleuler, also saw continuity with ordinary mental life as well as discontinuity: 'when we penetrate into the human secrets of our patients, the madness discloses the system upon which it is based, and we recognize insanity to be simply an unusual reaction to emotional problems which are in no wise foreign to ourselves' (Jung, 1960).

Jones (2004), like many others, has attributed the loss of interest in the meaning of madness to the uncoupling of psychotherapeutic approaches from mainstream psychiatry from the 1950s onwards, and with it the splitting off of clinical approaches based upon narrative, context and personal meaning from those focused on biological dysfunctions and drug treatments. Ciompi (1989) has described this as a 'disastrous splitting' into either biological or psychosocial reductionism, often caricatured as the difference between mindlessness and brainlessness. Here, we will consider the ways in which the brain is beginning to be considered as reciprocally influenced by and influencing the mind, in an intimately interconnected two-way process and attention will be given to the role of trauma, attachment and powerlessness in creating a process from which psychosis may arise.

Trauma

Recent work exploring the relationship between childhood trauma and adversity (especially abuse) and psychosis has provided evidence that these may well be contributory factors. It has been hypothesised that the relationship may operate through neurological mechanisms and thus that life events can contribute to not just the 'stress' but also the 'vulnerability' component of stress–vulnerability models. While the evidence is not unequivocal and the proposed models not thoroughly researched, leaving room for the possibility that constitutional vulnerability may still play a part, there are beginning to be indicators that trauma, childhood adversity and associated psychological mechanisms could significantly contribute to the development of psychosis.

A recent meta-analysis of 41 studies of childhood adversity and psychosis found that exposure to any form of childhood abuse, including neglect and bullying, substantially increased the risk of psychosis, with an odds ratio of 2.8. The authors estimated that if this relationship was assumed to be causal, removing these adversities would result in the number of people with psychosis being reduced by 33% (Varese et al, 2012). There are some indicators that the relationship may indeed be causal, with the relationship holding up in the 10 prospective studies included. One of these (Cutajar et al, 2010) found that a sample of people known to have been sexually abused as children were twice as likely as the general population to be diagnosed with a psychotic disorder between 12 and 43 years later. Although this may appear relatively low, the possible presence of sexual abuse in the general population comparison sample was not controlled for and people who disclose abuse are believed likely to be less severely affected by it (Barker-Collo & Read, 2003), thus potentially reducing the difference between the two groups. Sexual abuse is also just one form of adversity, and the existence of a dose–response relationship is also cited as an indication of a causal contribution of adverse experiences, with severity, frequency and number of types of adverse experience all having been found to be related to the probability of psychosis (Read *et al*, 2005).

Some theorists have suggested that the process through which trauma leads to psychotic experiences is dissociation, a psychological defence mechanism whereby painful aspects of experience are not integrated into consciousness but stored separately. Classic psychotic symptoms are thought to result when dissociated content intrudes into the executive self. Hallucinations may thus represent trauma flashbacks, or in the case of voices, dissociated parts of the self. Such dissociated parts could also result in the experience of such common delusions as thought withdrawal, thought insertion and delusions of control. Different aspects of trauma memories are also thought to be stored separately, so that the associated emotions may be retrieved from memory without their autobiographical context or memory of the events that caused them (Nadel & Jacobs, 1996). This could lead to the development of other forms of delusions, such as paranoia and delusions of reference, where a person misattributes the source of emotional experiences and attempts to develop an explanation to account for intrusive feelings of fear or persecution (Read *et al*, 2005; Moskowitz *et al*, 2009).

Attachment

While there is some evidence of a link between childhood adversity and psychosis, it is still unclear why some individuals might experience childhood adversity and go on to be diagnosed with psychosis, whereas for others it may lead to other forms of psychopathology or not result in contact with mental health services at all. There is also a need to account for psychosis occurring in individuals with no apparent history of adversity. One possible way of understanding this, which has received considerable theoretical and clinical interest, relates to the role of the attachment system.

Children are thought to develop attachment styles during their first year of life, depending on the way that their caregivers relate to them, with sensitive, responsive parenting being associated with secure attachment (Ainsworth *et al*, 1978). These styles have been found to be relatively stable throughout the lifespan and to influence the way that people manage emotions and relationships in adulthood. It may be through this pathway that early adverse experiences can to lead to later mental health difficulties, although this relationship is not absolute. Bowlby (1973) used a metaphor of branching railroad tracks to illustrate how developmental trajectories can change in response to significant life events and the quality of available relationships, with long-term consequences. There is evidence that attachment style can mediate the effects of abuse and trauma, such that secure attachment is associated with better coping and less severe symptoms (Shapiro & Levendosky, 1999).

Children who have been abused have been observed to fail to develop a coherent style for relating, resulting in an attachment style described as 'disorganised' (Van Ijzendoorn *et al*, 1999). This is characterised by states of mind concerning relationships which are incoherent, non-integrated and contradictory and is thought to be a precursor to dissociative experiences (Liotti, 1999). Disorganised attachment style is thought to originate when a parent is frightened or frightening, causing an irresolvable dilemma for the child, who will simultaneously experience that parent as a source of fear and wish to seek comfort and care from him or her (Main & Hesse, 1990). This has been observed to be related not just to frank abuse but to emotional misattunement between the caregiver and child and is thought to result from such parents having themselves experienced trauma, loss or other disruption to their own attachment system (Main & Hesse, 1990).

Disorganised attachment style is associated with a wide range of adult psychopathology and it has been theorised that this may result from its impact on mentalisation. This refers to the ability to reflect on experience and hold an intentional stance, understanding that experience and behaviour are mediated through mental states in both self and others. It has been suggested that the development of psychosis rather than other forms of distress may be linked to particularly severe mentalisation deficits, where people with psychosis have less ability to reconsider dissociative experience in the light of external or objective perspectives, or to deficits in particular subfunctions, such as source memory, where the source of events is more likely to be misattributed (Liotti & Gumley, 2008). At present, while there is some evidence of such mentalisation deficits in people diagnosed with schizophrenia (Sprong *et al*, 2007), more research is needed to establish the relationship between attachment disorganisation and psychosis.

Attachment theory provides a framework for understanding how people can be exposed to childhood adversity without experiencing mental health difficulties, through the insulating effect of secure attachments, and how life events could have contributed to the development of psychosis in people without clear trauma histories. Although it is not clear how disrupted attachment relationships might contribute specifically to the development of psychosis, it is worth considering that people using rehabilitation services are likely to have had negative experiences within their personal relationships. There is evidence to suggest that this may impact on how effectively they engage with services (Tait *et al*, 2004) and there are implications for how rehabilitation services can most productively relate to people. Berry & Drake (2010) identify the importance of staff being consistently available over long periods of time and offering the kind of sensitivity and responsiveness that characterises secure attachment relationships, balancing reassurance and encouragement of independence.

Attachment is conceptualised as a psychobiological system, implying that attachment relationships and styles will have consequences for neurobiological development. There is some evidence that attachment style can influence physiological responses to stress (Goldberg, 2000) and overreactivity and dysregulation of the hypothalamic–pituitary–adrenal (HPA) axis has been found in abused children. This has led to the development of a 'traumagenic neurodevelopmental model', which proposes that adverse life experiences can create vulnerability to psychosis through increased physiological sensitivity to subsequent stress (Read *et al*, 2005). In combination with evidence that psychotherapy changes structures and functions in the brain (Fuchs, 2004), this offers the intriguing possibility that seeking to develop an understanding of madness can be antipsychotic at multiple levels.

Victimisation and powerlessness

There is also considerable evidence that social inequality is correlated with psychosis, especially poverty, immigration and discrimination (Read, 2004). While increased rates of childhood abuse are associated with poverty (Van der Kolk *et al*, 2001), a unifying theme of all these experiences is being in a position of powerlessness (Bentall, 2006). The content of psychotic experiences often has themes of victimisation and powerlessness and clear links can often be seen with events in a person's life (see Case example 5.1). Beyond the individual level, associations have been found between paranoia and an external locus of control (a belief that factors

---

Case example 5.1 Just because you're paranoid doesn't mean people aren't out to get you...

Robert believed that he was the victim of an elaborate conspiracy, which he described as 'The Game', orchestrated by powerful figures, such as members of the government and celebrities. He received coded messages about his worthlessness through books and the television, which he took as signs that he was being played with. Robert felt completely helpless and unable to take any action that would free him from persecution. He thought this was punishment for having seriously injured someone in a pub fight as a young man.

Robert's early life was also characterised by experiences of persecution and helplessness. His father had abandoned his mother and their four children without financial support. His mother worked hard to pay the bills but this meant that she was not always around to take care of the children, so Robert often went to school without being fed or washed and in old clothes. He was teased and ostracised by other children for being poor. He had trouble concentrating and understanding his lessons and became something of a class clown. This led his teachers to view him as a troublemaker and, as his mum did not have time to get involved, he tended to be punished both at school and at home, rather than be given support for learning. It is possible to see how Robert's early life experience became dominated by themes of victimisation, incomprehension and persecution at the hands of powerful people, which later appeared as the dominant themes in his psychosis.

---

outside of yourself determine your life) (Bentall, 2006). The level of distress that people experience in relation to hearing voices is also related to the perceived power and control of those voices and this in turn has been found to reflect actual life experiences (Birchwood *et al*, 2000; Andrew *et al*, 2008).

Supporting the search for personal meaning

We have reviewed some of the emergent indicators that suggest madness may be causally related to confusing and overwhelming life events and that it is therefore worth considering people's descriptions of their experiences as considerably more than 'empty speech acts, whose informational content refers to neither world nor self', as delusions have been described (Berrios, 1991). They may instead contain some truth about the person's life, albeit transformed and distorted and requiring careful listening for understanding to emerge.

Although some people accept and value a biomedical frame for their experience, finding it comforting or reassuring (Dillon & May, 2002), many describe biomedical models of explanation as unhelpful or even harmful (Thomas & Bracken, 2004). While there are good reasons for being alive to the possibility of a connection between individuals' psychotic experiences and their personal history, the need, as described above, is for them to have a 'personally satisfactory' way of making sense of it, which may or may not be consistent with the clinician's preferred view.

This places both the clinician and the person experiencing madness in the role of explorers in uncharted territory, seeking a way of mapping the landscape of the person's internal world that will enable him or her to navigate it successfully. Although experienced clinicians may have an awareness of what kind of terrain they are likely to encounter and the rules that tend to apply, they have no knowledge of this particular world or what will work best for this particular person. This requires clinicians to adopt a posture of curious uncertainty and avoid 'beating the drums of logic' (Huszonek, 1987). It may help if clinicians freely express their confusion or uncertainty and ask the person to help them make (the person's) sense. Clinicians can also offer what they do know, the possible frameworks that are available to guide them, and encourage patients to investigate these, considering both the evidence that is available and how helpful they find this way of thinking about themselves. In this clinicians are influenced by the social constructionist stance of Michael White's narrative therapy (White & Epston, 1990), in which there are multiple possible truths or stories about a person's life and the focus is on supporting the development of a story that is enabling of living well with the experience. This could also include spiritual or occult frameworks or drawing on beliefs from other cultures, such as shamanism, where experiences such as hearing voices are seen as potentially valuable and transformatory (Randal *et al*, 2008). Groups can provide a useful format for sharing information and generating discussion and also provide a valuable opportunity to bring together people who are travelling a similar path. Many attest to the benefits of this, especially where a person with lived experience of psychosis is involved in leading the group (Straughan & Buckenham, 2006; Gillespie & Clarke, 2007), which enables learning from the experience of others. The recovery movement has given great emphasis to the power of recovery stories as a way of inspiring hope and sharing wisdom (Leibrich, 1999). One example, Roger Smith's (2004) *Stop Paddling, Start Sailing*, uses the metaphor of a river journey and so in that sense literally offers navigational advice. Many such stories are now available and easily accessible in book form and online as written documents or videos. We believe that there is great value for people in reflecting on multiple stories that illustrate how different people have found their own personal adaptation and adjustments (Roberts, 2010).

As a clinician, it can feel uncomfortable to contemplate supporting people to consider more unconventional or unscientific accounts of their experience and this has particularly raised dilemmas for us when we meet people who are apparently satisfied with their view of reality yet who, to us, appear to be living in highly impoverished and unnecessarily isolating ways. This has led to considerable debate in a clinical context about the extent to which clinicians are justified in imposing their values in determining what constitutes a 'satisfactory' life. In addressing this, we have found that through building trusting relationships, in which people feel heard and respected, we have been able to foster reflection and re-appraisal in people who were initially rejecting of offers of help. Drawing on techniques such as those used in motivational interviewing, where people are gently encouraged to reflect on the way their explanatory framework and the actions that flow from that may conflict with their values, we have found that people usually identify a desire to be more connected to others or meaningfully participate in society and can begin to re-evaluate their beliefs in that light. This may involve reviewing their understanding of their experience or, as we shall discuss further below, finding new ways of relating to those understandings so that they do not conflict with their ability to realise other valued aspects of their life.

Routes to understanding the meanings in madness

In supporting people experiencing madness to consider the ways in which it may be a meaningful response to their life context, we have begun with attempts to appreciate the person's inner world:

> the crux of therapy becomes the task of empathizing with the schizophrenic's perspective and attempting to understand its essential plausibility and validity ... the therapist in searching for kernels of truth is better able to construct an empathic appreciation of the patient's experience than by focusing on what appears distorted and unrealistic. (Josephs & Josephs, 1986)

Case example 5.2 In pursuit of the FBI

'A friend called me when he was having a tough time. He was clearly panicked and said that the FBI has bugged his apartment. He was also worried that if he left, they would follow him. That experience was very real for him. I knew it wouldn't be useful or respectful to tell him not to worry, that it was not really happening. Instead I asked him what we could do together to help him feel less afraid. I shared a story about a fear I'd often had of people reading my mind. I told him that this fear had gotten easier to deal with after remembering someone reading my diary and then being hospitalised. He said that his father had been a judge and that he'd felt like every move he made was being scrutinised. Slowly but surely he sounded sad rather than panicked. We talked about helping each other with old feelings and responses.'

From Copeland & Mead (2004: p. 39), with permission.

We have found it helpful to consider delusions 'unlabelled metaphors' (Bateson, 1973) and look for thematic associations, identifying resonance between psychotic and ordinary life experience and validating the common emotional response (Case example 5.2).

It is regarded as routine good practice to construct a comprehensive biographical picture from both the person her- or himself and all available sources, and this is essential in the process of collaborative enquiry into meaningful connections. However, there is considerable evidence that despite the high prevalence of abuse histories among people using mental health services, the majority are not asked about this and never disclose it and that asking leads to much higher rates of disclosure (Read, 2006). It is therefore important to ask specifically about experiences of abuse and trauma in creating the potential for developing a meaningful understanding of a person's experience. Clinicians often shy away from this, for fear of upsetting the person or believing that it will lead to false reports. However, the evidence suggests that such enquiries are welcomed (Friedman *et al*, 1992) and that people are more likely to under-report than over-report (Read, 2006), with people experiencing psychosis no more likely to make incorrect allegations than the general population (Darves-Bornoz *et al*, 1995). As it is important not just to ask about clear abuse but the emotional quality of relationships, we also draw on the Adult Attachment Interview (George *et al*, 1996), which asks about closeness and distance in family relationships and childhood experiences of being comforted, rejected, threatened, separation and loss. These can all give an indication of important relationship experiences that may not be revealed by asking only about abuse.

This information can help us develop hypotheses about the way in which people's psychotic experiences may be meaningfully connected to their life history, which can be explored with them. Various models exist to guide this process, such as the cognitive model described by Larkin & Morrison (2006) or Romme & Escher's (2000) Maastricht Hearing Voices Interview, which leads to the development of a 'construct' or an understanding of the purpose of the voices in someone's life, negotiated between interviewer and voice hearer. In offering people a new understanding, these hypotheses can support them to move beyond their experiences (see Case example 5.3). For some this will simply be through the process of reaching the understanding but for many others it is likely to be a starting point for identifying helpful therapeutic interventions. A description of 'trauma-informed' approaches to mental healthcare that has been offered by a recovery-focused organisation in the USA (Substance Abuse and Mental Health Services Administration, 2012) includes a focus on building trusting, collaborative relationships in which people who have experienced trauma can feel safe and in control. It also recommends the provision of trauma-specific services, based on Herman's (1997) three-stage model of recovery from trauma (stabilisation, remembrance and mourning, reconnection). This includes offering people psychoeducation and basic coping strategies such as grounding and relaxation in relation to trauma symptoms, which can provide the foundation for safely revisiting and processing traumatic memories and reinterpreting their meanings. This can allow people to begin to look beyond their trauma, finding new meanings in their life and suffering, and building connections with others. Offering people the opportunity to meet with others with similar experiences and think about how they might be able to use their experiences in constructive ways can be especially powerful in this final stage.

It is also important that clinicians view their hypothesis as just that, a tentative possible understanding that the person can choose to accept

---

Case example 5.3 Who's looking after whom?

Marianne was troubled by the presence of spirits in her life, who followed her everywhere she went. However, this meant that they would often get injured, getting trapped in closing doors, sat on or run over because other people could not see them, and Marianne found this very upsetting and felt very guilty. It seemed that the spirits were following her because they cared about her and wanted to look after her, but Marianne ended up having constantly to be on the lookout for them.

Marianne grew up with a single mum who had a drink problem and would often leave her and her younger brother with distant members of the extended family while she went on a drinking binge. Marianne remembered putting her fears to one side to focus on looking after her brother and while her mum was around trying to keep her safe while she was drinking. She was able to make the connection between having needed to be protective of others (even if they should have been protecting her) and her relationship with the spirits. She was able to give this responsibility back to them and focus on her own needs.

or reject. In attempting to reattribute meaning to unlabelled metaphors, clinicians may also seek to understand why it is that the labels have come off, how is it that the person cannot easily see the links her- or himself, and what it might mean to say that the person 'lacks insight'. It may be that the labels did not just fall off in some haphazard way; sometimes they appear to have been peeled off for good reason. For example, a detained patient struggling to get a tune out of the ward piano stated that 'they' must have broken his fingers when he was 'in captivity', and complains that as a consequence he can no longer reach the keys – rather than recognising that he was hopelessly out of practice, anxious and distracted, and still traumatised by his sojourn in the police station prior to admission. This and other examples (Case example 5.4) may illustrate that a denial of meaningful connections can itself be meaningful and purposeful.

Understanding that delusions can hold personally salient meanings, but at arm's length and thus be powerfully psychologically protective, may help to explain their intractability. In some way, thematically, people may be speaking about their life but in ways that are detached from immediate recognition, even from themselves. It also suggests that for some people becoming free of symptoms will not be an unambiguously positive process, as evidenced by the established link between insight and suicidality (Schwartz & Smith, 2004). Taken in context, it is understandable that

---

Case example 5.4 Who is Osmicron?

Over a considerable time of building trust, Mary grew more interested and willing to engage in trying to make sense her unusual experiences. She was persecuted by a magical creature which she called Osmicron, who was a malicious male that taunted her and sought to disrupt her life and relationships. From knowing something about her life, it appeared potentially meaningful to ask her to compare the characteristics of Osmicron with those of her father. She was able to list both, in adjacent columns on a single sheet of paper. The results were strikingly similar and raised the obvious possibility that she was 'haunted' by past experience of a traumatic relationship with her father, manifest as Osmicron. Remarkably, she could not see the similarities at all. When her attention was gently drawn to the striking parallels that she had recorded in almost the same words, instead of drawing the obvious conclusions she wondered instead whether Osmicron had made her father like that. Furthermore, in response to gentle questioning, she could say that despite all her experience, she still longed for her father to love her. Thus her lack of insight appeared understandable and purposeful also.

These discoveries, tentatively held, created a strong sense of understanding Mary and something of what her life had been about, and her continuing needs. Without requiring her to agree with the clinician's view of what her symptoms meant, it became more possible to draw alongside and successfully support her working towards recovery, which was achieved without either medication or agreement concerning diagnosis.

people would wish to preserve their delusional perspectives in preference to awakening to the reality of their lives, which would include an acceptance of having been mad. Interventions designed to challenge delusions are therefore likely to be met with resistance and have the potential to increase the person's subjective experience of distress. We have found that engagement may be assisted by a form of therapeutic collusion, not in offering any false agreement, but through respecting the person's belief structures as purposeful and valuable to them, and seeking to build trust and find common ground.

We have found it productive to try to reach agreement with people on what aspects of an experience are problematic, either in causing them distress or in conflicting with other values they may hold (we often pay particular attention to the need to live safely and respectfully alongside others, which is almost universally endorsed, although not necessarily reflected in behaviour). People can then engage in problem-solving around ways of coping with that experience that do not prevent them from getting on with their lives (see Case example 5.5). The focus is on the person's relationship with the experience rather than the experience itself. May (2004) describes how building such coping strategies can increase control and decrease the sense of powerlessness. People can be supported to gain mastery over their voices through a variety of means (see May, 2011, for a useful summary), including 'voice dialoguing' (Corstens *et al*, 2012), a method for directly engaging with voices in order to establish more productive communication. In her personal account (in Romme *et al*, 2009: p. 142) Eleanor Longden describes beginning to resist a terrifying dominant voice by refusing to do what it commanded, learning to listen to the emotional messages it contained and establishing a more compassionate and trusting relationship with it. Knight (2009) has investigated how people manage the experience of having beliefs that are not shared by others and written about a range of strategies people have used to increase their sense of control, such as wearing protective clothing, making

---

Case example 5.5 Dealing with the paparazzi

Jane was a resident on the rehabilitation unit and believed that she was a famous singer. This made her extremely anxious about going out, as she was sure she would be recognised and that journalists and members of the public would hassle her. This prevented her from moving forward in her rehabilitation, as she was unable to shop for herself or pursue the college course in which she was interested.

Conversations with Jane about how other celebrities who frequently had to deal with the paparazzi, such as Victoria Beckham and Kate Middleton, managed to get on with their lives helped her to identify strategies, such as wearing sunglasses and going out in clothes very different from her usual style, that would prevent her from being recognised.

contact with others who share their belief and using visualisation. Sharing awareness of such coping strategies with others is not a recommendation that people adopt these responses so much as an invitation to consider that it is possible to take action and develop control over what may otherwise seem like overwhelming experiences.

Knight (2009) also describes how having a life characterised by purpose and connection can enable people to live successfully with unusual beliefs and consequently focusing on how to develop these aspects of someone's life can be a useful strategy. If we understand delusions as in some way meeting people's emotional needs, identifying the function they are potentially serving could point us towards alternative strategies for fulfilling those needs, irrespective of whether the person shares the guiding formulation (see Case example 5.6). Supporting people to be part of their community, take on valued roles such as work or study, or gain a sense of achievement and recognition through creativity or sports are all possible means through which self-esteem can be increased and the need for psychotic experience diminished. This also illustrates that understanding madness is important not just for the person experiencing it but also for those seeking to help, even when such understandings are not shared.

Whose understanding is it anyway?

The word 'understanding' has multiple meanings and in this chapter we have primarily been concerned with its use as an intellectual process of comprehending or making sense of something. However, it is also used to describe a process of being compassionate or sympathetic, and in the case

---

Case example 5.6 Growing apart

Bob heard a voice that he believed to be his girlfriend Suzanne communicating with him telepathically. Bob did not find the voice distressing but described it as comforting and reassuring. However, if he became upset or anxious he would leave the ward in search of Suzanne, raising concerns about his safety.

Bob had experienced considerable instability in his childhood, with his father being in the army and frequently away from home and his mother having mental health problems that meant she could be both very physically and emotionally abusive of him but also clingy and dependent. It was hypothesised that Suzanne represented Bob's need for closeness and affection. Rather than challenging Bob about Suzanne's existence, he was supported to overcome his shyness and build social relationships in which he felt appreciated. As he grew in confidence, he began to find Suzanne intrusive and that she got in the way of other relationships. She faded into the background and eventually Bob announced that they had broken up as they had grown apart.

of madness we believe that the former can be highly influential in the latter. We have found that recovering a biographical perspective on psychotic symptoms can enable staff to maintain an awareness of the patient as a person, at times when a person's difficulties are particularly challenging and there is a risk of losing the perspective that symptoms may be attempted solutions to problems in a person's life. Using psychodynamic principles to help professionals understand the experiences of people with schizophrenia has been identified as good practice by the National Institute for Health and Clinical Excellence (2009) and we have found that supporting the development of more complex, psychologically informed formulations can help staff identify constructive alternative strategies in situations where they feel stuck. One useful forum for this is a weekly reflective practice group held on the rehabilitation ward and an example of such a discussion is shown in Case example 5.7.

Just as comprehension can lead to greater compassion among mental health professionals, it may also have the potential to do the same for their families and wider communities, re-engagement with whom should be supported by rehabilitation practice. This is evidenced by the highly successful 'open dialogue' approach used in Western Lapland (Seikkula *et al*, 2006), which uses an approach of meeting with people with psychosis together with their families to generate a dialogue that leads to common understandings of the meaning of the person's psychosis and more lucid expression. There is also evidence that there is less fear and prejudice associated with viewing psychosis as understandable emotional reactions to life events than with biogenetic explanations (Read *et al*, 2006). Thinking

---

Case example 5.7 You can lead a horse to water

The staff team asked to discuss a resident who was spending all his time in bed and refusing to talk to anyone who came into his room, pulling the covers over his head. At the outset of the discussion one of the nurses stated that this was due to negative symptoms and that he was under-medicated. The resident was on a depot antipsychotic and was refusing to try clozapine, which it had been hoped would address this problem. The staff were very frustrated that he would not accept this medication or join in with the programme of therapeutic activities. They thought he should be forced to take medication and get out of bed.

In discussing the resident's history it emerged that he had been sexually abused by two male members of the household while he was growing up. This led to an increased understanding of his wariness of other people and what the experience for him of having people enter his room without his consent might be like. It was also hypothesised that he might feel unworthy of the support that was available to him, or fear taking positive steps that would take him out of his comfort zone. These discussions enabled the staff team to be more empathetic and to maintain the patience to try gently to build trust with the resident.

about how we can use these findings in the service of the people using rehabilitation services requires us to shift our focus from engaging with the individual to intervening with their social context. Slade (2010) suggests that this kind of social activism may be an important role for future mental health professionals, but while it presents tantalising possibilities, it is one that is yet to be successfully established.

Conclusions

As colleagues and co-authors from different disciplines, we draw on different dominant paradigms of theory of the origins of psychosis. However, we hold a common position that it is worth being interested in the content of psychotic experience and how this might link to the person's life experiences. We have found Cutting's (1989) use of Gestalt theory to explain psychotic phenomena to be a useful bridging concept between our different positions on causation. Cutting proposes that in the early phase of psychosis, the Gestalt, or organising principles determining the meanings of perceptions, disintegrates, leading to a state of terror. Delusions emerge when the person attempts to reconstruct meanings. Numerous factors may contribute to a person's vulnerability to experience such fragmentation when under stress, including a disorganised and dissociated internal world or difficulties modulating arousal responses resulting from early relationship trauma or biogenetic vulnerabilities.

The meanings that are available in attempts to reconstruct a Gestalt are derived from people's life experiences; the process of attributing meaning to altered experience can reduce confusion and anxiety, and thus form a basis for psychotic reorganisation and reorientation. Exploring the meanings that are available to people to attribute to their altered experience through reflection on their life history can thus make the apparently nonsensical understandable, creating the potential for meaningful connection with others.

Evidence of what best supports people in recovery suggests that they benefit most from finding frameworks for understanding their experience that are personally satisfactory rather than necessarily those held by practitioners and theoreticians. In supporting people's own attempts to make sense of their experiences, it may be useful to offer theories and make them aware of what evidence is available, but people will need to consider not just whether ideas are true but whether they ring true for them and offer an understanding that supports well-being, engagement and moving forward in their lives.

For many people using rehabilitation services, painful and traumatic relationships and experiences have been part of the fabric of their lives, out of which they have needed to construct new meanings and guiding principles. The relationships and experiences that rehabilitation services offer people may be most effective when they seek to offer an alternative way of being in relation to others, one that is collaborative and respectful of what people have lived through and how it has impacted on them. Developing an understanding of a person in the context of their life, through creating empathy and a sense of commonality rather than alien experience, is likely to support this. Understanding that the experience of psychosis may be driven by emotional responses that are too difficult to bear also creates new possibilities for therapeutic supports, with a focus on developing people's sense of being effective in managing their relationship with their perceptual world. Out of these experiences of being validated and empowered, the potential for new, more constructive meanings can emerge, perhaps allowing madness to be left behind.

A note on case examples

The case examples given have been either derived from our clinical practice or credited to their original source. Where possible we have used examples with the prior consent of the people involved and in all cases we have sought to disguise the identity of those whose experience is described.

References

Ainsworth MDS, Blehar MC, Waters E, *et al* (1978) *Patterns of Attachment*. Lawrence Erlbaum.

Andrew EM, Gray NS, Snowden RJ (2008)The relationship between trauma and beliefs about hearing voices: a study of psychiatric and non-psychiatric voice hearers. *Psychological Medicine*, **38**: 1409–17.

Barker-Collo S, Read J (2003) Models of response to childhood sexual abuse: their implications for treatment. *Trauma, Violence and Abuse*, **4**: 95–111.

Bateson G (1973) *Steps to an Ecology of Mind*. Paladin.

Bentall R (2006) The environment and psychosis: rethinking the evidence. In *Trauma and Psychosis: New Directions for Theory and Therapy* (eds W Larkin, P Morrison): 7–22. Routledge.

Berrios G (1991) Delusions as 'wrong beliefs': a conceptual history. *British Journal of Psychiatry*, **159** (suppl 14): 6–13.

Berry J, Drake R (2010) Attachment theory in psychiatric rehabilitation: informing clinical practice. *Advances in Psychiatric Treatment*, **16**: 308–15.

Birchwood M, Meaden A, Trower P, *et al* (2000) The power and omnipotence of voices: subordination and entrapment by voices and significant others. *Psychological Medicine*, **30**: 337–44.

Bleuler E (1950) *Dementia Praecox of the Group of Schizophrenias* (trans J Zinkin). International University Press.

Bowlby J (1973) *Attachment and Loss: Separation, Anxiety and Anger*. Basic Books.

Ciompi L (1989) The dynamics of complex biological psychosocial systems. *British Journal of Psychiatry*, **155** (suppl 5): 15–21.

Copeland ME, Mead S (2004) *Wellness Recovery Action Plan and Peer Support*. Peach Press.

Corstens D, Longden E, May R (2012) Talking with voices: exploring what is expressed by the voices people hear. *Psychosis: Psychological, Social and Integrative Approaches*, **4**: 95–104.

Cutajar MC, Mullen PE, Ogloff JR, *et al* (2010) Psychopathology in a large cohort of sexually abused children followed up to 43 years. *Child Abuse and Neglect*, **34**: 813–22.

Cutting J (1989) Gestalt theory and psychiatry: discussion paper. *Journal of the Royal Society of Medicine*, **82**: 429–31.

Darves-Bornoz JM, Lempérière T, Degiovanni A, *et al* (1995) Sexual victimization in women with schizophrenia and bipolar disorder. *Social Psychiatry and Psychiatric Epidemiology*, **30**: 78–84.

Dillon J (2013) The Hearing Voices Movement: beyond critiquing the status quo. At http://www.jacquidillon.org/2081/blog/the-hearing-voices-movement-beyond-critiquing-the-status-quo (accessed 9 February 2013).

Dillon J, May R (2002) Reclaiming experience. *Clinical Psychology*, **17**: 25–77.

Friedman LS, Samet JH, Roberts MS, *et al* (1992) Inquiry about victimization experiences: a survey of patient preferences and physician practices. *Archives of Internal Medicine*, **152**: 1186–90.

Fuchs T (2004) Neurobiology and psychotherapy: an emerging dialogue. *Current Opinion in Psychiatry*, **17**: 479–85.

George C, Kaplan N, Main M (1996) Adult Attachment Interview (third edition). Paper at the Department of Psychology, University of California, Berkeley.

Gillespie M, Clarke A (2007) Recovery group for people with severe and enduring mental health problems. *Clinical Psychology Forum*, **172**: 15–18.

Goldberg S (2000) *Attachment and Development*. Arnold.

Herman JL (1997) *Trauma and Recovery: The Aftermath of Violence from Domestic Abuse to Political Terror*. Basic Books.

Huszonek JJ (1987) Establishing therapeutic contact with schizophrenics: a supervisory approach. *American Journal of Psychotherapy*, **41**: 185–93.

Jones K (2004) The historical context of therapeutic environments. In *From Toxic Institution to Therapeutic Environments* (eds P Campling, S Davies, G Farquharson): 3–11. Gaskell.

Josephs L, Josephs L (1986) Pursuing the kernel of truth in the psychotherapy of schizophrenia. *Psychoanalytic Psychology*, **3**: 105–19.

Jung CG (1960) The content of psychoses. In *Collected Works of C.G. Jung, Volume 3: Psychogenesis of Mental Disease* (eds H Read, G Adler, RFC Hull). Princeton University Press.

Knight T (2009) *Beyond Belief: Alternative Ways of Working with Delusions, Obsessions and Unusual Experiences*. Peter Lehmann Publishing.

Larkin W, Morrison AP (2006) Relationships between trauma and psychosis: from theory to therapy. In *Trauma and Psychosis: New Directions for Theory and Therapy* (eds W Larkin, P Morrison): 259–82. Routledge.

Leibrich J (ed.) (1999) *A Gift of Stories. Discovering How to Deal with Mental Illness*. University of Otago Press/Mental Health Commission.

Liotti, G (1999) Disorganization of attachment as a model for understanding dissociative psychopathology. In *Attachment Disorganization* (eds J Solomon, C George): 291–317. Guilford Press.

Liotti G, Gumley A (2008) An attachment perspective on schizophrenia: the role of disorganized attachment, dissociation and mentalization. In *Psychosis, Trauma and Dissociation: Emerging Perspectives on Severe Psychopathology* (eds A Moskowitz, I Schäfer, MJ Dorahy): 117–33. John Wiley.

Main M, Hesse E (1990) Parent's unresolved traumatic experiences are related to infant disorganization status: is frightened and/or frightening behaviour the linking mechanism? In *Attachment in the Pre-School Years* (eds MT Greenberg, D Cicchetti, EM Cummings): 161–82. University of Chicago Press.

May R (2004) Making sense of psychotic experiences and working towards recovery. In *Psychological Interventions in Early Psychosis* (eds J Gleeson, P McGorry): 245–60. Wiley.

May R (2011) Changing the power relationship with your voices. At http://rufusmay.com/index.php?option=com_content&task=view&id=98&Itemid=33 (accessed 20 June 2011).

Morrison AP, Hutton P, Shiers D, *et al* (2012) Antipsychotics: is it time to introduce patient choice? *British Journal of Psychiatry*, **201**: 83–4.

Moskowitz A, Read J, Farrelly S, *et al* (2009) Are psychotic symptoms traumatic in origin and dissociative in kind? In *Dissociation and the Dissociative Disorders: DSM-V and Beyond* (eds P Dell & J O'Neil): 521–33. Routledge.

Nadel L, Jacobs W (1996) The role of the hippocampus in PTSD, panic and phobia. In *The Hippocampus: Functions and Clinical Relevance* (ed N Kato): 455–63. Elsevier.

National Institute for Health and Clinical Excellence (2009) *Core Interventions in the Treatment and Management of Schizophrenia in Primary and Secondary Care (Update)*. NICE.

Randal P, Geekie J, Lambrecht I, *et al* (2008) Dissociation, psychosis and spirituality: whose voices are we hearing? In *Psychosis, Trauma and Dissociation: Emerging Perspectives on Severe Psychopathology* (eds A Moskowitz, I Schäfer, MJ Dorahy): 333–45. Wiley.

Read J (2004) Poverty, ethnicity and gender. In *Models of Madness* (eds J Read, L Mosher, R Bentall): 161–94. Brunner-Routledge.

Read J (2006) Breaking the silence. In *Trauma and Psychosis: New Directions for Theory and Therapy* (eds W Larkin, P Morrison): 195–221. Routledge.

Read J, van Os J, Morrison AP, *et al* (2005) Childhood trauma, psychosis and schizophrenia: a literature review with theoretical and clinical implications. *Acta Psychiatrica Scandinavica*, **112**: 330–50.

Read J, Haslam N, Sayce L, *et al* (2006) Prejudice and schizophrenia: a review of the 'mental illness is an illness like any other' approach. *Acta Psychiatrica Scandinavica*, **114**: 303–18.

Roberts G (2010) Recovery and personal narratives. In *Psychosis: Stories of Recovery and Hope* (eds H Cordle, J Fradgely, J Carson, *et al*): 43–63. Quay Books.

Romme M, Escher S (2000) *Making Sense of Voices: A Guide for Professionals Working with Voice Hearers*. Mind.

Romme M, Escher S, Dillon J, *et al* (2009) *Living with Voices: 50 Stories of Recovery*. PCCS Books.

Schwartz RC, Smith SD (2004) Suicidality and psychosis: the predictive potential of symptomatology and insight into illness. *Journal of Psychiatric Research,* **38**: 185–91.

Seikkula J, Alakare B, Aaltonen J, *et al* (2006) Five year experiences of first-episode non-affective psychosis in open-dialogue approach: treatment principles, follow-up outcomes and two case studies. *Psychotherapy Research*, **16**: 214–28.

Shapiro DL, Levendosky AA (1999) Adolescent survivors of childhood sexual abuse: the mediating role of attachment style and coping in psychological and interpersonal functioning. *Child Abuse and Neglect,* **23**: 1175–91.

Slade M (2009) *Personal Recovery and Mental Illness: A Guide for Mental Health Professionals*. Cambridge University Press.

Slade M (2010) Mental Illness and wellbeing: the central importance of positive psychology and recovery approaches. *BMC Health Services Research*, **10**: 26.

Smith R (2004) *Stop Paddling, Start Sailing: A Journey and Some Ideas*. Publish America.

Sprong M, Schothorst P, Vos E, *et al* (2007) Theory of mind in schizophrenia: meta-analysis. *British Journal of Psychiatry*, **191**: 5–13.

Straughan H, Buckenham M (2006) In-sight: an evaluation of user-led, recovery-based, holistic group training for bipolar disorder. *Journal of Public Mental Health*, **5**: 29–43.

Substance Abuse and Mental Health Services Administration (SAMSHA) (2012) *Assessing for and Addressing Trauma in Recovery Oriented Practice* (webinar). At http://www.samhsa.gov/index.aspx (accessed 29 December 2012).

Tait L, Birchwood M, Trower P (2004) Adapting to the challenge of psychosis: personal resilience and the use of sealing-over (avoidant) coping strategies. *British Journal of Psychiatry*, **185**: 410–15.

Tew J (2005) Power relations, social order and mental distress. In *Social Perspectives in Mental Health* (ed J Tew): 71–89. Jessica Kingsley.

Thomas P, Bracken P (2004) Critical psychiatry in practice. *Advances in Psychiatric Treatment*, **10**: 361–70.

97

Van der Kolk B, Hopper J, Crozier J (2001) Child abuse in America: prevalence and consequences. *Journal of Aggression, Maltreatment, and Trauma*, **4**: 9–31.

Van Ijzendoorn MH, Schuengel C, Bakermans-Kranenburg MJ (1999) Disorganized attachment in early childhood: meta-analysis of precursors, concomitants and sequelae. *Development and Psychopathology*, **11**: 225–49.

Varese F, Smeets F, Drukker M, *et al* (2012) Childhood adversities increase the risk of psychosis: a meta-analysis of patient-control, prospective- and cross-sectional cohort studies. *Schizophrenia Bulletin* (electronic version online, doi: 10.1093/schbul/sbs050).

White M, Epston D (1990) *Narrative Means to Therapeutic Ends*. WW Norton.

CHAPTER 6

First-person narratives

Jerome Carson

Introduction

One of the most significant developments in contemporary psychiatry has been the emergence of a burgeoning literature of inspiring first-person narratives (Carson, 2013a). These may be defined as 'a relatively brief report, usually focussed on one or a few aspects of lived experience of a person, who has one or more mental health challenges, or less commonly, a significant other of such a person' (Rudnick *et al*, 2011: p. 879). This upsurge has been partly stimulated by the recovery approach, described 'as a grassroots movement of the disenfranchised' (Resnick & Rosenheck, 2006: p. 121). In this chapter, I start off by outlining the importance of first-person narratives and outline my involvement in co-developing some of the first-person narrative base. Four examples are then presented, two written by mental health professionals who have also experienced mental health problems and two written by others with lived experience. The findings of two comprehensive reviews of the first-person narrative literature will be discussed, and a critique presented of the use by services of first-person literature, before I conclude by underlining the importance and value of this literature. I should state at the outset that this account is written by a professional, not from the perspective of someone with lived experience, which may of course limit the power of my own narrative account.

Broadly speaking, first-person narrative accounts can be broken into two categories. First, there are accounts written by mental health professionals, who have themselves experienced mental illnesses, such as the book *Wounded Healers*, edited by Vicki Rippere and Ruth Williams (Rippere & Williams, 1985). Second, there are personal or edited accounts about individuals with lived experience (Styron, 1990; Kaysen, 1993; LeCroy & Holschuh, 2012; Nizette *et al*, 2013). Hornstein (2011) lists over 700 titles. Several psychiatric journals publish first-person accounts, including *Psychiatric Services*, *Psychosis*, the *Psychiatric Rehabilitation Journal* and the *Schizophrenia Bulletin*. The last has been publishing such accounts (133 at the time of writing) since 1979. The first paper (DuVal, 1979) described a mother's worry that her child might grow up to develop schizophrenia and the steps she took to improve her parenting and his upbringing as she recovered. Geller (2000) reports that in the first 25 years of the publication of *Psychiatric Services* there were six first-person accounts, with only four in the second 25-year period. Yet between 1994 and 2000, there were 34 personal accounts and since 2000 there had, at the time of writing, been a further 46. A comprehensive review of this literature is beyond the scope of the present chapter; however, two published reviews will be considered (Andresen *et al*, 2003; Leamy *et al*, 2011). Many recovery-oriented groups and organisations have offered collections of personal accounts (see for example http://www.schizophreniadiaries.com; http://www.mentalhealth.org.uk; http://www.scottishrecovery.net; http://www.recoverydevon.co.uk; http://www.rethink.org).

The importance of first-person narratives

When the *Schizophrenia Bulletin* introduced its first 'first-person account' article (DuVal, 1979), it said such accounts were important for three main reasons:

1   It would help mental health professionals learn about the issues and difficulties confronted by consumers of services.
2   The accounts might give patients and their families a better sense of not being alone in dealing with the problems of mental illness.
3   There was a continuing need for experiences to be shared among mental health professionals, families and current and former patients.

Glenn Roberts argues that 'Narrative preserves individuality, distinctiveness and context' (2000: p. 438). He cites Greehalgh & Hurwitz, who state that 'at its most arid, modern medicine lacks a metric for existential qualities such as inner hurt, despair, hope, grief and moral pain, which frequently accompany and often constitute the illnesses from which people suffer' (Roberts, 2000: p. 433). The business of psychiatry is of course seeking to understand and relieve psychic pain, and stories and narratives may be the best way of making sense of this. Gail Hornstein uses first-person accounts as the core sources of her seminars in personality and abnormal psychology. She comments, 'Testimonies and first-person accounts have a crucial role to play – exposing the limits of psychiatry's explanations, helping to reframe fundamental psychological issues, and offering up new theories or methods' (Hornstein, 2010: p. 12). Rudnick and colleagues further suggest that first-person accounts 'may be an important way to promote learning from, and empathy with, people who have mental health challenges' (Rudnick *et al*, 2011: p. 879). Glenn Roberts makes the additional point that 'the fundamental value of first-person stories are that they put people first and underline the reality that the recovery journey is that of someone trying to get over their problems and on with their lives and our professional contribution is intermittent and of secondary importance' (G. Roberts, personal communication, 2011).

My story of personal involvement in helping develop the first-person narrative base

My work and career have been significantly influenced by engaging with the stories of those with whom I have worked. The first paper I co-authored with a service user was with Vic Stevenson (Stevenson & Carson, 1995). This was an account of Vic's time in Cane Hill asylum in Surrey. It is remarkable how the first-person narrative is missing from so many of the histories of asylum life (e.g. Valentine, 1996). There are exceptions: David Russell's account, *Scenes from Bedlam*, is one of the few such asylum histories that features 'the patient's voice' (Russell, 1997). It was a move to work in a different community mental health team (CMHT) in 2006 that led to my involvement with the recovery approach and an expansion of my engagement with first-person narratives.

The main factor in changing my own views about recovery was moving away from a deficit or dysfunction approach, towards looking more at patients' strengths. I had an idea to run a recovery group (Morgan & Carson, 2009). This was to be a forum for service users to give a presentation on a topic they were expert in or where they had a particular talent. Most of the presenters came from our local service, though occasionally we had outside presenters as well. I also started trying to incorporate principles from the recovery approach into my clinical work, most notably with Gordon McManus (McManus & Carson, 2012). He came up with his own definition of recovery, which he defined as 'coping with your illness and having a meaningful life'. Few definitions from mental health professionals have been as parsimonious.

This work led to a number of local initiatives based around the recovery approach. We developed recovery workshops and along with Michelle McNary and psychiatrists Frank Holloway and Paul Wolfson made a film about recovery (which can be viewed at http://www.slam.nhs.uk/patients-and-carers/patient-information/recovery; see also Carson *et al*, 2008, 2012). Commenting on the people interviewed for the film, Paul noted:

> Nearly all of them suffered from a major mental illness. Their symptoms ranged from mild to so intrusive that you could not help but admire them for being able to get up in the morning, never mind being prepared to share their insights about recovery. (Wolfson, 2008: p. 9)

We had a 'Recovery Oscars' ceremony, partly funded by the actor Matt Ward giving a charity performance of the play *St Nicholas* (Ward *et al*, 2010*a*). In partnership with local service user and journalist Sarah Morgan, we wrote a series of papers on 'recovery heroes'. I defined these as 'individuals whose journey of recovery can inspire both other service users and professionals alike' (Sen *et al*, 2009: p. 6). In addition to Dolly Sen, we featured Dr Peter Chadwick (Chadwick *et al*, 2009), Gordon McManus (McManus *et al*, 2009), Matt Ward (Ward *et al*, 2010*b*) and Margaret Muir (Muir *et al*, 2010). The idea of recovery heroes was not my own. Patricia

Deegan had talked about seeing service users as heroes (Deegan, 1996). Premila Trivedi had also talked about her own four personal recovery heroes at a local recovery training event and M. Scott Peck talks about the 'routine heroism of human beings' (Scott Peck, 1991). It is not just the South West Lambeth CMHT that has recovery heroes: every service has them. Indeed, Margaret Muir argues that every person coping with a mental illness is a hero (Muir *et al*, 2010).

This work culminated in the publication of a trilogy of books on recovery, each building on the others (Carson, 2013*a*). The first of these was *Psychosis Stories of Recovery and Hope* (Cordle *et al*, 2011), which was followed by *Mental Health Recovery Heroes Past and Present* (Davies *et al*, 2011). The final book in the trilogy was the story of Gordon McManus's descent into madness and his journey of recovery (McManus & Carson, 2012).

Four first-person narratives

The US clinical psychologist Dr Patricia Deegan has written what I consider to be the single most important paper on personal recovery (Deegan, 1996). One of her earlier papers (Deegan, 1988) was one of the first papers to be published on the subject of recovery. Further insights into her thinking and background can be gleaned from an interview with Professor Shirley Smoyak (Smoyak & Deegan, 1996). Deegan (1988) contrasts her own recovery from mental illness with that of a man with paraplegia. She talks of the paradox of recovery, 'that in accepting what we cannot do or be, we begin to discover who we can be and what we can do' (Deegan, 1988: p. 15). She suggests that the process of recovery starts with the experience of despair and then the transition to 'hope, willingness and responsible action' (p. 16). She argues that professionals need to 'embrace and accept our own woundedness and vulnerability as the first step toward understanding the experience of the disabled ... we discover we share a common humanity with the disabled and that we are not worlds apart' (p. 18).

Patricia Deegan's account is a remarkable story of recovery in its own right. As she reminds us, she was already on her third hospitalisation at the age of 18. She recounts being told by her psychiatrist, 'You have a disease called chronic schizophrenia. It is a disease that is like diabetes. If you take medications for the rest of your life and avoid stress, then maybe you can cope' (Deegan, 1996: p. 92). This, she says, 'crushed' her hopes and dreams for her life. Yet, 11 years later she qualified as a clinical psychologist. She was one of the first professionals to show how Martin Seligman's (1975) model of learned helplessness could be used as a way of understanding the behaviour of people with long-term mental health problems and not just reactive depression. Like Seligman, she has since gone on to promote positive approaches to well-being. Her personal experience has also enabled her to teach others how best to work with other patients and support their decisions and choices (Deegan *et al*, 2008). According to Deegan, the goal of recovery 'is to become the unique, awesome, never to be repeated human being that we are called to be' (Deegan, 1996: p. 92). More information is available on her website (http://www.patdeegan.com).

A second professional who has written about his own mental illness is Dr Peter Chadwick. In an early account (Chadwick, 1993), Peter describes the background to his psychotic episode in 1979, which led to him throwing himself in front of an oncoming bus. Amazingly, he survived, sustaining only minor injuries. He has been able to use his 'unusual position as a former patient, who has a doctorate and career in psychosis research, and hence is a peer professional or user academic, to straddle the chasm separating the insane from the sane and hence facilitate cross talk between them' (Chadwick, 2007: p. 166). Peter has tried to present a more positive image of psychosis, away from 'the deficit, dysfunction and diagnosis driven nature of much psychosis research' (Chadwick, 2012: p.144).

There are now several published anthologies of accounts of living with mental illnesses written from the perspective of the service user or lived experience (e.g. Barker *et al*, 1999; Leibrich, 1999; Chandler & Hayward, 2009; Davidson & Lynn, 2009). I focus on two written by individuals I have worked with, Dolly Sen and Andrew Voyce.

> I'm standing over my sleeping father with a knife in my hand. Because he is a demonic alien plotting my destruction he has to die.... That moment described was the culmination of decades of abuse at the hands of my father and his friends and several years of psychosis and depression. It was the worst point in my life.... But strangely enough it was the beginning of my recovery. (Sen, 2012: p. 154)

Dolly relates the story of her life and her battle with mental illness in her book *The World Is Full of Laughter* (Sen, 2002) and in the sequel, *Am I Still Laughing?* (Sen, 2006). She describes herself as a 'writer, director, artist, filmmaker, poet, performer, raconteur, playwright, mental health consultant, musician and public speaker' (Sen *et al*, 2009: p. 6). She has appeared on television and radio talking about mental illness. Her childhood was, by her own admission, not a happy one, with 'physical, emotional, mental and sexual abuse, racism, poverty, neglect and bullying' (Sen, 2002: p. 6). She developed a psychotic illness aged 14 and had four hospital admissions.

Dolly's publisher, Jason Pegler, believed she would recover, when few other people did. Her involvement with creative activities was also of benefit. She felt that many artists were particularly helpful, as 'they see a human being.... They don't see something that's broken, they see someone who can make poetry and write' (Sen *et al*, 2009: p. 7). According to Dolly,

> Recovery is a letter of hopes, dreams, songs, peace, hurt, chaos, transcendence, night and light. Recovery is to be able to dream and live those dreams. To shine my brightest and live my fullest. To seize the day without the weight of the past. To find the Dollyness of Dolly. (Sen, 2008: p. 11)

103

Andrew Voyce has spent nearly 40 years in the mental health system with over 10 admissions to Hellingly and Oakwood Hospitals (Voyce, 2011). One of his biggest complaints about his in-patient treatment was about depot injections. He experienced major problems with akathisia. He commented, 'the extreme restlessness, combined with sedation, which lasted for a week after the injection had been administered.... I couldn't concentrate to read or watch TV' (Voyce & Carson, 2013: p. 16). When he was discharged he would often stop his medication. He lived rough for many years (Voyce, 2009).

> I lived in bus shelters for five years.... I was lucky I did survive. As I was happily psychotic.... I felt protected by magical forces, that someone would come along and hypnotise me as I was getting ready to go to sleep and this would keep me warm during the cold nights. (Voyce & Carson, 2013: p. 16)

He also developed an interest in digital art as a way of describing and coming to terms with his mental health history. His latest book, *Side Effects*, is a graphic novel (Voyce *et al*, 2012).

These few illustrative stories offer a glimpse of the richness to be found in first-person narratives. They remind us that people live their lives in social and societal contexts and they illuminate personal perspectives on both treatment and recovery that are very different from that of a conventional case history. This offers a bridge and connection with their lived experience, their humanity, as a more secure basis for forming trusting and useful therapeutic relationships.

Learning from first-person accounts

There are several major published reviews of the first-person narrative literature linked to recovery, some of which have offered the foundations for national orientations to service development (Lapsley *et al*, 2002; Scottish Recovery Network, 2006). I will discuss two further influential reviews that have led to structured understandings of recovery processes. Andresen *et al* (2003) looked at 'consumer accounts of recovery'. Two of the most significant findings to emerge from their review were a delineation of the components of the recovery process and the identification of five discrete stages. They focused on four key components described in the personal accounts they reviewed. *Hope* was the most prominent and consistent factor. This can be seen as coming from the individuals themselves or as being triggered by a significant other, role model or peer. The second major component was *redefining identity* as a response to the loss of a sense of identity following the onset of mental illness. As one service user commented, 'the key is to know yourself, know your identity and to know the difference between the two'. The third component was *finding meaning in life*. For one person, their 'life's suffering led to their life's work'. The source of meaning could vary not just between individuals but also over time for one individual. The final element was *taking responsibility for recovery*. The authors describe this as self-management of wellness and medication, making autonomous life choices, being accountable for your actions and taking risks.

They developed their identification of five stages in recovery as a model of successive achievements and experiences in the recovery process. Stage 1 they describe as *moratorium*, characterised by denial, confusion and social withdrawal, a time when it may appear nothing is going on but in which the person is preparing for change. The second stage they called *awareness*. Here the person considers that a better life may be possible. They describe the third stage as *preparation*, in which individuals start working on their own recovery. It is in the fourth stage, *rebuilding*, that most work takes place. It involves taking risks, experiencing setbacks and trying again. The final stage, *growth*, is the outcome of the recovery process. While people may not be entirely free of symptoms at this stage, they know how to manage their illness and stay well through building self-understanding, resources and resilience. Using this narrative-based model of personal recovery, the authors went on to develop the Stages of Recovery Instrument (STORI) and the Self-Identified Stages of Recovery Scale, as quantitative measures of progress in recovery (Andresen *et al*, 2006).

The second review, by Leamy *et al* (2011), looked at 97 papers on personal recovery. The authors identified three interlinked superordinate categories: characteristics of the recovery journey, recovery processes and recovery stages. The last two are similar to what Andresen *et al* (2003) identified. The authors also identified 13 characteristics of the recovery journey, which are presented, ranked according to prevalence, in Table 6.1.

Table 6.1 Characteristics of the recovery journey

Recovery as ...	Proportion of studies that report that characteristic
An active process	50%
As an individual and unique process	29%
As a non-linear process	24%
As a journey	20%
As stages/phases	17%
As a struggle	16%
As multi-dimensional	15%
As a gradual process	15%
As life changing	13%
As not meaning cure	10%
As helped by a supportive, healing environment	7%
As possible without professional intervention	7%
As a trial and error process	7%

After Leamy *et al* (2011)

Table 6.2 Recovery processes

Aspect of recovery	Proportion of studies that report that aspect of recovery
Connectedness	86%
Support from others	61%
Peer support	45%
Being part of the community	40%
Relationships	38%
Hope and optimism about the future	79%
Belief in the possibility of recovery	34%
Motivation to change	17%
Hope-inspiring relationships	14%
Positive thinking and valuing success	11%
Having dreams and aspirations	8%
Identity	75%
Rebuilding/redefining a positive sense of identity	66%
Overcoming stigma	46%
Dimensions of identity	9%
Meaning in life	66%
Quality of life	65%
Meaningful life and social role	46%
Spirituality	41%
Rebuilding life	22%
Meaningful life and social goals	17%
Empowerment	91%
Personal responsibility	91%
Control over life	90%
Focusing on strengths	16%

After Leamy *et al* (2011)

From this extensive review, Leamy *et al* (2011) identified five main recovery processes (see Table 6.2), four of which were very similar to the Andresen *et al*'s (2003) categories, to which they added a dimension related to social connections. These were *connectedness, hope and optimism about the future, identity, meaning in life* and *empowerment,* allowing the acronym CHIME. Finally, they mapped 13 studies onto the transtheoretical model of change developed by Prochaska & DiClimente (1982), again noting similarities and overlapping categories and processes involved in personal change. However, there was little consensus regarding the number of recovery phases and it is important to regard such condensed and structured models as offering only a map of the territory on which people take a huge variety of different personal recovery journeys.

Critique of the use of first-person narratives by services

The Social Perspectives Network published a set of papers presented at a conference on recovery provocatively entitled *Whose Recovery Is It Anyway?* (Social Perspectives Network, 2007). Costa *et al* (2012) in a challenging paper argue that mental health services have used consumer/survivor stories to promote themselves as agents of recovery. Indeed, they suggest that this is a form of 'disability tourism' or 'patient porn':

> By pornographic we mean that, while some people reveal their most intimate personal details, others achieve relief through passive watching, while still others profit from the collaboration of those in the front line in compromised positions. (Costa *et al*, 2012: p. 86).

They believe that services are able to use patients' stories without having to really change how they operate and that such accounts are being abused for the benefit of professionals. The resulting narrative is that if patients take their medication, and heed the advice of their service providers, along with hard work and perseverance, that they 'can be cured' (p. 89). The authors are especially wary of politically correct qualitative researchers who 'have discovered how to be really effective at stealing stories for their own academic gain' (p. 91). They provide a number of tips for service users considering a professional's invitation to share their story. First, they say that service users can refuse to share their stories. They then give a series of questions service users should consider:

- Who will benefit from telling the story?
- What purpose does sharing your story serve?
- How will services use stories for organisational change?
- Do they intend to pay you?

Lastly, Costa *et al* (2012: p. 93) say that service users should not forget that the story will be on the internet forever and potentially available to future employers and landlords (see http://wp.me/p4aZsh-2q). They conclude, 'For the longest time, the mental health system wasn't interested in our stories. Our stories, after all, were the stories of mad people and therefore not credible' (p. 95).

As we move towards valuing and engaging with personal stories we would do well to respect and respond to these sensitivities, primarily about authority and ownership. We might rephrase the Social Perspectives Network question as 'Whose Stories Are They Anyway?' and consider how best to manage the ethical and personal issues involved in sharing them (Recovery Devon, 2013).

Conclusions

Collections of first-person narratives in psychiatry have existed for many years. There is no doubt though that the recovery approach, 'grounded in the developing service user literature of real stories, of real people, battling heroically against mental illness' (Carson, 2013b), has given this area additional momentum. Recovery privileges the stories of individuals with lived experience and in many ways the 'recovery movement' can be seen to have a narrative foundation. First-person accounts are critical in helping mental health professionals understand the lived experience of mental illness, and its effects on both sufferers and carers. This is something that is very hard to comprehend without seeing it from the sufferer's perspective. Accounts written by mental health professionals who have themselves experienced mental illness may have an additional potency and remind us 'that there but for the grace of God go I'; they also narrow the gap between 'them and us'. A knowledge of this literature can help clinicians point out to sufferers and their carers that they are not alone. Such accounts will help educate future professionals about the lived experience of mental illness and how vulnerabilities, triggers, symptoms, treatment and progress are all played out through personally salient perspectives.

Personal stories and support for telling your story are also core components in emerging recovery education curricula and constitute the foundation of peer support. Listening to such stories can touch, inspire, inform and guide clinicians in the continuing struggle to form helpful, hopeful and supportive relationships with those they seek to help (Wasow & Moore, 2007).

References

Andresen R, Oades L, Caputi P (2003) The experience of recovery from schizophrenia: towards an empirically validated stage model. *Australian and New Zealand Journal of Psychiatry*, **37**: 586–94.

Andresen R, Caputi P, Oades L (2006) Stages of Recovery Instrument: development of a measure of recovery from severe mental illness. *Australia and New Zealand Journal of Psychiatry*, **40**: 972–80.

Barker P, Campbell P, Davidson B (eds) (1999) *From the Ashes of Experience: Reflections on Madness, Survival and Growth*. Whurr.

Carson J, Holloway F, Wolfson P, *et al* (eds) (2008) *Recovery Journeys: Stories of Coping with Mental Health Problems*. South London and Maudsley NHS Foundation Trust.

Carson J (2013a) Recovery and clinical psychology: one psychologist's journey. *Clinical Psychology Forum*, **252**: 22–6.

Carson J (2013b) Revolution: what revolution? *Mental Health Today*, May/June: 21.

Carson J, McNary M, Holloway F, *et al* (2012) The making of a film about recovery. *Mental Health and Social Inclusion*, **16**: 72–8.

Chadwick P (1993) The stepladder to the impossible: a first-hand phenomenological account of a schizoaffective psychotic crisis. *Journal of Mental Health*, **2**: 239–50.

Chadwick P (2007) Peer professional first person account: schizophrenia from the inside – phenomenology and the integration of causes and meanings. *Schizophrenia Bulletin*, **33**: 166–73.

Chadwick P (2012) Does a psychotic episode ever do anybody any good? In *From Communism to Schizophrenia and Beyond: One Man's Long March to Recovery* (eds G McManus, J Carson): 142–52. Whiting & Birch.

Chadwick P, Morgan S, Fradgley J, *et al* (2009) Recovery heroes – a profile of Peter Chadwick. *A Life in the Day*, **13** (3): 6–9.

Chandler R, Hayward P (eds) (2009) *Voicing Psychotic Experiences: A Reconsideration of Recovery and Diversity*. Pavilion.

Cordle H, Fradgley J, Carson J, *et al* (eds) (2011) *Psychosis Stories of Recovery and Hope*. Quay Books.

Costa L, Voronka J, Landry D, *et al* (2012) Recovering our stories: a small act of resistance. *Studies in Social Justice*, **6**: 85–101.

Davidson L, Lynn L (eds) (2009) *Beyond the Storms: Reflections on Personal Recovery in Devon*. Devon Partnership NHS Trust.

Davies S, Wakely E, Morgan S, *et al* (eds) (2011) *Mental Health Recovery Heroes Past and Present*. Pavilion.

Deegan P (1988) Recovery: the lived experience of rehabilitation. *Psychosocial Rehabilitation Journal*, **11** (4): 11–19.

Deegan P (1996) Recovery as journey of the heart. *Psychiatric Rehabilitation Journal*, **19**: 91–7.

Deegan P, Rapp C, Holter M, *et al* (2008) A program to support shared decision making in an outpatient psychiatric medication clinic. *Psychiatric Services*, **59**: 603–5.

DuVal M (1979) First person account: giving love … and schizophrenia. *Schizophrenia Bulletin*, **5**: 631–6.

Geller J (2000) Personal accounts: first-person accounts in the journal's second 25 years. *Psychiatric Services*, **51**: 713–16.

Hornstein G (2010) Teaching mental health using first-person accounts of madness. *Higher Education Academy Psychology Network Newsletter*, **57**: 12.

Hornstein G (2011) *Bibliography of First-Person Narratives of Madness in English* (5th edn). At http://www.gailhornstein.com/files/Bibliography_of_First_Person_Narratives_of_Madness_5th_edition.pdf (accessed December 2014).

Kaysen S (1993) *Girl Interrupted*. Random House.

Lapsley H, Nikora L, Black R (2002) *Kia Mauri Tau: Narratives of Recovery from Disabling Mental Health Problems*. University of Waikato.

Leamy M, Bird V, Le Boutillier C, *et al* (2011) Conceptual framework for personal recovery in mental health: systematic review and narrative synthesis. *British Journal of Psychiatry*, **199**: 445–52.

LeCroy C, Holschuh J (eds) (2012) *First Person Accounts of Mental Illness and Recovery*. Wiley.

Leibrich J (1999) *A Gift of Stories*. University of Otago Press.

McManus G, Carson J (eds) (2012) *From Communism to Schizophrenia and Beyond: One Man's Long March to Recovery*. Whiting & Birch.

McManus G, Morgan S, Fradgley J, *et al* (2009) Recovery heroes – a profile of Gordon McManus. *A Life in the Day*, **13** (3): 16–19.

Morgan S, Carson J (2009) The recovery group: a service user and professional perspective. *Groupwork*, **19**: 26–39.

Muir M, Cordle H, Carson J (2010) Recovery heroes – a profile of Margaret Muir. *Mental Health and Social Inclusion*, **14** (2): 7–11.

Nizette D, McAllister M, Marks P (eds) (2013) *Stories in Mental Health: Reflection, Enquiry, Action*. Elsevier.

Prochaska J, DiClimente C (1982) Transtheoretical therapy: toward a more integrative model of change. *Psychology and Psychotherapy Theory Research and Practice*, **19**: 276–88.

Recovery Devon (2013) Stories of personal recovery: examples and guidance on collecting stories. At http://www.recoverydevon.co.uk/index.php/stories-of-recovery http://www.recoverydevon.co.uk/index.php/creative-cafe/the-stories-gathered-so-far (accessed December 2014).

Resnick S, Rosenheck R (2006) Recovery and positive psychology: parallel themes and potential synergies. *Psychiatric Services*, **57**: 120–3.

Rippere V, Williams R (eds) (1985) *Wounded Healers: Mental Health Workers Experience of Depression*. Wiley.

Roberts G (2000) Narrative and severe mental illness: what place do stories have in an evidence-based world. *Advances in Psychiatric Treatment*, **6**: 432–41.

Rudnick A, Rofè T, Virtzberg-Rofè D, *et al* (2011) Supported reporting of first person accounts: assisting people who have mental health challenges in writing and publishing reports about their lived experience. *Schizophrenia Bulletin*, **37**: 879–81.

Russell D (1997) *Scenes from Bedlam: A History of Caring for the Mentally Disordered at Bethlem Royal Hospital and the Maudsley*. Ballière Tindall.

Scott Peck M (1991) Foreword. In *The Path of the Everyday Hero* (eds L Catford, M Ray): ix–xii. Jeremy P. Tarcher/Puttnam.

Scottish Recovery Network (2006) *Journeys of Recovery: Stories of Hope and Recovery from Long Term Mental Health Problems*. Scottish Recovery Network.

Seligman M (1975) *Helplessness: On Depression, Development and Death*. Freeman.

Sen D (2002) *The World is Full of Laughter*. Chipmunka Publishing.

Sen D (2006) *Am I Still Laughing?* Chipmunka Publishing.

Sen D (2008) Dolly's story. In *Recovery Journeys: Stories of Coping with Mental Health Problems* (eds J Carson, F Holloway, P Wolfson, M McNary): 11–12. South London and Maudsley NHS Foundation Trust.

Sen D (2012) Recovery: what I have learned from my own journey of recovery. In *From Communism to Schizophrenia and Beyond: One Man's Long March to Recovery* (eds G McManus, J Carson): 153–64. Whiting and Birch.

Sen D, Morgan S, Fradgley J, *et al* (2009) Recovery heroes – a profile of Dolly Sen. *A Life in the Day*, **13** (3): 6–8.

Smoyak S, Deegan P (1996) Blending two realities into a unique perspective. *Journal of Psychosocial Nursing*, **34** (9): 39–46.

Social Perspectives Network (2007) *Whose Recovery Is It Anyway?* London: Social Perspectives Network.

Stevenson V, Carson J (1995) The pastoral myth of the mental hospital: a personal account. *International Journal of Social Psychiatry*, **41**: 147–51.

Styron W (1990) *Darkness Visible: A Memoir of Madness*. Vintage Books.

Valentine R (1996) *Asylum, Hospital, Haven: A History of Horton Hospital*. Riverside Mental Health Trust.

Voyce A (2009) *The Durham Light and Other Stories: A Personal History of Homelessness and Schizophrenia*. Chipmunka Press.

Voyce A (2011) The Voyce of experience. In *Psychosis Stories of Recovery and Hope* (eds H Cordle, J Fradgley, J Carson, *et al*): 64–73. Quay Books.

Voyce A, Carson J (2013) Andrew Voyce in conversation with Jerome Carson. *Mental Health and Social Inclusion*, **17**: 14–19.

Voyce A, Cordle H, Hovlind O (2012) *Side Effects*. Recovery.

Ward M, Chander A, Robinson S, *et al* (2010a) It's a one man show. *Mental Health Today*, March: 32–3.

Ward M, Cordle H, Fradgley J, *et al* (2010b) Recovery heroes – a profile of Matthew Ward. *Mental Health and Social Inclusion*, **14**: 6–10.

Wasow M, Moore S (2007) Then and now. *Psychiatric Services*, **58**: 1039–40.

Wolfson P (2008) Auditioning for recovery. In *Recovery Journeys: Stories of Coping with Mental Health Problems* (eds J Carson, F Holloway, P Wolfson, *et al*): 9–10. South London and Maudsley NHS Foundation Trust.

Part 2

Treatment approaches

CHAPTER 7

Treatment approaches: overview

Sridevi Kalidindi, Frank Holloway, Helen Killaspy and
Glenn Roberts

Introduction

In this part of the book the next eight chapters discuss approaches to
treatment in rehabilitation practice. What does treatment mean for
people with longer-term psychoses who find themselves in rehabilitation
settings? The challenge is great, but the rewards greater. All our authors
underline the key importance of forming good therapeutic relationships.
An overwhelming sense of hope, despite the challenges, comes through
strongly in all the contributions, as our authors answer the question posed.
Together, they provide the reader with a formidable array of therapeutic
approaches.

This group of people experience complex, multiple and severe issues
that affect their ability to live safely and independently in the community.
Good treatment necessitates addressing needs by using interventions that
are informed by the best evidence. A longer period of engagement may be
required than is usual just to facilitate access, and treatments may need to
be used particularly creatively and flexibly. The ability to build up a trusting
and compassionate working relationship and ensure person-centred practice
is central to success. This requires supporting service users to identify their
strengths, their resources and their goals. It is necessary to work alongside
them, their families and key people in other services to enable holistic,
incremental, 'long-view' care and progress. The 'whole system' approach
advocated throughout this book seeks to use everyone within the extended
team, working towards common goals alongside the service user. The aim
is increasing self-management of the service user's condition(s) and greater
independence, with occasional setbacks being understood to be par for the
course and an opportunity for learning.

To expand further on the 'person-centred' premise, this is about meeting people at whatever point they are on their journey, engaging them,
endeavouring to understand them and formulating with them and their
significant others an individualised, bespoke or tailor-made plan. Having
knowledge of a person's narrative, maintaining continuity and ensuring
that necessary support is not taken away before the person is ready are all
important. The authors in Part 2 uniformly emphasise the importance of

treatment as 'working with' people as agents in their recovery rather than merely 'doing to' a passive recipient of care.

The staff team

The staff team is key to effective treatment. The necessary skills, spanning biopsychosocial aspects as well as service development and more managerial skills for senior staff, are discussed in a recent report from the Royal College of Psychiatrists' Faculty of Rehabilitation and Social Psychiatry (Kalidindi *et al*, 2012). Specialist training for staff, certain attitudes, being able to stay well as individuals and as a whole team themselves, providing mutual support for one another and receiving good supervision are all necessary ingredients to sustain good work and a consistently hopeful demeanour. Employers should be considerate of the welfare of their staff, in order that staff can in turn provide good care for service users. This basic fact came to the fore very strongly in the inquiry into systematic failures of care identified at Mid-Staffordshire NHS Trust, an acute hospital (Francis, 2013). These failures have greatly shaken people's faith in the care system. There is some evidence that improving staff well-being is likely to have a positive impact on patients' experiences of care (Maben *et al*, 2012).

Rehabilitation in practice

Chapter 8, 'Rehabilitation at the coalface', focuses on the practicalities of helping people improve their skills. It describes a wide range of methods, informed by psychological theory and occupational therapy theory, that can be employed with service users, depending on their needs and presentation. The broad framework is of engagement, the establishment of a rationale for rehabilitative work and then an exploration of practical approaches to facilitating change. The authors advocate the use of techniques derived from motivational interviewing (Miller & Rollnick, 2013) as a means of effecting behavioural and lifestyle change.

Cognitive therapies

People with a diagnosis of schizophrenia experience two distinct kinds of cognitive difficulties: poor communication due to delusional thinking or disorganised language; and cognitive problems in memory, concentration and attention. Both aspects have been addressed in the development of a specific psychological therapy, cognitive–behavioural therapy for psychosis (CBTp) and cognitive remediation therapy (CRT). These are described in Chapter 9, 'Cognitive approaches'. Both CBTp and CRT work to transfer therapeutic gains into real-life situations such as attending a social activity. CBTp focuses on emotional responses to symptom content, and its primary outcome is a reduction in symptoms and distress. CRT aims to improve cognition and thereby increase functional outcome.

CBTp is a 'formulation-based' therapy that, according to the authors of Chapter 9, aims 'to develop a personal account of the development and maintenance of currently distressing experiences that is less threatening than the beliefs that are currently held'. CBTp practice, like all high-quality psychological therapies, puts great emphasis on the importance of supervision. The evidence to date predominantly provides support for CBTp as an intervention for individuals suffering from 'treatment-resistant' psychosis in a chronic but stable phase.

CRT involves supervised practice of cognitive tasks of graded difficulty, presented in a paper-and-pencil format or using a computer. CRT programmes adopting a more strategic approach achieve better functional outcomes than methods simply requiring the practice of cognitive skills (McGurk et al, 2007; Wykes et al, 2011). This is postulated to be due to allowing transfer of training from individual cognitive remediation tasks to other aspects of everyday functioning. Of particular relevance is that CRT using a strategy-based method alongside a rehabilitation programme such as supported employment produced significantly improved functional outcomes (Wykes et al, 2011).

Working with families

There is an extensive literature on the impact of a family member developing severe mental illness on the family as a whole, particularly primary caregivers, who are usually parents or spouses. Mainstream mental health services often have difficulty working well with families, despite relatives' potentially key role in supporting a service user in their recovery. As a consequence, many people entering rehabilitation services have become alienated from their families. Chapter 10, 'Family interventions', describes best practice in working with families, which can be at various levels of intensity, from family-sensitive practice, to the structured provision of family education and support, and on to formal family intervention. Family intervention has been shown to be of benefit for many years, but it has rarely been available in routine practice, at least until recently.

Feeling loved, needed and part of a family forms the basis of many people's lives: the majority of service users want family members to be involved in their care. Family intervention can enable those relationships to continue and in a more positive way; it has good outcomes both clinically and fiscally. The evidence base continues to grow but is well summarised in the full psychosis and schizophrenia guideline from the National Institute for Health and Care Excellence (National Collaborating Centre for Mental Health, 2014).

The importance of cultural variations in family involvement is rightly highlighted, as is the need for recovery for families themselves. Of note, when asked, family members state that professionals get in the way of their own recovery in two main ways: by poor communication and issues of confidentiality impeding carers' access to services.

Challenging behaviour

Some people within rehabilitation services are described as exhibiting 'challenging behaviour', a socially determined construct 'which describes those extreme behaviours that fall well outside the usually accepted ideas of "normal" behaviour', as Shawn Mitchell and Sanjith Kamath say in Chapter 11, 'Working with challenging behaviour'. They offer a theoretical and practical approach to this complex issue. It emphasises the value of the formulation as an empirical approach to understanding the causes of an individual challenging behaviour within a biopsychosocial framework and identifying potential ways of addressing the behaviour that can be tested. Importantly, the authors address the staff and ward issues that must be attended to for work to be successful and be maintained consistently to a high standard by a team. In an area where the evidence base has far to go, this chapter provides expert guidance on how to approach and successfully treat challenging behaviour in a complex patient group.

Substance misuse

In the past active substance misuse was commonly an exclusion for entry into rehabilitation services, but that approach can no longer be justified. Dual diagnosis has been identified as 'the most challenging clinical problem that we face' (Department of Health, 2004). Chapter 12, 'Working with coexisting substance misuse has an opening epigraph with a helpful counterbalancing statement: 'Seeing opportunities for change and believing that these can be achieved makes a big difference' (Kipping & Simpson, 2010), which sets the scene for how to support people who are complex and challenging to work with to achieve recovery.

At least a third of people with schizophrenia or other psychotic disorders also have problems with substances (Carra *et al*, 2012) (so-called dual diagnosis). In the past there was a skills gap for mental health staff surrounding substance misuse, which had been exacerbated by the separation between substance misuse and psychiatric services but has been addressed in some services by mandatory training in dual diagnosis. Comorbid substance misuse exacerbates the risks associated with mental illness, clouds the clinical picture and results in increasing complexity in care planning. One of the key lessons from Chapter 12 is that 'assessment, if conducted skilfully, can also be an intervention, promoting reflection and a decision for change'. As well as covering the underlying theory based on the cycle of change (Prochaska & DiClemente, 1986) and motivational interviewing (Miller & Rollnick, 2013), practical methods of how to work well with the group of people are described. The key message is that by working with the person's priorities, changes may be produced that can then enable progress in other areas too.

Creativity

A classic paper by Davidson & Strauss (1992) described processes by which people living with severe mental illness experienced recovery by rediscovering 'a sense of self'. Frequently, recovery narratives describe creativity as a key element in this process. Chapter 13, 'Creative therapies and creativity', describes a range of specific therapies and their evidence base and a number of projects that allow people with severe mental health problems the opportunity to express themselves through artistic media. Specific therapies include art therapy, drama therapy, music therapy and dance movement psychotherapy: their strength lies partly in offering a different way to engage with people and to contribute to the healing in those unable or not wishing to verbalise their difficulties and experiences. The chapter also demonstrates the importance of the third sector (non-government organisations) working alongside the statutory services.

Medication

By definition, people in contact with specialist rehabilitation services have, for whatever reason, not done well within less specialist services. Commonly, previous psychopharmacological treatments have been refused or not worked well. Chapter 14, 'Management of medication when treatment is failing', offers a detailed account of the pharmacological management of treatment resistance in schizophrenia, the commonest diagnosis among people in contact with rehabilitation services. Clozapine is the only medication with proven superiority to other antipsychotics but does come with a very significant burden of side-effects. Management of the side-effects of clozapine is key to ensuring that the service user can benefit from this medication for long enough to see positive changes in terms of symptom load, associated distress, reduced suicide risk and improved level of functioning. Some people do very well indeed on clozapine and are able to achieve more independence, for example a move from a 24-hour residential care home to independent living, with or without domiciliary support. There is a significant problem for patients and prescribers when clozapine is ineffective or poorly tolerated. The authors' specialist experience is distilled into a usable format, with treatment at the very edges of the evidence base being covered.

Coming off medication, with the doctor's (usually reluctant) support, can be a part of therapeutic risk-taking. People do this anyway, so it is better for this to happen in a planned fashion, working alongside the individual. This enables a quick detection of symptoms and signs when they do recur, which it is important in working to ensure that the service user can also see and then consider the options for treatment at each point, including changes in medication. Advanced directives are pertinent here. Everyone can learn from the process of medication reduction, including the doctor: it may lead to clarity over the lowest therapeutic dose of medication for an individual, which may result in fewer side-effects and support the service user in moving further towards recovery. There are, however, service and resource implications of a relapse which can lead to costly hospital admissions, as well as the human cost to the service user and significant others; in addition, a hospital admission due to relapse may be seen by commissioners to indicate a failure of staff.

Physical healthcare

Last in this part of the book, but most certainly not least, the monitoring and management of physical health conditions are discussed in Chapter 15, 'Physical healthcare'. Treatment or facilitation of physical health treatment is increasingly recognised as being absolutely the remit of psychiatrists as the doctors in the multidisciplinary team, although it is in reality the business of everyone on the clinical team. The inequities in physical health outcomes, including the threefold excess mortality in those with severe mental illness compared with the general population (Laursen *et al*, 2007) and the 15- to 30-year reduced life expectancy (Vreeland, 2007), are stark statistics. The reasons why the mortality gap exists, what the main physical health problems are (such as those related to smoking, obesity and diabetes mellitus), the recommended monitoring and the role of psychiatric services in providing and facilitating physical healthcare are discussed. Examples of effective physical health interventions in rehabilitation and recovery settings are also to be learnt from.

References

Carra G, Johnson S, Bebbington P, *et al* (2012) The lifetime and past-year prevalence of dual diagnosis in people with schizophrenia across Europe: findings from the European Schizophrenia Cohort (EuroSC). *European Archives of Psychiatry and Clinical Neuroscience*, **262**: 607–16.

Davidson L, Strauss JS (1992) Sense of self in recovery from psychosis. *British Journal of Medical Psychology*, **65**: 131–45.

Department of Health (2004) *The National Service Framework for Mental Health – Five Years On*. Department of Health.

Francis R (2013) *Report of the Mid-Staffordshire NHS Foundation Trust Public Inquiry. Chaired by Robert Francis QC* (HC 947). TSO (The Stationery Office).

Kalidindi S, Killaspy H, Edwards T (2012) *Community Psychosis Services: The Role of Community Mental Health Rehabilitation Teams* (Faculty of Rehabilitation and Social Psychiatry Report FR/RS/07). Royal College of Psychiatrists.

Kipping C, Simpson L (2010) Contrasting maintenance and recovery approaches to the care of people with dual diagnosis. *Advances in Dual Diagnosis*, **1**: 15–18.

Laursen TM, Munk-Olsen T, Nordentoft M, *et al* (2007) Increased mortality among patients admitted with major psychiatric disorders: a register-based study comparing mortality in unipolar depressive disorder, bipolar affective disorder, schizoaffective disorder, and schizophrenia. *Journal of Clinical Psychiatry*, **68**: 899–907.

Maben J, Peccei R, Adams M, *et al* (2012) *Patients' Experiences of Care and the Influence of Staff Motivation, Affect and Wellbeing* (Final Report, NIHR Service Delivery and Organisation programme). At http://www.nets.nihr.ac.uk/__data/assets/pdf_file/0008/85094/FR-08-1819-213.pdf (accessed 24 December 2013).

McGurk SR, Twamley EW, Sitzer DI, *et al* (2007) A meta-analysis of cognitive remediation in schizophrenia. *American Journal of Psychiatry*, **164**: 1791–802.

Miller WR, Rollnick S (2013) *Motivational Interviewing: Helping People Change* (3rd edn). Guilford Press.

National Collaborating Centre for Mental Health (2014) *Psychosis and Schizophrenia in Adults. The NICE Guideline on Treatment and Management, Updated Edition 2014.* British Psychological Association.

Prochaska J, DiClemente C (1986) Towards a comprehensive model of change. In *Treating Addictive Behaviours: Processes of Change* (eds W Miller, N Heather): 3–27. Plenum.

Vreeland B (2007) Bridging the gap between mental and physical health: a multidisciplinary approach. *Journal of Clinical Psychiatry*, **68** (suppl 4): 26–33.

Wykes T, Huddy V, Cellard C, *et al* (2011) A meta-analysis of cognitive remediation for schizophrenia: methodology and effect sizes. *American Journal of Psychiatry,* **168**: 472–85.

CHAPTER 8

Rehabilitation at the coalface: practical approaches to helping people improve their functional skills

Simon Tobitt, Thérèse Jenkins and Sridevi Kalidindi

Introduction

The 'coalface' for the chapter authors comes from working in mental health rehabilitation services (in-patient and community) in the UK National Health Service. This involves working with service users with complex clinical presentations – more than half have more than one significant psychiatric diagnosis. This clinical context is further complicated by: behaviours risking harm to self, to others and from others; relatively greater physical health problems, resulting in an excess mortality of up to three times that of the general population (Laursen *et al*, 2007); and working with complex social factors, such as current adversity, social isolation and stigma.

In this chapter, practical ways in which to help service users improve their functional skills are shared. The term 'functional skills' is commonplace in rehabilitation settings. 'Functional skills' are defined by the concept of need. Needs-assessment approaches aim to identify need across a range of domains. Need can arise from the service user struggling in a given domain of functioning (Brewin *et al*, 1987; Slade *et al*, 1999). Therefore, identified need can indicate that intervention is required by rehabilitation clinicians to support the person improving 'functional skills'. Box 8.1 summarises the skills areas with which rehabilitation clinicians are frequently working, and is based on the needs-assessment literature.

This straightforward definition of functioning in relation to identified needs is, though, an oversimplification. Slade *et al* (1999) suggest that what is identified as a need depends on whose viewpoint is considered: service user, carer or clinician. They may concur, or there may be differing perspectives. The recovery approach recognises that what is most meaningful to the service user should shape the agenda (Slade, 2009). Brewin *et al* (1987) make a distinction in assessing functioning between lack of competence (the skill has been lost or not acquired) and lack of performance (the skill's performance is affected by psychological factors such as motivation, negative affect or lack of opportunity to perform).

Box 8.1 Summary of skills areas with which rehabilitation clinicians work

- Food preparation
- Shopping
- Managing money
- Budgeting and paying household bills
- Looking after the home environment
- Attending to personal care, appearance and health
- Access and use of community-based amenities and transport
- Accessing communication and information technology
- Occupation in personally meaningful activity (e.g. employment, interests)
- Engaging in satisfying social relationships
- Numeracy and literacy
- Maintaining or changing behaviour to match personal desires and optimise health and well-being
- Staying safe/reducing risk of harm
- Decision-making, problem-solving and planning

The spirit in which ideas are shared is to provide options for the reader. The authors draw on different theoretical approaches, rather than a single model or framework. So, the ideas may be useful for some service users in some situations. Implementation will require clinicians to draw on evolved qualities of flexibility, adaptability and being experimental. The chapter is structured along the chronology of rehabilitative work: starting with engagement; moving on to establishing a rationale for skills work; then exploring practical approaches for facilitating change. This structure aims to help thinking about an individual piece of clinical work, and is applicable to service users at different stages of their recovery.

Engagement

The starting point for any clinician supporting someone to overcome problems with functional skills is developing a working relationship. A therapeutic approach drawn on at several points in this chapter is motivational interviewing. Miller & Rollnick (2013) emphasise that engagement is continuous through all phases of therapeutic work, not just the beginning. Motivational interviewing is based on the principles of a person-centred approach, commonly identified with substance misuse work, but is more broadly applicable to any behavioural or lifestyle change. Personal recovery (Slade, 2009) is now central to the orientation of rehabilitation services. In the initial stages of rehabilitative work, hope is a core element of recovery that the clinician needs to convey to the service user. Hope is the belief that change is possible (different from making a promise). It is in opposition to a past attitude of pessimism about the possible progress service users could make, which was experienced as 'spirit breaking' (Deegan, quoted in Slade, 2009). Putting the 'personal' into personal recovery is also essential in the early stages. Service users are more likely to invest in forging a relationship with a clinician if therapeutic work is going to address their priorities and desires. An enticing agenda is going to be a personally meaningful one, not one set by the clinician. A recovery orientation also endorses working on life goals alongside the service user managing mental health issues. Therefore failure to achieve the abolition of symptoms does not have to hold a person back from getting back into life or from undertaking functional skills work.

The recovery orientation challenges traditional notions of professional expertise. Respect is rightly paid to the perspective of the service user, as 'expert by experience' (Slade, 2009). An approach based on their experience and learning so far in their recovery journey will be the best foundation for moving forward. This does not negate professional expertise ('expert by training'). In motivational interviewing, the 'righting reflex' is discussed (Miller & Rollnick, 2013): if the professional adopts an over-directive style in voicing arguments for change in the service user's life, the service user is more likely to respond by defending the existing position.

Rehabilitation services are frequently working with service users who present with psychosis. In the current case-load of our team, approximately 85% of service users have a diagnosis of schizophrenia, bipolar disorder or schizoaffective disorder. This can present unique challenges to engaging service users. The engagement principles used in cognitive–behavioural therapy (CBT) for psychosis (Chadwick *et al*, 1996; Chadwick, 2006) are informative for engagement in rehabilitative work. Initial CBT sessions are as open as the service user feels comfortable with, to enable talking freely. Feedback on any concerns the person has and how he or she finds the sessions with you is encouraged. Employing active listening skills will show service users you are interested in their understandings and ideas: paying close attention to their priorities, using the language they do to describe their experiences (rather than imposing a professional jargon), and demonstrating your listening through accurate reflections. Clinicians can empathise with the emotion of service users' psychotic experiences, without influencing their conviction in their distressing beliefs. As part of trusting you, service users may need to feel heard in discussing their experiences within the mental health services. If they ask for your advice, this is best shared tentatively in the early stages.

Rehabilitation teams frequently work with people in complex networks: the service user; the family and other informal sources of support; the accommodation placement staff; and the multidisciplinary rehabilitation team itself. Engagement can include others in this system, where the service user consents. Working with the system has strengths: if others are instrumental in the functional skill area, it is probably helpful to have them involved in the process. This reduces misunderstandings about what the work is about in the wider system. It also provides potential 'co-therapists', and improves the opportunities for practice and therefore generalisation. It positively models interdependence within the support network.

Establishing a rationale for skills work

Picking up from the previous section, recovery-oriented working means working on goals arising from the service user's priorities. If this can be done, there is no need to establish a rationale: it is what the service user wants, and she or he will readily and willingly use support to achieve these desires. This is not always straightforward in rehabilitation settings. First, motivational issues for service users mean they can have mixed feelings (ambivalence) about recovery expectations, or even lack a sense about the direction in which their personal recovery lies. Additionally, the work of rehabilitation teams and clinicians with service users can be influenced by criminal, mental health and mental capacity legal frameworks. In these situations the need for change or response is influenced by authorities outside the working relationship. This is recognised in the recovery literature: Slade (2009) differentiates recovery goals (the service user's dream and aspirations) from treatment goals (arising from societal requirements and professional obligations imposed on clinicians).

Motivational interviewing can be used when the clinician is faced with ambivalence about behavioural change (Miller & Rollnick, 2013). Ambivalence is familiar to professionals who have struggled with changing their own habits (or failing to change!). Miller & Rollnick make a distinction between 'change talk' (self-expressed argument for change) and 'sustain talk' (argument to maintain the status quo). Where the balance in the service user's language is more towards change, this is associated with a higher likelihood of change. Within motivational interviewing, different types of change talk have been identified: desire ('I want', 'I hope'), ability ('I can', 'I'm able to'), reason ('It would mean') and need ('I must', 'I have to'). Clinicians can be attuned to which types of change talk are present, which absent, and use this to inform exploratory questions. The clinician should listen attentively for change talk voiced by the service user. At a natural conclusion, the clinician can summarise for the service user the user's arguments for change. Miller & Rollnick (2013) use the metaphor of collecting up the service user's change talk, and arranging it as a 'bouquet' of his or her articulated rationale for change.

The clinician should ask questions that elaborate the change talk, affirm the service user's attitude towards change and provide reflections and summaries which echo the change talk. Where the balance in the service user's language is against change, motivational interviewing provides ideas for working to support her or him. If there is minimal change talk, the clinician can show curiosity about this. The clinician can be attentive to

Table 8.1 Framework of a decisional balance

Making the change		Keeping things the same	
Advantages	Disadvantages	Advantages	Disadvantages
1.	1.	1.	1.
2.	2.	2.	2.
etc.			

the service user voicing issues about confidence or ability to change, where skills work or other resources may be suggested. In a non-blaming tone, the clinician can reflect back the negative consequences of not changing where the service user mentions these.

Where there is discrepancy between the present situation and service users' views of themselves and/or their future, this can be helpful in exploring change. It needs to be done with caution since exposing such discrepancy may render the service user's esteem vulnerable or elicit defensiveness (which would be counterproductive). Therefore, the clinician needs to respond gently and empathically, and at first explore the discrepancy rather than recruit it as an argument for change.

Decisional balance can be a useful tool in rehabilitation work (see Table 8.1). In motivational interviewing (Miller & Rollnick, 2013) decisional balance is used only where the clinician wants to remain neutral rather than promote change. However, it can prove helpful with rehabilitation service users for several reasons. First, some service users tend to acquiesce to a professional's suggestions, but without an established rationale for change the person does not then show commitment. Likewise, where a rationale has been established it avoids post-decisional regret, where the change is less easy to undo (e.g. moving placement, financial outlay required). Lastly, where cognitive deficits are part of the service user's problems, the decisional balance can aid this cognitively complex task.

In some situations 'sustain talk' will be dominant – even where negative consequences to the service user seem evident to all. In such situations, clinicians can remain alert to any 'change talk' and revisit desire for change at occasional intervals. It is important to remember the 'righting reflex' mentioned above, and the danger of the clinician forcing the case for change, which is counterproductive. Motivational interviewing emphasises, as do the authors, that the service user's autonomy and right to make a personal choice have to be respected (Miller & Rollnick, 2013).

Practical approaches for change

Throughout this chapter different therapeutic approaches and ideas are shared. Integration is endorsed by some of the approaches' originators (e.g. Miller & Rollnick, 2013). Rehabilitation clinicians can artfully draw on these resources in their clinical work. There are some cautions, though, to note about integrative practice. First, it is advisable to use one idea for one element of work and in implementation give it fair opportunity to have the intended effects. Service users may be overwhelmed by overly complex interventions. Clinicians too can get lost if they make their interventions too complex or get frustrated where they rashly switch between approaches. Second, in terms of assessing the effects of an intervention, it can be helpful to measure pre- (before), during and post- (after) your intervention. This could be by using: an appropriate standardised questionnaire; a simple yes/no report; a rating on a scale of the service user's performance of a functional skill; or an observational measure (e.g. how often John does his own laundry, how often Jane goes out). By taking these measures before and after, you and the service user can discern whether the intervention has brought about change in the desired direction.

Lastly, it is important to emphasise the common professional obligation to work within the scope of one's competency. If the ideas shared here are new to a professional, then they should be discussed in clinical supervision before implementation is attempted. A supervisor will need to support and have oversight of the development of any new competency.

Using existing strengths and resources

Hope is an essential part of recovery. The clinician's ability to encourage service users to identify their current strengths and resources will contribute to them feeling hopeful about the future. Clinicians will rarely understand what living with a mental health problem is like. Therefore, finding ways of assessing and encouraging service users to share their strengths and resources is important. Within our team, assessments such as an interests checklist or a functional checklist are used. An interests checklist will indicate activities a service user has previously engaged in, which can guide the clinician in working with that person towards re-establishing old skills. The checklist also gives the clinician an idea of the service user's current engagement or interest in certain activities, which can be either explored further or built upon. Completing a 'life chart' or 'timeline' with service users provides a visual tool that demonstrates to them the positives and resources used during difficult times, as well as reflecting on the past and their resilience.

The Occupational Self Assessment (Baron *et al*, 2006) is an evaluation tool and outcome measure used by occupational therapists. It is a client-centred assessment, which gives voice to the service user's views. It is a two-part self-rating form. Section 1 includes a series of statements about occupational competence. The service user responds to these statements, indicating a level of performance for each item. In section 2, the service user establishes priorities for therapy, which can be translated into therapy goals.

'Telling my story' groups are a popular method for encouraging service users to provide accounts of their lives and experiences. Describing their journey can bring understanding and insight into service users' current circumstances. Communicating their life story allows them to reflect on how far they have come and the difficulties they have overcome. Clinicians can contribute to service users' sense of their own resources by including regular feedback during interactions, done in a way that highlights the person's strengths (Creek, 2002).

The use of a motivational interviewing approach (Miller & Rollnick, 2013) provides verbal affirmations of a person's efforts and any gains, no matter how small. This can work to change behaviour in a desired direction. This verbal reinforcement – or simply 'praise' – aims to elicit more progress in the same direction. To be effective, praise needs to be authentically expressed by the clinician to the service user, and timely in relation to the service user's effort and gain made.

In a solution-focused therapy (SFT) approach (Lipchik, 2002) the focus is shifted off the problem. Instead, a way forward is found by: using 'problem-free' talk; focusing on the person's strengths and resources; identifying what change has happened already in his or her life; and noting exceptions to the problem (times when the problem is not there, there less, or the person is actively coping). SFT uses questions to invoke an imagined future without problems. The 'miracle question' is employed to get an understanding of how, with all obstacles removed, the service user sees life without these problems. Use of scaling questions can help the person understand what has happened and what progress has been made already, and what the person thinks needs to happen to edge further up the scale in the desired direction of change.

Identifying a positive self-identity separate from the diagnosis and illness experience is a significant aspect of personal recovery. The clinician can play a role in amplifying this positive sense of self. As Slade (2009) notes, hope is more than optimism (positive expectations). Hope is also about perceived external resources and internal resources (which overlaps with the concept of 'agency') to move forward in personal recovery.

Goal-setting

The identification of personal recovery goals needs to be led by the client, and clinicians must offer support in all goal domains in ways that the service user agrees would be helpful (Lloyd et al, 2008). Goal-setting helps service users to think about their ambitions and break these down into manageable steps. Goal-setting is useful in almost all functional skills domains. It will involve the clinician reviewing goals with the service user and being flexible in changing course if the service user wishes (Repper & Perkins, 2003).

Goal-setting formats are widely used by occupational therapists, but are also encouraged as part of the Care Programme Approach (CPA) as well as informally. Occupational therapists can support service users with setting and reviewing goals where there is occupational deprivation, lack of motivation, an inappropriate environment or a skill deficit. Goals should be negotiated between the clinician and service user, as this facilitates partnership and encourages involvement of the service user. It is advised that goals are individualised, user-centred, realistic and challenging.

In our service, we have developed a simple handout to help service users clarify their goals. This uses the SMART acronym, with guiding questions; there are different interpretations of what SMART signifies. Our version is: Specific (Is your goal detailed enough for you to see what to do next?), Measurable (What will tell you that you have achieved your goal?), Attainable (Are there any obstacles that might get in the way of you achieving your goal?), Relevant (Why is it important to you to achieve this goal) and Timed (How much time do you estimate you will need to achieve this goal?).

A change plan is a particular type of goal, arising from motivational work (Miller & Rollnick, 2013), concerning behaviour or lifestyle change. When the person has worked through any ambivalence about change and reached a decision to change (see 'Establishing a rationale for skills work', above), then it is time to make a change plan. Wherever possible, the service user should generate ideas for the plan, with clinicians making suggestions as necessary, in support. A collaborative process to develop the plan has a greater chance of resulting in positive change. There may be one clear change plan or options of different plans, or the service user may have no clear plan. If more than one option exists, the service user may have a view about the best approach. The change plan moves from intention to change to more specifics: the service user voicing commitment; defining the steps towards the change; identifying the 'when' and 'how'; and troubleshooting any obstacles encountered or foreseen.

In working with change, the groundwork done of engagement and attention to ambivalence pays dividends, as wavering commitment and any slip-ups can be overcome by revising the rationale for the work. Setbacks and slip-ups should be normalised as part of the change process, not treated as a catastrophe. If appropriate, the change plan can be adjusted to incorporate any unforeseen factors.

Acceptance and commitment therapy (ACT; Harris, 2009) emphasises the importance of establishing the service user's values prior to goal-setting work. Where establishing goals with a service user feels a struggle, looking at values may usefully reignite the work. Harris (2009) defines values as 'leading principles that can guide and motivate us as we move through life' – what we stand for, how we want to behave. The metaphor of a compass is used, which sets direction and enables one to keep on track on life's journey. Understanding a person's values tells you what motivates, inspires and sustains him or her as a person.

Behaving in line with one's values brings a sense of integrity to a person's life. Identifying personal values can be done through questions: 'What do you care most about in life?', 'What matters most to you?' It can be done by exploring self-perceptions. As a child, what did the service user imagine for his or her future? If they were to imagine their 80th birthday, and people making speeches about their life – what would these speeches say they stood for, about their role in life? Who are their role models in public life, and what is it they find so inspiring about these people? There are values card sorts freely available (e.g. Miller & Rollnick, 2013: ch. 7) with examples of values on the cards like 'Adventure', 'Belonging', 'Creativity', 'Duty'. The card sort can be used in different ways, such as identifying the 'Top 5' values with which the service user identifies.

Monitoring and scheduling activity

Humans engage in activity and benefit both themselves and others by active participation (Creek, 2002). Scheduling and monitoring help service users to focus on meaningful activity as part of their routine. They should focus on activities that are meaningful and fulfilling to them and clinicians should be able to assist them in making appropriate choices so that individual need is satisfied (Reed, 1984, cited in Di Bona, 2000). An interests checklist allows service users to identify interests past and present and to choose activities they would like to re-engage in or engage in for the first time. Leisure satisfaction scales allow people to indicate whether their needs are being satisfied through their current leisure pursuits.

Planning can benefit service users with problems of motivation, disorganisation and indecisiveness, as well as allowing them to take control over their life (Creek, 2002). Timetables are a useful method of allowing service users to document their daily living skills, activities and roles within a weekly/monthly format. Hemphill *et al* (1991) offer some useful considerations. First, explore all possible activities available in the home and community environment. Then, taking note of preferences, interests and values will help an individual in making choices. Finally, the activity can be initiated.

Information-sharing

Information-sharing is a common component of family work (Kuipers *et al*, 2006) and of motivational interviewing (Miller & Rollnick, 2013). The practice goes by other names as well, such as psychoeducation. In terms of functional skills work, information-sharing can be helpful in supporting the service user make informed decisions about treatments or occupational activities, about health behaviours (e.g. diet, drug use, self-managing chronic health conditions) or about how to stay safe/reduce risk.

Miller & Rollnick (2013) provide a useful elicit–provide–elicit framework for information-sharing. First, the person's information needs are elicited, discussing what they know already, establishing any gaps, and asking if they would like more information on a topic. By eliciting first, the clinician shows respect for service users' existing knowledge, which increases their receptiveness to information imparted. Second, information is provided that most closely fits the service user's expressed priorities. It is best to select sources of information in everyday language and of a manageable length, as it is better to start small and provide more later than to overwhelm a service user. During the information-sharing, the professional should allow plenty of opportunities for questions, comments and reflections. The professional should then check how the information fits with service users' experiences. Lastly, the professional elicits their response to the information, and whether they need further information.

Following this model can avoid some of the pitfalls of information-sharing: talking down to service users, attempting to fill their heads with too many facts, and imposing professional theories or jargon. Furthermore, it should be clear that information-sharing is an activity in which the clinician is encouraging as much participation as possible, and far from a didactic worker-to-client monologue.

Information-sharing may be brief and spontaneous (a one-sentence response) or the focus of a couple of dedicated sessions. Information may be verbal or written. Verbal information has the advantage of being seamless in the discussion. Written information has the advantage that it can be taken away, kept for the future and shared with others in the support network; it may particularly suit less chatty individuals. Information should always be from a trustworthy source. In the UK national mental health charities offer such information, often freely available to download from their websites. Not all internet-based information is likely to be helpful though, or indeed accurate. Service users may struggle to retain information, so clinicians should be tolerant to revision.

In family work for psychosis (Kuipers *et al*, 2006) information-sharing is often specific to diagnosis, covering areas like the associated symptoms, theories about cause, prognosis and available treatments. This can be done individually too. It should be interactive; it is crucial that service users talk of their experiences. Recovery-oriented working recognises that different models of mental illness exist: biomedical, psychological, social and cultural (Slade, 2009). Clinicians need to be sympathetic to different perspectives, not impose one idea, and tolerate being unable to provide absolute certainty and clear-cut answers.

Problem-solving

Problem-solving is a technique identified with family work and CBT (Falloon *et al*, 2007; Grey, 2010) but is also described in the recovery literature (Repper & Perkins, 2003). Problem-solving is a tool that can be used in many functional skills areas, including managing money and other household issues, and relationship and social difficulties. Problem-solving and decision-making are functional skills in themselves, so clinicians should aim to enable the service user to problem-solve independently.

There are several reasons why structured problem-solving can be useful (Falloon *et al*, 2007). Service users in emotional distress can encounter problem-solving difficulties, or can be impulsive in acting on the most immediate solution. Cognitive deficits experienced by people with psychosis can impair problem-solving. A structured tool can help overcome these difficulties. A stepped problem-solving approach and its fundamental principles are described in Table 8.2.

Graded exposure

Many service users suffer from anxieties that prevent them from engaging in meaningful routines and therefore impact on their socialisation. Graded exposure is an intervention that can be used to help service users overcome fears that stop them from doing what they want to do (Repper & Perkins, 2003). The obvious functional skills domains where graded exposure may be helpful are social and community-oriented goals, but it may be applicable in other areas where anxiety is a barrier to achieving improved functioning.

Table 8.2 A stepped problem-solving approach

Steps	Principles
1. Define the problem	The emphasis in this step is on moving from a broad to a specific sense of the problem. The clinician can play a role in identifying whether there is one problem, a complex but interconnected problem, or a series of discrete problems which could be problem-solved separately
2. Think of solutions ('brainstorming')	The emphasis here is on encouraging creativity, permitting solutions no matter how silly, and avoiding a premature focus on one solution. The clinician should take note of whether solutions are in the service user's realm of control, particularly for those with a tendency to externalise responsibility to others to solve their problems
3. Consider advantages and disadvantages of each solution	Each solution is evaluated in terms of advantages and then disadvantages. It can be helpful to appreciate the advantages of all solutions first, before dismissing any
4. Decide on a plan	In our experience, service users often adopt a combination of solutions rather than a single solution, but it depends on the problem. Sometimes in thinking through advantages and disadvantages, questions are raised, to which answers need to be sought first. The clinician should helpfully differentiate solutions that are short-term stop-gaps and those with more long-term effects. When it comes to deciding on a plan or goal see our section 'Goal-setting' for creating a step-by-step plan
5. Action and review	The clinician can play a motivating role in encouraging action. For both parties, it can be helpful to adopt an experimental approach to action, as an opportunity to learn and report back for reflection in the next session, rather than a pass/fail test

By its nature it provides service users with the opportunity for gradual change, by adapting or adjusting a certain activity. It allows service users to explore skills, progress and achieve. This approach is also relevant in the context of a 'graded return', related to people returning to activities after a relapse. Where possible, a return to the role(s) they previously held will be preferable (Repper & Perkins, 2003).

Graded exposure is a behavioural intervention and a fundamental of CBT (Butler, 1989; Kennerley, 1997). Its theoretical basis is that anxiety has been learned through association with a particular stimulus or situation, and through graded exposure to the anxiety-provoking situation, the anxiety and the learned association diminish. It is essential to bear in mind that this is an intervention that can exacerbate anxiety if not done properly – the grading must be set and paced by the service user. It is also essential for it to work towards a meaningful goal for the service user; there is no incentive to face fears if there is no ultimate desired outcome. A framework for undertaking graded exposure is presented in Table 8.3.

Coping strategies

There is much literature on the subject of coping strategies and an in-depth discussion of this work is beyond the scope of this chapter. Earlier literature focused on reactions to stressors (Lazarus & Folkman, 1984); the later literature also discussed strategies to be used when stressors are not present, in order to reduce the likelihood of them occurring (Aspinwall & Taylor, 1997; Schwarzer & Taubert, 2002).

Imparting relevant skills to service users and supporting them to develop and regularly use them can have a significant impact on levels of distress and function. There are three broad types of coping strategies (Weiten & Lloyd, 2008). Appraisal-focused strategies involve patients modifying their thinking, such as altering their goals or denying the problem. Problem-focused strategies attempt to get to the core of the problem by gathering relevant information on the difficulty and developing skills to manage them. This has the function of trying to remove the source of stress. Emotion-focused strategies aim to reduce the distress felt in relation to difficulties. They can, for example, involve distraction techniques such as counting backwards in 3s from 100, or being mindful of one's surroundings, which can have the effect of stopping rumination on distressing thoughts.

As can be expected, coping strategies may be adaptive, improving function, or maladaptive, which may reduce symptoms in the short term but in fact strengthen and maintain the disorder. Maladaptive coping strategies include the use of illicit drugs or alcohol to alleviate immediate distress. Adaptive coping strategies can include: active preventive strategies such as accessing social support and engaging in hobbies or other activities; mental distraction techniques; and relaxation or mindfulness techniques.

A good method can be to work collaboratively with the client to ascertain what coping strategies are currently used and then to discuss whether

Table 8.3 A framework for undertaking graded exposure

Steps	Principles
Explain the vicious cycle of avoidance	It is important to provide a theory for how the person's fear/anxiety is maintained and how this vicious cycle can be broken. The anxiety (emotions and thoughts) leads to avoidance behaviour; the avoidance feeds back to increase fear/anxiety when the stimulus/situation is contemplated. This cycle is broken by behaving in a new way, through gradual exposure to the fear
Identify the feared stimulus or situation	Sometimes this will be obvious, when the service user clearly identifies a stimulus or situation. It is worth exploring recent experiences of the problem and breaking them down to identify the source of anxiety where this is not directly identified, and also to ensure the clinician does not to jump to erroneous conclusions in seemingly straightforward scenarios
Develop a hierarchy of target tasks	Work with the service user to identify a hierarchy of anxiety-provoking targets and tasks, from least anxiety-provoking (e.g. walking past the outside of the supermarket with a trusted person) to the most (e.g. spending a half-hour shopping on a busy Saturday morning alone). The ordering of the hierarchy can be established by rating perceived anxiety for each target on a scale of 0–100. The target tasks can vary on different variables: intensity, proximity to situation/stimulus, duration of time, whether accompanied or alone, etc.
Develop coping skills for managing anxiety during exposure	Anxiety is about overestimating danger and underestimating ability to cope. By identifying and rehearsing some anxiety-management techniques, the service user's ability to cope is increased. Examples might include deep-breathing techniques and having ready challenges to likely anxious thoughts
Start with the least anxiety-provoking target	It may take a few or many exposures with the least anxiety-provoking target before the service user feels more confident. It is essential to let the service user set the pace; pressurising someone to move to the next stage risks exacerbating anxiety, which will mean the intervention fails, and is unethical. The clinician and any co-therapists from the service user's support network can play the role of praising the effort and reminding the service user of the rationale for the intervention
Continue to the next stage of the hierarchy	When the service user feels ready to face the next level of challenge, he or she can move to the next target identified in the hierarchy, until confident with that, and so on to the next level

they are adaptive or maladaptive, in language that is jargon-free. Further potential strategies can be suggested by the clinician, with a final list being made of strategies the client may find useful. This can be kept in written form, perhaps as part of a 'staying well' plan, which can be referred to whenever necessary. The idea of employing some of these methods to minimise and avoid stressful situations, before they arise, should be promoted. Practising techniques with a clinician can also be highly relevant and practising them when all is calm means that when distress levels do become high, the methods are more readily put into action.

Modelling and role-play

Modelling is not something we use explicitly in our clinical work. This is not to dismiss its value and power as a learning mechanism. Certainly, it is important for clinicians to keep in mind that in their interactional style in direct work with service users, they will be acting as a model with regard to communication and social skills, and through verbalisations may be modelling self-management of emotions and cognitive skills such as decision-making and problem-solving. In practical skills learning, clinicians can often be demonstrating a skill. In this situation, it can be helpful to verbalise each step as well as physically to demonstrate it. This increases opportunities for learning and for the service user to internalise the skill. Complex skills may need breaking down into smaller steps.

Role-play is more of an intentional intervention. The clinician may demonstrate positive communication or behaviour based on circumstances where the service user has experienced problems or distressing emotion. The service user can then practise or replicate the behaviour shown. Clinician and service user may also engage in role-play by practising communication or behaviour with each other and the service user then practises this as homework. There can be value in service users role-playing themselves, but also role-playing the other person, if they are happy to do this. Drama groups will use a similar format, with the added benefit of peers interacting, practising and demonstrating positive skills.

Peer support workers can be particularly effective role models. It can inspire hope for service users to work with those who have gone through a similar experience and are now in recovery. Peers offer support, information and hope (Repper & Perkins, 2003), as well as providing role models for service users. Peer support workers are now being employed within workplaces and in the voluntary sector for the value they can add to a workforce based on their own 'lived experiences' (see Chapter 21, 'Peer support in mental health services').

Befrienders, mentors and support workers are also widely used to engage service users in activities and occupations through modelling. Other forms of role-modelling are occupational therapy/activity groups, which are available in the community as well as in-patient settings. Groups are activity-based and are usually focused around leisure pursuits or an activity of daily living (ADL). Groups can help service users to develop new skills or re-establish old skills. Occupational therapists are encouraged to spend time doing activities with service users as a way of modelling and teaching (Cook & Birrell 2007).

Conclusions

Engagement, assessment and developing clear and achievable goals that are relevant to the service user are all complex processes that require sensitivity, skill and persistence. Specific therapeutic methods such as those outlined above should be employed at the discretion of the clinician, working in collaboration with the service user. Identifying when a client is ready for a particular approach and working with the person are complex but potentially highly rewarding clinical tasks.

References

Aspinwall LG, Taylor SE (1997) A stitch in time: self-regulation and preventive coping. *Psychological Bulletin*, **121**: 417–36.

Baron K, Kielhofner G, Iyenger A, *et al* (2006) *The Occupational Self Assessment (OSA) Version 2.2*. Model of Human Occupation Clearinghouse, University of Illinois at Chicago.

Brewin CR, Wing JK, Mangen SP, *et al* (1987) Principles and practice of measuring needs in long-term mentally ill: the MRC Needs for Care Assessment. *Psychological Medicine*, **17**: 971–81.

Butler G (1989) Phobic disorders. In *Cognitive Behaviour Therapy for Psychiatric Problems: A Practical Guide* (eds K Hawton, PM Salkovskis, J Kirk, *et al*): 97–128. Oxford University Press.

Chadwick P (2006) *Person-based Cognitive Therapy for Distressing Psychosis*. John Wiley.

Chadwick P, Birchwood M, Trower P (1996) *Cognitive Therapy for Delusions, Voices and Paranoia*. John Wiley.

Cook S, Birrell M (2007) Defining an occupational therapy intervention for people with psychosis. *British Journal of Occupational Therapy*, **70**: 96–106.

Creek J (2002) *Occupational Therapy and Mental Health*. Churchill Livingstone.

Di Bona L (2000) What are the benefits of leisure? An exploration using the leisure satisfaction scale. *British Journal of Occupational Therapy*, **63**: 50–8.

Falloon IRH, Barbieri L, Boggian I, *et al* (2007) Problem solving training for schizophrenia: rationale and review. *Journal of Mental Health*, **16**: 553–68.

Grey S (2010) Problem solving groups for psychiatric inpatients: a practical guide. In *Psychological Groupwork with Acute Psychiatric Inpatients* (eds J Radcliffe, K Hajek, J Carson, *et al*): 191–213. Whiting & Birch.

Harris R (2009) *ACT Made Simple*. New Harbinger Publications.

Hemphill B, Peterson C, Werner P (1991) *Rehabilitation in Mental Health: Goals and Objectives for Independent Living*. SLACK Inc.

Kennerley H (1997) *Overcoming Anxiety: A Self-help Guide Using Cognitive Behavioural Techniques*. Robinson Publishing.

Kuipers E, Leff J, Lam D (2006) *Family Work for Schizophrenia: A Practical Guide* (2nd edn). Royal College of Psychiatrists/Gaskell.

Laursen TM, Munk-Olsen T, Nordentoft M, *et al* (2007) Increased mortality among patients admitted with major psychiatric disorders: a register-based study comparing mortality in unipolar depressive disorder, bipolar affective disorder, schizoaffective disorder, and schizophrenia. *Journal of Clinical Psychiatry*, **68**: 899–907.

Lazarus RS, Folkman S (1984) *Stress, Appraisal, and Coping*. Springer.

Lipchik E (2002) *Beyond Technique in Solution-Focused Therapy*. Guilford Press.

Lloyd C, Wagorn G, Williams P (2008) Conceptualising recovery in mental health rehabilitation. *British Journal of Occupational Therapy*, **71**: 321–8.

Miller WR, Rollnick S (2013) *Motivational Interviewing: Helping People Change* (3rd edn). Guilford Press.

Repper J, Perkins R (2003) *Social Inclusion and Recovery: A Model for Mental Health Practice.* Baillière Tindall/Elsevier.

Schwarzer R, Taubert S (2002) Tenacious goal pursuits and striving toward personal growth. In *Beyond Coping: Meeting Goals, Visions and Challenges* (ed E Frydenberg): 19–36. Oxford University Press.

Slade M (2009) *Personal Recovery and Mental Illness.* Cambridge University Press.

Slade M, Thornicroft G, Loftus L, *et al* (1999) *Camberwell Assessment of Need.* Royal College of Psychiatrists/Gaskell.

Weiten W, Lloyd MA (2008) *Psychology Applied to Modern Life* (9th edn). Wadsworth Cengage Learning.

CHAPTER 9

Cognitive approaches: cognitive–behavioural therapy and cognitive remediation therapy

Craig Steel, Til Wykes and Rumina Taylor

Introduction

The cognitive underpinnings of schizophrenia took some time to be recognised, despite the phenomenology including cognition as a main distinguishing factor in all diagnostic descriptions over the past 100 years. Thinking was described as problematic because of two issues: poor communication, engendered through either delusional thinking or the problems of understanding syntactically or semantically disorganised language; and the cognitive problems in memory, concentration and attention described by patients, or cognitive disorganisation or loose associations as described by Kraepelin and Bleuler. It is only relatively recently that these phenomena have been the focus of targeted treatments in psychology, in the form of cognitive–behavioural therapy for psychosis (CBTp) and cognitive remediation therapy (CRT). These approaches take their roots in the two different aspects of poor cognition but have now begun to move together under the guise of metacognition. Both ascribe the problems of cognition as part of the disorder and this has now been recognised in the new version of the *Diagnostic and Statistical Manual* (DSM-5; American Psychiatric Association, 2013).

This chapter sets out the two broad psychological approaches, their similarities and differences. The evidence base for both therapies is similar, as are their effect sizes (Wykes *et al*, 2008, 2011). At the time of writing, CBTp is firmly recommended within evidence-based guidelines for the treatment of schizophrenia. CRT has not yet achieved this level of recognition, although a recently published national guideline, from Scotland, states that: 'Cognitive remediation therapy may be considered for individuals diagnosed with schizophrenia who have persisting problems associated with cognitive difficulties' (Scottish Intercollegiate Guidelines Network, 2013).

Historical context

Although single case reports of psychological interventions for psychosis date back more than 50 years (e.g. Beck, 1952), significant developments in this area did not occur until the 1980s. Early behavioural interventions were aimed at symptom management and were predominantly embedded within the traditional psychiatric view of schizophrenia. However, the development of cognitive–behavioural models for affective disorders had a significant impact on psychosis research during the late 1990s. This work highlighted the extent to which the development and maintenance of symptoms could be understood with reference to psychological processes. The traditional view that schizophrenia symptom content should be ignored was challenged and therapists began to examine the content of psychotic symptoms directly and to use this dialogue as a basis for collaborative discussion. At the same time, single case studies examining behavioural strategies to allow individuals to improve their attention for a few seconds through to carrying out conversations (with divided-attention techniques developed in experimental psychology) provided optimism that individuals with previously poor engagement could after intervention be engaged in meaningful dialogue.

CBTp and CRT do not differ by just a capital letter. They developed in different ways, with CBTp considering first and foremost the emotional responses to symptom content and CRT considering the problem as driven by cognitive processes. However, both consider the dialogue and relationship with the client, as well as celebrating and reinforcing activities where therapeutic gains are transferred into real-life gains, such as going to the shops or attending a social activity. The primary goals are different: with CBTp, it is the reduction in symptoms or distress; with CRT, it is the improvement of cognitive domains such as memory and attention. The following descriptions enter into more detail on each of the approaches. Both have their place in the psychological treatment armamentarium.

Cognitive–behavioural therapy schizophrenia

The cognitive approach on which CBTp is based assumes that it is not experiences which distress an individual but rather how these experiences are appraised. Thus, being ignored is upsetting only if people believe they are being ignored for reasons that are negative, such as being disliked.

Paul Chadwick and Max Birchwood applied the same principle to the experience of hearing voices (Chadwick & Birchwood, 1994, 1995). They showed that the distressing affect and behaviour arising from hallucinations were not simply the result of the content of the voices, but reflected the voice hearer's appraisal of the voices. In particular, individuals who believed their voice originated from a powerful source, which had malevolent intent towards them, were particularly likely to suffer distress.

Two influential cognitive models of the positive symptoms of psychosis have since been proposed by Philippa Garety and colleagues and Tony Morrison (Garety *et al*, 2001; Morrison, 2001). Both incorporate the role of negative core beliefs, hypervigilance for threat, scanning for confirmatory evidence and safety behaviours. In essence they concur that a psychotic presentation may evolve out of the presence of unusual experiences, with a critical factor being how these experiences are interpreted. Such experiences may include hearing voices, strong déjà vu, dissociative experiences such as derealisation and intrusive thoughts or images. Psychosis is associated with such experiences being interpreted as negative, threatening and external, which leads to hypervigilance and safety behaviours. For example, an individual who 'hears a voice' and decides that this perceptual experience is due to a lack of sleep is likely to have a more benign outcome than an individual who decides that the Devil is angry with her or him. A major strength of these models is that they integrate a wide range of psychological processes and therefore provide a flexible framework within which to formulate the heterogeneous range of presentations associated with psychosis.

Clinical researchers have advocated the potential for an individualised formulation based on a cognitive–behavioural approach to schizophrenia (e.g. Morrison, 2002; Kingdon & Turkington, 2005). Such an approach, as for other disorders, is based on the integration of developmental experiences with current beliefs and behaviours. The aim is to derive a personal account of the development and maintenance of currently distressing experiences that is less threatening than the beliefs that are currently held. This approach can be useful for people suffering from schizophrenia, who are often limited to two forms of disempowering belief, namely 'It is all true, people are out to get me' or 'I am insane. I cannot trust my thoughts. I must take medication forever'.

Engagement in the therapeutic process is highly emphasised as it is anticipated that the patient may not trust healthcare professionals and may withhold important clinical information. A non-judgemental stance is recommended, with the therapist proactively alleviating some of the patient's potential anxieties, for example by stating 'I am not here to assess whether you need in-patient treatment'. Over a number of sessions a cognitive–behavioural formulation is developed that highlights the key links between current thoughts, feelings and behaviours, and how current beliefs are maintained. The historical development of currently distressing beliefs is also included. The focus of therapy then moves gently into an intervention phase. For some patients, simply gaining a different perspective on how they have come to hold their current beliefs is an intervention in itself. For others, more specific interventions may include cognitive restructuring, or experimenting with new behaviours in order to gather information regarding the validity of their current beliefs. For example, not doing what a voice tells you to do in order to find out if their negative predictions are accurate. Throughout, the therapist adopts a non-expert position and collaborates with the patient by helping to set up new tests in order to gather new relevant information. This represents a generic formulation-based approach to working with the wide range of symptoms associated with a diagnosis of schizophrenia. However, more recent work has focused on developing targeted shorter interventions for specific symptoms and presentations, such as comorbid symptoms of post-traumatic stress disorder, sleep problems or depression.

Does CBTp work?

During the mid-1990s a small number of mainly UK-based researchers conducted the first clinical trials in CBTp. The encouraging results led to clinical trials being conducted in other countries and to large randomised controlled trials being funded. The rapid growth in the number of studies aimed at evaluating CBTp led to an increasing number of meta-analyses. A comprehensive review by Wykes *et al* (2008) incorporated a large enough sample of trials to be able to explore factors associated with outcome. Thirty-four trials met inclusion criteria, with 22 of these being individual CBTp aimed at the positive symptoms of psychosis. The overall effect size[1] for CBTp was moderate, and was broadly similar (around 0.4) whether outcome was assessed in relation to positive symptoms, negative symptoms, mood or social functioning.

The evidence to date predominantly provides support for CBTp as an intervention for individuals suffering from 'treatment-resistant' psychosis in a chronic but stable phase. Relatively little is known about the effectiveness of CBTp for other phases of the disorder. Also, little is known about which elements of CBTp are the most important in producing change, and there are few markers as to who benefits most from this intervention.

What are the critical ingredients of CBT for schizophrenia?

Treatment characteristics

Given the somewhat generic nature of CBTp for schizophrenia, compared with a protocol-driven approach, such as cognitive therapy for panic disorder (Clark *et al*, 1999), it is of interest to determine what elements of therapy are important. Morrison & Barratt (2010) conducted a Delphi study with a panel of experts, in which they established seven themes within the therapeutic process that were considered important by at least 80% of the panel. These themes were termed engagement, assessment and model, structure and principles, formulation, homework, change strategies and therapist assumptions. The last includes a position adopted by therapists, whereby any belief reported by a patient is taken seriously as one possible explanation of recent experiences.

Researchers have developed adherence measures for use in clinical trials. These are designed to ensure trial therapists are including the

---

1. Effect size is the difference between the mean scores of an experimental group and a control group divided by the standard deviation of the scores – it provides a measure of the importance of the difference rather than its statistical significance.

relevant components of therapy into their intervention, and doing so with an adequate level of competence. The Cognitive Therapy for Psychosis Adherence Scale (Startup *et al*, 2002) has recently been revised. Factor analysis suggests three distinct elements to the therapy process, namely engagement/assessment work, relapse prevention work and formulation/ schema work (Rollinson *et al*, 2008). One report suggests that a high level of clinical supervision is associated with an enhanced outcome (Steel *et al*, 2012).

Patient characteristics

An improved outcome in CBTp is reported with older (Haddock *et al*, 2006) and female (Brabban *et al*, 2009) participants. Another key variable is the chronicity of illness, where a higher number of recent admissions has been associated with an improved response to CBTp (Garety *et al*, 1997). However, to date, such reports are based on the outcomes of specific trials, and there has been no meta-analysis in relation to these variables.

Cognitive remediation therapy for schizophrenia

For more than 100 years, cognition has been recognised as an issue for people with a diagnosis of schizophrenia and was part of making a diagnosis in both the Kraepelinian and Bleulerian models. Cognitive deficits are evident during the course of the disorder in the areas of attention (Elvevag *et al*, 2000; Pukrop *et al*, 2003), working and long-term memory (explicit but not implicit memory; Addington & Addington, 1999; Cirillo & Seidman, 2003) and executive functioning (Morris *et al*, 1995; Moelter *et al*, 2001). The variability of intellectual abilities in schizophrenia is wide, although approximately 40% of patients show a decline in IQ of 10 points or more after the illness begins (Leeson *et al*, 2009). Studies have also identified IQ deficits in persons who later develop schizophrenia before the onset of the illness (Seidman *et al*, 2006), supporting the neurodevelopment model, which argues that some symptoms and cognitive deficits precede the onset of psychosis (Murray *et al*, 1992). Zubin & Spring's (1977) vulnerability–stress model suggests that those with a diagnosis of schizophrenia have a number of vulnerabilities that increase the likelihood of symptoms emerging when they are faced with stress, and cognitive difficulties have been seen as vulnerability factors for the disorder (Wykes & Reeder, 2005). However, the link between cognition and symptoms is relatively weak, with small associations emerging between increased negative symptoms and poorer cognition but very few between impairments and positive symptoms (Wykes *et al*, 2011).

It is only recently that cognitive deficits have become a target for intervention, spurred on by the revelation that these impairments affect quality of life (Savilla *et al*, 2008; Maat *et al*, 2012) and limit the rate of recovery following rehabilitation (Nuechterlein *et al*, 2012). Service users also report cognitive difficulties to be distressing. The most important reason for providing interventions for deficits has been the strong and significant associations between cognitive difficulties and functional outcome (Green, 1996; Green *et al*, 2000). A range of cognitive domains have been found to be associated with community functioning, social problem-solving, psychosocial skill acquisition and occupational functioning.

Unemployment is a central feature of the social disability that accompanies schizophrenia, with rates of employment rarely getting above 10% (McGurk *et al*, 2009), despite employment being important for recovery. Cognitive deficits are rate limiters even when individuals are provided with the best rehabilitation, as they restrict an individual's ability to acquire skills from such programmes, which subsequently affects functioning. The importance of cognition in schizophrenia has been realised and this has led to a standardised neuropsychological test battery being agreed for the assessment of cognitive ability in schizophrenia, the Measurement and Treatment Research to Improve Cognition in Schizophrenia (MATRICS; Green *et al*, 2004).

What is cognitive remediation therapy?

Presently, there are no drugs specifically approved for the treatment of cognitive impairments, although several are being assessed in clinical trials. Non-pharmacological treatments for cognitive impairments have been designed which come under the umbrella term 'cognitive remediation'. CRT for schizophrenia aims to improve cognition and thereby increase functional outcome (Wykes *et al*, 2007). It has been more formally defined as 'a behavioural-training based intervention that aims to improve cognitive processes (attention, memory, executive function, social cognition, or metacognition) with the goal of durability and generalization' (Cognitive Remediation Experts Workshop, Florence, Italy, April 2010).

Does it work?

Research from clinical studies has shown that CRT, consisting of cognitive training, whether computer-assisted or using paper-and-pencil methods, does work. Several meta-analyses have shown cognitive improvements with CRT and there is some evidence from neuroimaging studies of accompanying neural changes in key frontal and temporal brain areas (see Kurtz, 2012, for a review). A meta-analysis by Wykes *et al* (2011) of 40 studies showed a moderate effect for cognition (0.45) that lasted after therapy had stopped. Therapy had only a small effect on symptoms which did not last. However, there was a moderate effect on functioning outcomes (0.42). This study also showed that the results were consistent even in the most methodologically rigorous studies and so are robust.

What are the critical ingredients of CRT?

Treatment characteristics

Despite there now being an agreed definition of CRT, treatments continue to differ in their theoretical underpinnings, their mode of delivery and in the cognitive functions they target. Most CRT programmes are designed to be carried out with the support of a therapist on an individual basis, although some include a group component to improve social cognition (e.g. Bell *et al*, 2001). Some use paper-and-pencil methods, whereas others rely on computer presentation. The majority vary in terms of the recommended number of sessions, the length of these sessions, as well as their frequency. However, such treatment factors were not found to influence cognition following CRT in a recent meta-analysis (Wykes *et al*, 2011). Wykes & Reeder (2005) examined the effect of the presence of a therapist in CRT and found the average effect size for cognitive change to be almost twice as large when the therapist was an active component. Medalia & Richardson (2005) also found the level of training the therapist received to affect CRT treatment success. More recently, Huddy *et al* (2012) showed that the relationship between the therapist and participant is important for patient satisfaction and outcome. In their study, clients who rated the alliance with their therapist more favourably remained in therapy longer and were more likely to improve on their main cognitive complaint.

Therapeutic approaches to cognitive remediation have differed, although all have included positive reinforcement for correct behaviour. Some programmes have used adaptive strategies such as environmental aids, for example signs, labels and electronic devices designed to cue appropriate behaviours (Velligan *et al*, 2000). Some have taught compensatory strategies to provide individuals with alternative ways to achieve their goals, such as developing their thinking skills or explicitly teaching certain strategies. Others have employed the use of repeated practice or rehearsal learning of tasks with the emphasis on maintaining high levels of accuracy as tasks become increasingly difficult (Kurtz, 2012).

It is not the case that strategic procedures do not involve practice; rather, in this approach strategies to complete the task are discussed prior to practising the tasks and participants are then encouraged to try these in their everyday life. Strategic programmes have been argued to provide more choice to the client as to how they wish to complete the task in hand, which may be crucial for improvement as an individual then owns the process and may be more likely to use it again (Wykes & Reeder, 2005). Indeed, recent meta-analyses (McGurk *et al*, 2007; Wykes *et al*, 2011) have shown that CRT programmes that adopt a more strategic approach achieve significantly better functional outcomes when compared with drill and practice methods. This may be because these types of therapies more easily allow a transfer of training from the individual cognitive remediation tasks to everyday functioning. In line with this was the recent finding that when CRT is provided together with a rehabilitation programme such as supported employment, there are significantly better functional outcomes for those CRT packages that adopt a strategy-based method (Wykes *et al*, 2011).

Patient characteristics

Effect sizes reported by meta-analyses are relatively homogeneous, although modest. Although cognitive improvements are ultimately desired from CRT programmes, these need to translate to functional outcomes so that service users can lead a more valued life, characterised by integration within the community and recovery (Cella *et al*, 2012). It is possible the effects of CRT might be improved through better knowledge of individual responses to treatments. This would allow identification of factors to refine treatment approaches and improve the effectiveness of CRT. Research has begun to look at within-group differences in cognitive change and response to CRT as well as predictors of a positive outcome to the intervention. Participant characteristics have been found to influence the success of therapy. For example, Fiszdon *et al* (2006) divided patients into three groups based on their pattern of premorbid and current deficits, and their cognitive remediation outcomes were examined. Those with 'compromised' intellect (consistently low intellectual functioning) benefited from CRT by achieving substantial increases in test scores, but they had difficulty in generalising these gains to novel neuropsychological tests, unlike those in the 'preserved' and 'deteriorated' intellect groups, who were more successful. Age has also been shown to influence outcome, with younger participants (aged under 40 years) achieving greater benefits in negative symptoms, cognitive flexibility and planning following cognitive remediation when compared with older adults (aged 40 years or more) (Wykes *et al*, 2009). Studies have shown an association between high levels of participant intrinsic motivation and a positive response to CRT (Choi & Medalia, 2005; Medalia & Richardson, 2005). One study found levels of intrinsic motivation to predict vocational outcomes for those with schizophrenia and schizoaffective disorder participating in a 6-month work rehabilitation programme that included CRT (Saperstein *et al*, 2011). The meta-analysis conducted by Wykes *et al* (2011) found those with more symptoms experienced less improvement in cognition following therapy, although they did make some gains, suggesting even those with high levels of psychopathology can benefit.

Metacognitive remediation

Some cognitive remediation programmes with a strategic approach incorporate a number of training principles such as self-instruction and self-monitoring on the basis of evidence from early 'laboratory' studies which showed such techniques to be beneficial in improving cognition and teaching new skills to people with schizophrenia (see Wykes, 2000, for a review). More recently, such training principles have been suggested to target metacognitive skills (Wykes & Reeder, 2005). Metacognition refers to 'thinking about thinking' (Flavell, 1979) and has frequently been divided into two subcomponents: knowledge about cognition and regulation of cognition (Schraw & Dennison, 1994).

Wykes & Reeder (2005) have emphasised the importance of a client transferring skills learnt in CRT to everyday life to produce gains in functioning. They have suggested metacognitive knowledge and effective metacognitive regulation are crucial for this transfer. People need to learn about their own cognitive strengths and weaknesses and understand with which situations they are likely to have difficulties, to know what to do to make some improvements (i.e. to have metacognitive knowledge) and to monitor and regulate their thinking in order to make these changes (i.e. to use metacognitive regulation). Deficits in metacognitive capacity in schizophrenia have been linked to cognitive impairments (Lysaker et al, 2008), particularly in executive functioning, and metacognition has been shown to be a predictor of learning in those with schizophrenia. For example, during one CRT training programme, patients with preserved metacognition were found to improve more in the learning paradigm than those with reduced metacognitive abilities (Tas et al, 2012). Studies have shown a mediator role for metacognition between cognitive deficits and functioning (Koren et al, 2006; Stratta et al, 2009; Lysaker et al, 2010). Studies have also more specifically highlighted the importance of metacognition in bridging the gap between improved cognition and functional gain within CRT (Reeder et al, 2004, 2006; Eack et al, 2011). Metacognition therefore might be the connection between cognition and functional outcome. Many have suggested that deficits in metacognition play a fundamental role in the persistence of psychosocial dysfunction in schizophrenia and that remediation interventions that directly target such skills are needed (Stratta et al, 2009; Gumley, 2011).

Some clinical and research groups have started to target metacognition more specifically by incorporating the development of metacognitive skills into existing cognitive remediation programmes. For example, in Wykes and colleagues' paper-and-pencil and computerised CRT programmes, clients completed 40 individual sessions of cognitive remediation, at least 3 days a week, with a therapist who encouraged a metacognitive and strategic information-processing approach (Wykes et al, 2007). During sessions the therapist discussed with the client which cognitive functions were being used in tasks and which strategies they found helpful in supporting their cognitive difficulties. The use of strategies has an important role in improving metacognition. It allows people to learn about their own cognitive strengths and weaknesses and understand in which situations they are likely to have difficulties and to know what to do to make some improvements. Using strategies also facilitates monitoring and regulation of thinking in order to make these changes. Over the course of therapy, participants learn which strategies are particularly helpful to them. These strategies can subsequently be used not just within the programme, but also in many aspects of the client's everyday life with the development of metacognitive knowledge and regulation (Wykes & Reeder, 2005).

The computerised version itself additionally facilitated metacognition in a number of ways. Participants were asked to estimate how difficult they would find a task and how long they thought it would take to complete. They were then asked to rate how difficult they actually found the task at the end, and to compare their predicted completion time with their actual time. The therapist could further support the development of metacognition by discussing these predictions with the client.

Keefe *et al* (2012) in a feasibility study included 'bridging groups' to their CRT condition. Patients completed 40 sessions of computerised CRT over 12 weeks, supplemented with weekly structured group sessions where participants met to discuss newly acquired cognitive skills and how these could be applied to everyday tasks. This new pilot approach to cognitive remediation was found to be feasible and efficacious. Others have continued to offer cognitive remediation alongside other psychosocial interventions to support the transfer of skills from therapy to everyday functioning. Bowie *et al* (2012) found improvements in functional competence to be greater and more durable in a combined treatment condition of functional adaptation skills training and CRT.

Where do CBTp and CRT overlap?

So far we have described the two cognitive therapies independently and therapies are usually promoted by distinct groups of clinical researchers and practitioners. As has been discussed, the main focus of CBTp is to target the psychological processes associated with the maintenance of emotional distress, whereas CRT targets cognitive deficits. The former is usually associated with a formulation-based approach, whereas the latter mainly uses training methodologies in order to enhance functioning.

There is some evidence that they do in indeed target different processes. Penadés *et al* (2006) randomised individuals to receive either CBTp or CRT and discovered that the outcomes differed. Those receiving CBTp improved on depression and anxiety and those receiving CRT had an overall improvement on neurocognition (mean effect size 0.5), particularly in verbal and non-verbal memory and executive function. The CRT group demonstrated clinically meaningful improvements in social functioning. CBTp also produced a slight improvement in working memory, suggesting overlap as well as distinctive qualities, with gains remaining at 6-month follow-up.

They are both psychological therapies, so of course both rely on engagement with the therapeutic process. Also, both aim to modify specific psychological processes in order to enhance outcome. There have been several recent developments that may represent a common ground between these two approaches. Typically, these new developments have been positioned under the umbrella term of cognitive–behavioural therapy, as the main goal is still to target emotional distress. However, the interventions tend to target specific psychological processes using an approach based on training and practice rather than through gaining insight.

Recent research where CBT and CRT may overlap

Perhaps the most significant development within this area is the metacognitive training (MCT) programme developed by Moritz & Woodward (2007), within which metacognition is defined as 'thinking about thinking'. MCT targets typical cognitive errors and problem-solving biases in schizophrenia. There is evidence that these disturbances may separately or in combination culminate in the formation of beliefs that may become delusions. The main objective of the training is to raise patients' awareness of these cognitive distortions and to prompt them to critically reflect on, complement and alter their current repertoire of problem-solving skills. These processes are the targets of a number of training modules. The training is delivered by a healthcare specialist, working with a group of 3–10 patients with a schizophrenia spectrum disorder. It comprises eight modules with the following targets: *attributional style* (module 1), *a jumping-to-conclusions bias* (modules 2 and 7), *a bias against disconfirmatory evidence* (module 3), *problems in social cognition* (modules 4 and 6), *overconfidence in memory errors* (module 5) and *depressive cognitive patterns* (module 8). Studies have indicated that MCT is associated with improvements in delusional distress as well as cognitive processes such as memory and reasoning biases (Moritz *et al*, 2011).

Another specific area of cognitive functioning that has been the target of a training programme is social cognition (including facial affect recognition, social cue perception, 'theory of mind' and attributional style). This approach is based on research that identifies deficits in social cognitive skills within individuals diagnosed with schizophrenia, and associated this with poor functional outcome (Penn *et al*, 2005). David Penn and colleagues developed the Social Cognition and Interaction Training (SCIT) programme, a group-based intervention delivered weekly over 6 months, with the purpose of improving both social cognition and social functioning among persons with schizophrenia spectrum disorders. SCIT comprises three phases: emotion training, figuring out situations, and integration. The programme has evolved and been used in a number of clinical trials (e.g. Horan *et al*, 2008, 2011). A meta-analysis (Kurtz & Richardson, 2011) suggests that social cognition training programmes have been successful in modifying facial affect recognition and theory of mind, but have not had an impact on social cue perception, attributional style, or levels of psychotic symptoms.

The process of attention has also been the subject of a training programme within a small body of work conducted by Wells and colleagues. Attention training (ATT; Wells, 1990) has been reported within a single case study in which a patient was trained to attend to external stimuli rather than auditory hallucinations, with some encouraging results (Valmaggia *et al*, 2007).

There has also been a focus on reasoning, based on previous research suggesting that people diagnosed with schizophrenia use less information than others when making decisions. Ross *et al* (2011) have developed a brief training package directly aimed at encouraging patients to consider more information before making decisions. There was a significant increase in data-gathering after the training module; however, the potential for longer-term impact on symptoms and distress was not assessed.

The role of bias within the interpretation of ambiguous material is central to the cognitive–behavioural model for anxiety disorders (Mathews & MacLeod, 1994). Recent research has focused on the direct modification of bias through the use of a training paradigm. Cognitive bias modification (CBM) is achieved through repeated exposure to ambiguous scenarios (often via headphones in a laboratory), in which it is argued that the (negative) anxiety bias is activated before the resolution of the ambiguity (MacLeod & Mathews, 2012). A positive resolution means that the predicted (anxious) outcome is not accurate, and repeated exposure to this will result in an update of the bias. While this approach has mainly been developed for use with patients suffering from anxiety only, a recent study suggests that the method may be used with individuals diagnosed with schizophrenia who are also suffering from comorbid anxiety (Steel *et al*, 2010).

A theoretical paper by Brewin (2006) has led to the development of a new treatment for depression, competitive memory training (CoMeT). This intervention focuses on helping patients enhance the recall of meaningful positive memories, especially at times when they may be vulnerable to the experience of highly vivid and salient negative memories. The approach involves repeated practice of positive memory recall in order to strengthen the association between relevant cues and the positive memory. A recent study has used this intervention with individuals suffering from schizophrenia and auditory hallucinations and produced a significant decrease in depression (van der Gaag *et al*, 2012).

The combination of CBT and CRT for schizophrenia

Wykes *et al* (2007) showed that CRT seemed to improve auditory hallucinations and this was predicted by the improvement in cognitive flexibility. This suggests that CRT alone has the potential to alleviate some positive symptoms. In fact, the anecdotes from service users that prompted these analyses were 'I can't fill in this form [on self-reported auditory hallucinations] because I don't hear voices any more ... I have too much to think about now'.

More recently there have been suggestions that combining the approaches of CRT and CBTp may accelerate improvements in symptoms. This is based on the assumption that CRT builds the cognitive skills needed for CBTp. Drake *et al* (2014) carried out a study in patients with first-episode psychosis who were randomised either to CRT or to a social therapy (to control for social contact) and were then provided with CBTp. The hypothesis was that people in the CRT + CBTp group would achieve better symptomatic outcomes. However, this was not the case. What they actually found was similar levels of symptoms at the end of the trial, though these were achieved with far fewer sessions in the CRT + CBTp group. These results suggest cost-effectiveness, as CRT requires a lower level of therapist training than CBTp. The formulation achieved at the end of CBTp was also rated as more sophisticated in the CRT + CBTp group, suggesting that CRT had indeed improved engagement and understanding. This combination therapy seems to offer much for recovery that could be implemented within mental health services relatively easily.

Conclusions

We have described both therapies and their current use around the world. Both have sound theoretical bases and appear to promote recovery. Experts in the field are now able to consider which people are likely to be helped by either or both treatments and can begin to tailor treatments to individuals. There is, for instance, evidence that treatment should be targeted during periods when individuals have all their needs met, for example housing and daily living support. When these are in place, individuals can consider other aspects of their lives. Cognitive therapies (CBTp and CRT) have much to offer people experiencing psychosis. These therapies are continuing to evolve, with the next step being the elaboration of specific treatments that improve social cognition.

The current evidence suggests a cost-effective implementation of cognitive therapies:

- CRT should be provided to everyone who has evidence of cognitive difficulties (and this is the majority of individuals with a diagnosis of schizophrenia)
- CBTp should be provided to those who can concentrate for reasonable periods of time and can therefore engage with the therapist.

References

Addington J, Addington D (1999) Neurocognitive and social functioning in schizophrenia. *Schizophrenia Bulletin*, **25**: 173–82.

American Psychiatric Association (2013) *Diagnostic and Statistical Manual* (5th edn) (DSM-5). American Psychiatric Association Press.

Beck AT (1952) Successful outpatient psychotherapy of a chronic schizophrenic with a delusion based on borrowed guilt. *Journal for the Study of Interpersonal Processes*, **15**: 305–12.

Bell M, Bryson G, Greig T, *et al* (2001) Neurocognitive enhancement therapy with work therapy: effects on neuropsychological test performance. *Archives of General Psychiatry*, **58**: 763–8.

Bowie CR, McGurk SR, Mausbach B, *et al* (2012) Combined cognitive remediation and functional skills training for schizophrenia: effects on cognition, functional competence, and real-world behavior. *American Journal of Psychiatry*, **169**: 710–18.

Brabban A, Tai S, Turkington D (2009) Predictors of outcome in brief cognitive-behavior therapy for schizophrenia. *Schizophrenia Bulletin*, **35**: 859–64.

Brewin CR (2006) Understanding cognitive behaviour therapy: a retrieval competition account. *Behaviour Research and Therapy*, **44**: 765–84.

Cella M, Huddy V, Reeder C, *et al* (2012) Cognitive remediation therapy for schizophrenia. *Minerva Psichiatrica*, **53**: 185–96.

Chadwick P, Birchwood MJ (1994) The omnipotence of voices: a cognitive approach to auditory hallucinations. *British Journal of Psychiatry*, **164**: 190–201.

Chadwick P, Birchwood M (1995) The omnipotence of voices II: the beliefs about voices questionnaire. *British Journal of Psychiatry*, **166**: 773–6.

Choi J, Medalia A (2005) Factors associated with a positive response to cognitive remediation in a community psychiatric sample. *Psychiatric Services*, **56**: 602–4.

Cirillo MA, Seidman LJ (2003) Verbal declarative memory dysfunction in schizophrenia: from clinical assessment to genetics and brain mechanisms. *Neuropsychology Review*, **13**: 44–77.

Clark DM, Salkovskis PM, Hackmann A, *et al* (1999) Brief cognitive therapy for panic disorder. *Journal of Consulting and Clinical Psychology*, **67**: 583–9.

Drake RJ, Day CJ, Picucci R, *et al* (2014) A naturalistic, randomized, controlled trial combining cognitive remediation with cognitive–behavioural therapy after first episode schizophrenia. *Psychological Medicine*, **44**: 1889–99.

Eack SM, Pogue-Geile MF, Greenwald DP, *et al* (2011) Mechanisms of functional improvement in a 2-year trial of cognitive enhancement therapy for early schizophrenia. *Psychological Medicine*, **41**: 1253–61.

Elvevag B, Weinberger DR, Suter JC, *et al* (2000) Continuous performance test and schizophrenia: a test of stimulus–response compatibility, working memory, response readiness, or none of the above? *American Journal of Psychiatry*, **157**: 772–80.

Fiszdon JM, Choi J, Bryson GJ, *et al* (2006) Impact of intellectual status on response to cognitive task training in patients with schizophrenia. *Schizophrenia Research*, **87**: 261–9.

Flavell JH (1979) Meta-cognition and cognitive monitoring: a new area of cognitive-developmental inquiry. *American Psychologist*, **34**: 906–11.

Garety PA, Fowler D, Kuipers E, *et al* (1997) London–East Anglia randomised controlled trial of cognitive–behavioural therapy for psychosis. II: Predictors of outcome. *British Journal of Psychiatry*, **171**: 420–6.

Garety PA, Kuipers E, Fowler D, *et al* (2001) A cognitive model of the positive symptoms of psychosis. *Psychological Medicine*, **31**: 189–95.

Green MF (1996) What are the functional consequences of neurocognitive deficits in schizophrenia. *American Journal of Psychiatry*, **153**: 321–30.

Green MF, Kern RS, Braff DL, *et al* (2000) Neurocognitive deficits and functional outcome in schizophrenia: are we measuring the 'right stuff'? *Schizophrenia Bulletin*, **26**: 119–36.

Green MF, Kern RS, Heaton RK (2004) Longitudinal studies of cognition and functional outcome in schizophrenia: implications for MATRICS. *Schizophrenia Research*, **72**: 41–51.

Gumley A (2011) Metacognition, affect regulation and symptom expression: a transdiagnostic perspective. *Psychiatry Research*, **190**: 72–8.

Haddock G, Lewis SW, Bentall RP, *et al* (2006) Influence of age on outcome of psychological treatments in first-episode psychosis. *British Journal of Psychiatry*, **188**: 250–4.

Horan WP, Kern RS, Green MF, *et al* (2008) Social cognitive skills training for individuals with schizophrenia: emerging evidence. *American Journal of Psychiatric Rehabilitation*, **11**: 205–52.

Horan WP, Kern R, Tripp C, *et al* (2011) Efficacy and specificity of social cognitive skills training for outpatients with psychotic disorders. *Journal of Psychiatric Research*, **45**: 1113–22.

Huddy V, Reeder C, Kontis D, *et al* (2012) The effect of working alliance on adherence and outcome in cognitive remediation therapy. *Journal of Nervous and Mental Disease*, **200**: 614–19.

Keefe RSE, Vinogradov S, Medalia A, *et al* (2012) Feasibility and pilot efficacy results from the multisite cognitive remediation in the schizophrenia trials network (CRSTN) randomized controlled trial. *Journal of Clinical Psychiatry*, **73**: 1016–22.

Kingdon D, Turkington D (2005) *Cognitive Therapy for Schizophrenia*. Guilford Press.

Koren D, Seidman LJ, Goldsmith M, *et al* (2006) Real-world cognitive- and metacognitive-dysfunction in schizophrenia: a new approach for measuring (and remediating) more 'right stuff'. *Schizophrenia Bulletin*, **32**: 310–26.

Kurtz M (2012) Cognitive remediation for schizophrenia: current status, biological correlates and predictors of response. *Expert Review of Neurotherapeutics*, **12**: 813–21.

Kurtz M, Richardson CL (2011) Social cognitive training for schizophrenia: a meta-analytic investigation of controlled research. *Schizophrenia Bulletin*, **38**: 1092–104.

Leeson VC, Sharma P, Harrison M, *et al* (2009) IQ trajectory, cognitive reserve, and clinical outcome following a first episode of psychosis: a 3-year longitudinal study. *Schizophrenia Bulletin*, **37**: 768–77.

Lysaker PH, Warman DM, Dimaggio G, *et al* (2008) Metacognition in schizophrenia. Associations with multiple assessments of executive function. *Journal of Nervous and Mental Disease*, **196**: 384–9.

Lysaker PH, Shea AM, Buck KD, *et al* (2010) Metacognition as a mediator of the effects of impairments in neurocognition on social function in schizophrenia spectrum disorders. *Acta Psychiatrica Scandinavica*, **122**: 405–13.

Maat A, Fett AK, Derks E, *et al* (2012) Social cognition and quality of life in schizophrenia. *Schizophrenia Research*, **137**: 212–18.

MacLeod C, Mathews A (2012) Cognitive bias modification approaches to anxiety. *Annual Review of Clinical Psychology*, **8**: 189–217.

Mathews A, MacLeod C (1994) Cognitive approaches to emotion and emotional disorders. *Annual Review of Psychology*, **45**: 25–50.

McGurk SR, Twamley EW, Sitzer DI, *et al* (2007) A meta-analysis of cognitive remediation in schizophrenia. *American Journal of Psychiatry*, **164**: 1791–802.

McGurk SR, Mueser KT, DeRosa J, *et al* (2009) Work, recovery, and comorbidity in schizophrenia: a randomised controlled trial of cognitive remediation. *Schizophrenia Bulletin*, **35**: 319–35.

Medalia A, Richardson R (2005) What predicts a good response to cognitive remediation interventions? *Schizophrenia Bulletin*, **31**: 942–53.

Moelter ST, Hill SK, Ragland JD, *et al* (2001) Controlled and automatic processing during animal word list generation in schizophrenia. *Neuropsychology*, **15**: 502–9.

Moritz S, Woodward TS (2007) Metacognitive training in schizophrenia: from basic research to knowledge translation and intervention. *Current Opinion in Psychiatry*, **20**: 619–25.

Moritz S, Veckenstedt R, Randjbar S, *et al* (2011) Antipsychotic treatment beyond antipsychotics: metacognitive intervention for schizophrenia patients improves delusional symptoms. *Psychological Medicine*, **41**: 1823–32.

Morris RG, Rushe T, Woodruffe PWR, *et al* (1995) Problem solving in schizophrenia: a specific deficit in planning ability. *Schizophrenia Research*, **14**: 235–46.

Morrison AP (2001) The interpretation of intrusions in psychosis: an integrative cognitive approach to psychotic symptoms. *Behavioural and Cognitive Psychotherapy*, **29**: 257–76.

Morrison AP (ed) (2002) *A Casebook of Cognitive Therapy for Psychosis*. Routledge.

Morrison AP, Barratt S (2010) What are the components of CBT for psychosis? A Delphi study. *Schizophrenia Bulletin,* **36**: 136–42.

Murray RM, O'Callaghan E, Castle DJ, *et al* (1992) A neurodevelopmental approach to the classification of schizophrenia. *Schizophrenia Bulletin,* **18**: 319–32.

Nuechterlein KH, Subotnik KL, Ventura J, *et al* (2012) The puzzle of schizophrenia: tracking the core role of cognitive deficits. *Development and Psychopathology,* **24**: 529–36.

Penadés R, Catalán R, Salamero M, *et al* (2006) Cognitive remediation therapy for outpatients with chronic schizophrenia: a controlled and randomized study. *Schizophrenia Research,* **87**: 323–31.

Penn, D, Roberts D, Munt E, *et al* (2005) A pilot study of social cognition and interaction training (SCIT) for schizophrenia. *Schizophrenia Research,* **80**: 357–9.

Pukrop R, Matuschek E, Ruhrmann S, *et al* (2003) Dimensions of working memory dysfunction in schizophrenia. *Schizophrenia Research,* **62**: 259–68.

Reeder C, Newton E, Frangou S, *et al* (2004) Which executive skills should we target to affect social functioning and symptom change? A study of a cognitive remediation therapy program. *Schizophrenia Bulletin,* **30**: 87–100.

Reeder C, Smedley N, Butt K, *et al* (2006) Cognitive predictors of social functioning improvements following cognitive remediation for schizophrenia. *Schizophrenia Bulletin,* **32** (suppl 1): S123–31.

Rollinson R, Smith B, Steel C, *et al* (2008) Measuring adherence in CBT for psychosis: a psychometric analysis of an adherence scale. *Behavioural and Cognitive Psychotherapy,* **36**: 163–78.

Ross K, Freeman D, Dunn G, *et al* (2011) A randomized experimental investigation of reasoning training for people with delusions. *Schizophrenia Bulletin,* **37**: 324–33.

Saperstein AM, Fiszdon JM, Morris DB (2011) Intrinsic motivation as a predictor of work outcome after vocational rehabilitation in schizophrenia. *Journal of Nervous and Mental Disease,* **199**: 672–7.

Savilla K, Kettler L, Galletly C (2008) Relationships between cognitive deficits, symptoms and quality of life in schizophrenia. *Australian and New Zealand Journal of Psychiatry,* **42**: 496–504.

Schraw G, Dennison RS (1994) Assessing metacognitive awareness. *Contemporary Educational Psychology,* **19**: 460–75.

Scottish Intercollegiate Guidelines Network (2013) *Management of Schizophrenia*. SIGN.

Seidman LJ, Buka SL, Goldstein JM, *et al* (2006) Intellectual decline in schizophrenia: evidence from a prospective birth cohort 28 year follow-up study. *Journal of Clinical and Experimental Neuropsychology,* **28**: 225–42.

Startup M, Jackson M, Pearce E (2002) Assessing therapist adherence to cognitive behaviour therapy for psychosis. *Behavioural and Cognitive Psychotherapy,* **30**: 329–39.

Steel C, Wykes T, Ruddle A, *et al* (2010) Can we harness computerised cognitive bias modification to treat anxiety in schizophrenia? A first step highlighting the role of mental imagery. *Psychiatry Research,* **178**: 451–5.

Steel C, Tarrier N, Stahl D, *et al* (2012) Cognitive behaviour therapy for psychosis: the impact of therapist training and supervision. *Psychotherapy and Psychosomatics,* **81**: 194–5.

Stratta P, Daneluzzo E, Riccardi I, *et al* (2009) Metacognitive ability and social functioning are related in persons with schizophrenic disorder. *Schizophrenia Research,* **108**: 301–2.

Tas C, Brown EC, Esen-Danaci A, *et al* (2012) Intrinsic motivation and metacognition as predictors of learning potential in patients with remitted schizophrenia. *Journal of Psychiatric Research,* **46**: 1086–92.

Valmaggia LR, Bouman TK, Schuurman L (2007) Attention training with auditory hallucinations: a case study. *Cognitive and Behavioral Practice,* **14**: 127–33.

van der Gaag M, van Oosterhout B, Daalman K, *et al* (2012) Initial evaluation of the effects of competitive memory training (COMET) on depression in schizophrenia-spectrum patients with persistent auditory verbal hallucinations: a randomized controlled trial. *British Journal of Clinical Psychology*, **51**: 158–71.

Velligan DI, Bow-Thomas CC, Huntzinger C, *et al* (2000) Randomised controlled trial of the use of compensatory strategies to enhance adaptive functioning in outpatients with schizophrenia. *American Journal of Psychiatry*, **157**: 1317–23.

Wells A (1990) Panic disorder in association with relaxation induced anxiety: an attentional training approach to treatment. *Behavior Therapy*, **21**: 273–80.

Wykes T (2000) Cognitive rehabilitation and remediation in schizophrenia. In *Cognition in Schizophrenia. Impairments, Importance, and Treatment Strategies* (eds T Sharma, P Harvey): 332–51. Oxford University Press.

Wykes T, Reeder C (2005) *Cognitive Remediation Therapy for Schizophrenia*. Routledge.

Wykes T, Reeder C, Landau S, *et al* (2007) Cognitive remediation therapy in schizophrenia. *British Journal of Psychiatry*, **190**: 421–7.

Wykes T, Steel C, Everitt B, *et al* (2008) Cognitive behaviour therapy for schizophrenia: effect sizes, clinical models, and methodological rigor. *Schizophrenia Bulletin*, **10**: 1–15.

Wykes T, Reeder C, Landau S, *et al* (2009) Does age matter? Effects of cognitive rehabilitation across the age span. *Schizophrenia Research*, **113**: 252–8.

Wykes T, Huddy V, Cellard C, *et al* (2011) A meta-analysis of cognitive remediation for schizophrenia: methodology and effect sizes. *American Journal of Psychiatry*, **168**: 472–85.

Zubin J, Spring B (1977) Vulnerability – a new view of schizophrenia. *Journal of Abnormal Psychology*, **86**: 103–26.

CHAPTER 10

Family interventions

Gráinne Fadden

Introduction

It remains one of the greatest anomalies in mental healthcare that an intervention with a robust evidence base, family intervention, has not been widely adopted in practice. The evidence for the effectiveness of family intervention for serious mental health problems has been known for over 30 years, and this approach has been consistently and repeatedly recommended in reviews, meta-analyses and guidelines (Pitschel-Walz *et al*, 2001; Pfammatter *et al*, 2006; National Institute for Health and Clinical Excellence, 2009; Dixon *et al*, 2010; Pharoah *et al*, 2010). Its effectiveness in terms of reductions in relapse and hospitalisation rates, reductions of stress for family members and reduced costs of care is highlighted in all of these.

There is now a greater recognition of the key role played by family and social networks in the recovery of those who experience mental health difficulties. However, the fact that the family is still commonly viewed as peripheral rather than core suggests that the central shift in thinking required to ensure that the importance of family, community networks, and cultural and kinship relationships is recognised has not yet taken place. In the first edition of this book, Fadden (2006a) identified factors contributing to the lack of adoption of family-based care such as lack of staff training and a perception of threat if a more collaborative model of care is adopted. As implementation issues persist, it really is time to take stock and think about what can be done to radicalise thinking, as the time lag for development to adoption of family interventions has gone well beyond the average for adopting new practices. There are various estimates of how long it takes to embed healthcare programmes into practice, ranging from 1 year (Bradley *et al*, 2004) to 17 years (Chaffin & Friedrich, 2004). Ensuring that service provision to families is common practice appears to be extremely complex in that it is now over 30 years since the evidence became available.

Levels of family work

One of the difficulties that clinicians and those responsible for commissioning, funding and managing services struggle with is agreeing on the range of services to make available to families so that their needs can be met in a comprehensive manner. Confusion exists about a number of issues: How is family work defined? How much family work should be offered in order to achieve maximum results? What benefits do different types of family work offer? What should be offered to families at different points in time? The terminology in the literature can be confusing for those unfamiliar with the complexity of different modes of family work. This results in questions about, for example, whether offering educational groups is enough, or when individual family sessions should be offered. This section 'translates' the research findings to provide clarity for those who are responsible for delivering services, both at a clinical and at a managerial level.

In 1982, Beels & McFarlane wrote of Utopian-style services where a range of family interventions of proven effectiveness would be available to those with severe mental health problems – brief crisis-oriented intervention for those recently diagnosed with psychosis, an individual family psychoeducational approach where this was indicated, and multi-family groups for those who would benefit from interaction with others in a similar situation. The idea of families being able to access what they need at different points in time is attractive but must be mapped against service constraints in terms of both fiscal limitations and, often more importantly, the skill level of clinicians delivering services to families.

It may be helpful to think of different levels of family work, although it is important not to suppose that all families have to progress through a series of levels of help or, equally, that families go through different levels in a linear order. Fig. 10.1 summarises the three main levels of support that families benefit from and each is described below in more detail.

Level 1. Family-sensitive practice

In the past, many mental health workers felt that their responsibility was to the person with the mental health difficulty, and the predominance of intrapsychic therapeutic models reinforced this view. In the Meriden Programme (a National Health Service body promoting family-sensitive mental health services) we come across numerous examples of families reporting that they are not recognised in services, and this is evidenced in testimonials from families on the website (http://www. meridenfamilyprogramme.com). One woman described her experiences of visiting her daughter on an in-patient ward: 'I thought – I must be a ghost. It was as if I was invisible. Nobody seemed to see me. Nobody spoke to me or asked me how I was.'

In order to progress from individually focused mental health services, those who have been attempting to implement services for families talk of family-focused or family-friendly services as a fundamental first step (Farhall *et al*, 1998; Fadden & Birchwood, 2002; Stanbridge & Burbach, 2007; Cohen *et al*, 2008). Family-sensitive practice refers to a culture that

---

Level 1. Family-sensitive, family-friendly or family-focused practice
Refers to the ethos of the service and the way in which families are treated
Helpful in facilitating engagement of families in therapeutic interventions

---

Level 2. Family education
Brief educational sessions usually delivered in group sessions provided by
statutory or voluntary agencies or self-help groups
Person with mental health problem is usually not involved
Reduces stress in families but has no impact on relapse

Level 3. Formal family intervention
Evidence-based approaches incorporating information-sharing, relapse prevention
strategies, communication and problem-solving skills training
Person with mental health problem must be involved to ensure effectiveness; delivered
either to individual families or groups of families (multi-family groups)
Results in reductions in relapse and hospitalisation

Fig. 10.1 Levels of family intervention

considers all family members in terms of the impact of mental health problems and involves them collaboratively in treatment.

This idea of services that are understanding and respectful of families and their experiences and that are proactive and non-judgemental in their approach is the first stage described in the heuristic proposed by Cohen *et al* (2008) in helping to determine what services families should receive. Some have suggested that brief training to large numbers of staff aimed at increasing awareness of the needs of carers and families may result in the less complex needs of a large number of families being met (Stanbridge & Burbach, 2007). However, evaluation of this type of brief training suggests that it does not result in attitudinal or behavioural change in relation to families, and that more extensive training is required for this to be achieved (Farhall *et al*, 1998). It would appear that family-sensitive attitudes and practices are a necessary but not sufficient condition for the development of effective family services.

Family-sensitive practice includes the provision of some initial information to families, and signposting them to other sources of support such as local carer support services. It is also likely that if services are family friendly from the outset, engagement of families in more detailed interventions will be more successful. Absence of this family-friendly culture frequently leads to complaints to services and poor relationships between clinicians and families.

Level 2. Family education and support

In the USA, brief educational groups with family members are referred to as 'family education', whereas in Europe the terms 'carer education and support' or 'family psychoeducational groups' are often used. Education and support groups provide information to family members and this is delivered by health professionals and/or trained family members. Of course, clinicians will frequently provide some information to some family members on an individual basis too. Table 10.1 describes a selection of level 2 services developed through voluntary or self-help organisations. The person with the mental health problem generally does not attend these groups, and what sometimes causes confusion in terminology is that some educational groups for those with mental health difficulties invite in relatives to some sessions (Rummel-Kluge & Kissling, 2008). The variations in format and terminology contribute to the lack of clarity and make it difficult for clinicians and managers to know what they should be offering.

Table 10.1 Examples of level 2 family intervention services

Country	Name of course	No. of sessions	Frequency	Trainers
Australia	Well Ways	8 (3 hours)	Weekly; 3-month follow-up for 1 year	Trained family members (2 together)
Canada	Strengthening Families Together	10 (2 hours)	Weekly	Trained family members (2 together)
Europe	Prospect (Eufami)	10 (2 hours)	Weekly	Trained family members
UK	Carers' Education and Support Programme	11 (3 hours)	Weekly	Professionals and trained family members
USA	Family to Family	12 (2 hours)	Weekly	Trained family members
WFSAD	Reason to Hope	8 (2.5 hours)	Variable 3-day workshop or weekly	Two trained family members or one trained family member and a trained professional

WFSAD, developed by the World Fellowship for Schizophrenia and Allied Disorders and applied in different countries.

Family education and support groups usually have the following features:

- They provide a relaxed and safe environment for family members
- The service user usually does not attend
- Families share experiences with people who are in a similar situation
- Mutual respect, understanding and empathy are encouraged
- Emotions, thoughts and concerns are shared
- Family members gain ideas and strategies from others
- Those attending are free to talk and to be listened to
- Confidentiality is respected
- There is freedom to express views about inadequate local services
- Carers value them and feel supported, and drop-out rates are low
- Carer stress and feelings of stigma and isolation are reduced
- Carers feel more positive towards services where the support groups are facilitated through the services
- They work best if group members are similar in terms of type of problem or age group (e.g. early psychosis groups; bipolar disorder groups)

Outcomes of these groups include increased knowledge, increased feelings of competence, and reductions in worry and depression (Johnson, 2007). This is extremely important and valuable, as surveys of carer stress have repeatedly shown the negative impact of caring on the health of family members of those with mental health problems. The Royal College of General Practitioners (2013) has recommended routine screening of carers for depression, as family members generally present to general practitioners with conditions related to the stress of caring.

In one of the few randomised controlled trials of family education groups, participants showed significantly greater improvements in problem-focused coping, increased acceptance of the family member's illness, reduced distress and improved problem-solving, but no reduction in subjective burden or in relapse rates of the person with the disorder (Dixon et al, 2011). While groups such as this have many benefits, the main limitation is the absence of benefit for the person with the disorder (Abramowitz & Coursey, 1989; Glynn et al, 1993; Johnson, 2007; Dixon et al, 2011). Another limitation of any kind of group intervention is that a high proportion of people do not wish to attend groups and have a preference for individual family support. Also, there may also be insufficient numbers in a geographical area at a given time to make a group viable.

In summary, these groups can be a valuable part of services to families and can help to identify those who could benefit from more detailed help, but they are not sufficient in themselves. A simple way of remembering the impact of different approaches is that input to relatives benefits relatives, but if you want to support the recovery of service users, they must be involved in the family intervention.

Level 3. Formal family interventions

In the 1980s a number of research studies were published describing the outcomes of randomised controlled trials that clearly demonstrated the effectiveness of psychoeducational family interventions in terms of reductions in relapse rates and hospitalisations (Falloon *et al*, 1982; Leff *et al*, 1982; Tarrier *et al*, 1988). These used similar approaches, emphasising factors such as the provision of information to families, relapse prevention, encouraging effective communication among family members and helping families to develop practical ways of problem-solving and dealing with difficulties they faced. The efficacy of this type of approach has been confirmed by numerous studies since these early trials, and positive outcomes have been confirmed in meta-analyses (Pfammatter *et al*, 2006; Pharoah *et al*, 2010). Reviews of the research conclude that psycho-educational family interventions are essential to schizophrenia treatment (Pitschel-Walz *et al*, 2001), should be available to the majority of those suffering from schizophrenia (Bustillo *et al*, 2001) and should be offered to people with schizophrenia who are in contact with carers (Pilling *et al*, 2002).

The most common mode of delivery of family intervention is individual family work, although in some parts of the USA and Scandinavia multi-family groups are common. This involves bringing together groups of families (with the service user). Multi-family groups have been shown to be effective (McFarlane, 2002), particularly for those with positive symptoms.

While the earlier studies were carried out with people with long-term disorders, it is now clear that these approaches are also effective in early psychosis. In a systematic review of cognitive–behavioural therapy and family work in psychosis, Bird *et al* (2010) concluded that it was the family intervention that resulted in reduced relapse rates. What is also clear is that service users value the involvement of their families in their care, both in the early stages of psychosis (Lester *et al*, 2011) and in situations where the difficulty has been present for longer (Cohen *et al*, 2013). In the latter study, the first systematic report on preferences expressed by service users for involvement of their families, 78% wanted family members to be involved in their care. The evidence from these studies certainly challenges the views frequently heard in services that clients are reluctant to engage in family approaches and are concerned about confidentiality issues.

It is not clear whether multi-family groups are effective in early psychosis. The study by Rossberg *et al* (2010) demonstrated that while there were fewer dropouts in the group attending multi-family groups, these participants showed less improvement than those in the control group and had significantly longer duration of psychotic symptoms during the follow-up period.

Principles and content of family work

In the first edition of this book, Fadden (2006a) described the core principles of effective family work. They include the following:

- a genuinely positive attitude towards families and an absence of labelling
- proactive engagement of families
- acknowledgement of the skill and expertise of the family
- understanding the intention behind the actions taken by families rather than superficially judging their actions
- recognition that every family has its own culture.

In spite of all that has been written about what the content of family work should be, it is interesting that there still appears to be a lack of knowledge of this among practising clinicians and managers. This is evidenced by the number of enquiries we get through the Meriden Family Programme for clarification of what should be offered to families. Services struggling to implement family work also talk about offering 'informal family work' or 'low-intensity family work', although there is no evidence of the effectiveness of this or clarity about what it consists of. There should no longer be any confusion about the content of evidence-based family intervention following the publication of the detailed family work competencies, covering psychosis and bipolar disorder (Roth & Pilling, 2013). There have also been books published that contain detailed clinical descriptions of family work in different contexts, including working in in-patient settings, with siblings, in early psychosis settings and with different cultural groups (e.g. Lobban & Barrowclough, 2009; French *et al*, 2010).

Box 10.1 Content of psychoeducational family interventions

- Establishment of a positive, respectful, collaborative working relationship between family and clinician
- Agreement that the service user and key family members will meet together with the clinician
- Information-sharing, and an agreement about issues relating to confidentiality
- Time and space for discussion of emotional issues and personal reactions to the mental health problem and its management
- Support for family members in the achievement of personal goals
- Focus on the management of practical, day-to-day issues
- Enhancement of family problem-solving skills
- Agreement on relapse prevention strategies and developing 'Staying Well' plans
- Development of effective communication patterns
- Agreement on the ongoing nature of the relationship between family and mental health services

---

Case example 10.1 Level 3 family intervention

Tony, now 42, has experienced episodes of bipolar disorder since his late teens. Between episodes, he functions well, and is in stable employment. His wife, Alison, finds the situation stressful, especially managing their two teenage children. Fourteen-year-old Louise has become increasingly quiet, not wanting to meet friends, and 16-year-old Tom is argumentative, frequently shouting at his parents. Things came to a head when he didn't return home one night, and his parents were frantic with worry. He returned the next day saying he had stayed with a friend and didn't know what all the fuss was about.

Tony's care coordinator felt that family work would be helpful and everyone agreed to take part. Even at the initial engagement session the family were surprised about how much they learned about how others in the family were feeling. Individual interviews revealed that Tony felt very guilty about his episodes of being unwell and tried to compensate by not setting limits on the children's behaviour. Alison felt she was becoming depressed herself and found it a struggle to keep all sides going. Tom felt his dad never wanted to spend time with him. Louise complained that her mother was always tired and expected her to do too much around the house. Each set an individual goal: Alison wanted some quiet time for herself each week, Tony wanted to keep his work under control and to limit the hours he worked, Tom wanted to spend time with his dad doing something like going to a football match and Louise wanted to go shopping with her mum.

The information-sharing sessions allowed Tony to explain what it was like to experience episodes of depression and also what it was like to feel 'high'. A 'Staying Well' plan was developed where all of the family were clear about early signs of relapse, with Tony making it clear that he didn't want to be over-monitored, which he felt Alison had done previously. The communication skills aspect of the family work was the part that the family found most beneficial, as they felt they were able to express what they had been feeling and what issues were between them. This led to them being able to resolve some long-standing issues such as Tony's guilt that he had gambled quite a bit of money during a hypomanic episode, which had led to both he and Alison working longer hours and spending less time with the children. Although regular meetings have finished, the family are aware that they can meet up with the care coordinator, who has offered them family work if things become difficult again.

These publications contain case examples with a focus on recovery. The process of family work is described in detail over time, which is helpful for clinicians keen to get a sense of what these approaches are like in practice.

A summary of the core content of psychoeducational family interventions is given in Box 10.1 and see Case example 10.1. The essential elements that were described when these approaches were developed remain central. These include an emphasis on relapse prevention strategies, communication skills and strategies to deal with current difficulties. As this way of working with families has developed over time, there has been a shift in relation to information-sharing. When some of these family approaches were developed, the focus was on professionals providing information to families, suggesting a one-way exchange, or that professionals had more expertise than the family. There is now a greater recognition of the knowledge and skills of service users and family members in relation to their own recovery, with professionals and the family working together to reach a shared understanding.

There is also greater emphasis on the need for time to process all of the emotional reactions of different family members to their experiences, including their feelings towards services about the availability or, more commonly, the lack of availability of different treatment approaches and the contact that service users and family members have with services. There is now recognition that some of these experiences can be as traumatic as the actual experience of mental health difficulties. For example, many relatives describe the trauma of seeing a son, daughter, husband or wife taken away in handcuffs, and admitted to hospital under a section of the Mental Health Act. Others talk of the stress of attending ward rounds and having to discuss family matters in front of a large group of professionals, many of whom have not even been introduced to them.

In the past, services to families were often disjointed. It is now recognised that all elements of the service need to work together if the needs of the family and the service user are to be met. There is little point in a relapse prevention plan being agreed with the family if all those in the relevant part of the service, including out-of-hours services, are not clear about their responsibilities in relation to how they should respond to crises.

Adapting family approaches for those with varied needs

Much of the literature on family work refers generically to families. There are a number of areas where the needs of families are not being met in a comprehensive manner, or where there are special considerations.

The needs of children and siblings

Many children support parents with ongoing mental health problems, but are less likely than adults to receive support in their own right. There is often a lack of clarity in services as to where the responsibility lies for addressing their needs. Staff in adult services frequently feel ill-equipped to provide services to children, and child and adolescent services will not see these children because they are not perceived as having problems that would warrant a referral to their services.

The result is that children in these roles, who often take on substantial responsibilities that are not age appropriate, such as monitoring of a parent's medication, do not receive help and support. Great sensitivity is required in adapting family approaches when there are young children in the family, and where issues are complex. For example, it can be difficult for a child to acknowledge recognising early-warning signs of relapse if this may result in a parent being hospitalised, especially if the child may then have to go into care. There are issues where parents are separated, and where staff do not keep one parent informed of what is happening if the other parent is admitted to hospital, because of concerns about breaches of confidentiality.

There are a number of publications on this topic that readers will find helpful. *Patients as Parents*, first published by the Royal College of Psychiatrists in 2002, has been revised (Royal College of Psychiatrists, 2011) and is helpful in prompting clinicians to reflect on their awareness of the needs of children whose parents are receiving services. Falkov (2013) has produced a detailed handbook that builds on previous work and provides a detailed guide on how to help children in these situations. It includes an interactive CD–ROM and is an excellent resource. The 'Think Family' UK government initiative (Social Care Institute for Excellence, 2011) highlights the need for all services to adopt whole-family approaches, and its website has a range of useful resources.

There is also a growing awareness of the needs of siblings with psychosis, some of which is driven by the fact that in early-psychosis services many service users have younger brothers and sisters. There is now an awareness of their needs and what helps, and many resources have been developed specifically for siblings, with interventions specifically tailored to their needs (Smith *et al*, 2009, 2010; Sin *et al*, 2012, 2013).

Families in forensic settings

Families of those in forensic rehabilitation services also have special needs, and services are as yet underdeveloped (MacInnes, 2000), with very little family intervention being offered (Geelan & Nickford, 1999). This is in spite of the fact that those in forensic settings have regular contact with their families. Absalom *et al* (2010) reported that up to 72% of people in forensic units have at least monthly contact with family members. In addition to the difficulties experienced by those in mainstream mental health services, they often have different stresses, such as living far away from the forensic unit, the double stigma of mental health issues and the crime that was committed and the fact that frequently the crime has been committed within the family. They can be exposed to violence and often receive less support from family, friends and professionals.

Family work in these circumstances requires effort and imagination in overcoming the many obstacles, such as restrictions on leave away from the unit and lack of family-friendly facilities. This is emotionally demanding work and staff need to be well trained, have appropriate supervisory structures in place and be given the opportunity to co-work. While as yet there is an absence of trials of implementing family work in forensic settings, there are reports of behavioural family therapy in particular being implemented (Peddie, 2009; Atchinson *et al*, 2010) and these have indicated that it may be possible to transfer the efficacy of family interventions to those with mental health problems in forensic settings (Richards *et al*, 2009).

Substance misuse

Supporting families where the service user has coexisting substance misuse is challenging, as there is often an increased range, severity and complexity of symptoms. Families can become critical of service users if, for example, they are unwilling to change or give up their cannabis or other drug use. Family approaches consisting of psychoeducation, goal-setting and the development of communication and problem-solving skills can reduce the stress in families (Gottlieb *et al*, 2012). It is clear that working with families with these dual difficulties requires flexibility and skill in order to deal with the complex interactions in the family (Barrowclough, 2003; Lowens *et al*, 2009). Family motivational interviewing, which combines aspects of motivational interviewing, psychoeducation and family interventions, has also shown promising results (Smeerdijk *et al*, 2009).

Families from diverse cultures

The issue of culture has already been mentioned and the needs of families from Black and minority ethnic groups requires special attention. Stigma and the effects of racism impact on family members as well as service users, with many families describing the experience of stigma by association. Awareness of different cultural models is essential and any interventions need to be culturally sensitive (Rosenfarb *et al*, 2006). For example, the concept of 'carer' is not meaningful in some cultures and needs to be replaced with an appreciation of the role of kinship networks and the obligations of members of the extended family. Literal interpretation of concepts developed for research purposes, such as the description of family members as being 'over-involved' from the 'expressed emotion' literature, are unhelpful in general, but particularly so in diverse cultural groups. In many communities, close involvement of the extended family is the norm when one individual is experiencing difficulties and anything other than this would be considered unacceptable.

Accessible translation and interpretation services are essential to work with families from diverse cultures, as are the use of a variety of media – video- and audiotapes, local radio – and working through community groups. Clearly, family work in this area also has to take account of spiritual and cultural beliefs about causation and recovery (Onwumere *et al*, 2009).

Implementation of family work

The lack of widespread availability of family work in routine services in spite of the strong evidence base was identified in the 1990s (Fadden, 1997) and remains the biggest challenge in this area (Kuipers, 2011). The ethos and culture of adult mental health services have for the most part been focused narrowly on meeting the needs of individuals. It is reflected in all aspects of the system, with paperwork and recording methods frequently not reflecting the needs of families. For example, there is often nowhere to record family work, or to indicate whether or not the service user has children, or to note whether the family has been offered any services. Lack of training and confidence of staff are also major obstacles (Brooker *et al*, 2003; Fadden, 2006*b*).

There has been for some time a clear recognition that the effective implementation of family work requires a systems approach, where the issue is addressed at an organisational level, with close involvement of management and those charged with operationalising services (Smith & Velleman, 2002; Fadden *et al*, 2004; Kelly & Newstead, 2004). In the absence of this focus on organisational issues, it is unlikely that the culture will change, or that those trained will be able to put their newly acquired skills into practice (Fadden & Heelis, 2011).

There is now an extensive literature on what is effective in terms of supporting the implementation of family work (Fadden, 2009; Fadden *et al*, 2010; Fadden & Heelis, 2011; Burbach, 2012):

- having a clear strategy and implementation plan
- training of staff and the development of ongoing supervision structures
- additional support for those newly trained in family work, to build confidence
- appointing product champions
- clarity about the role of management at all levels
- the involvement of family members in a range of roles in services
- ensuring that there is a 'critical mass' of people trained.

For those wanting an overview of strategies at all levels – from policy-makers through management to clinicians and 'carer consultants' – the book produced by the World Fellowship for Schizophrenia and Allied Disorders is a good starting point (Froggatt *et al*, 2007: pp. 10–21).

Policy – an effective driver

The rights of family members and those in caring roles have been recognised in UK government policy at least since 1995 (Department of Health, 1995, 2000). Legislation has emphasised the needs of those who provide regular and substantial care, and has helped local authorities to provide services to carers. One of the most significant factors supporting the rights of carers was the publication of the National Service Framework for Mental Health (Department of Health, 1999), in which standard 6 refers to the right of carers to have their own assessment and care plan. The associated policy implementation guide (Department of Health, 2002) offers guidance on how mental health carer support services can be developed and sustained.

The guidelines for schizophrenia (2009) and for bipolar disorder (2006) from the National Institute for Health and Clinical Excellence both recommend the availability of family interventions in primary and secondary care. The 'Think Family' initiative has already been referred to (Social Care Institute for Excellence, 2011) and the latest 'Triangle of Care' programme (Worthington *et al*, 2013) for developing collaborative relationships with families in in-patient settings is beginning to have an impact on the response to families in crisis.

Policy is now forcing a change in terms of the attention paid to the needs of families, although there is often insufficient attention paid to the implementation of policy and guidelines. Evaluations of the implementation of the guidelines produced by the National Institute for Health and Clinical Excellence have demonstrated that their implementation in clinical practice is poor (Berry & Haddock, 2008; Prytys *et al*, 2011; Lewis *et al*, 2012).

Families and recovery

When families are mentioned in the context of recovery it is generally in terms of how family and friends can support the recovery of the service user (Topor *et al*, 2006). Machin & Repper (2013) identify four main areas where families could learn skills to support someone's recovery – recovery planning, building on strengths, developing helpful relationships, and handing back control. In order to fulfil these roles, they suggest that services should offer a range of supports to families, including the following:

- identifying carers
- tackling stigma and discrimination
- understanding the impact of caring
- delivering family interventions
- developing carer peer support
- offering education, not therapy

Taking this a step further, there is now a growing recognition that the concept of recovery is also important for families in their own right. They can be traumatised by coping with odd behaviour, by some of their contacts with services, or by seeing loved ones hospitalised against their will or taken away by police. Many are worn down by years of caring. The Scottish Recovery Movement (Bradstreet & McBrierty, 2012) has been active in drawing attention to the recovery needs of family members and in collaboration with the Sussex Partnership Trust has recently published the first book of recovery narratives for carers, which is an excellent resource for understanding the experiences of family members (Chandler *et al*, 2013).

Fadden & Heelis (further details available from the author) conducted a qualitative study of family members' understanding of the concept of recovery and its applicability to their circumstances. Twelve participants caring for a relative with a serious mental health problem, primarily schizophrenia or bipolar disorder, for an average of 17.6 years, were interviewed. Interestingly, the family members generally did not see the concept of recovery as relating to them, and some struggled with the idea of 'recovering from' a loved one or their actions. They preferred concepts such as regaining control, accepting, coping and moving on with their own lives. All but one mentioned that a particular turning point, such as a health scare, or realising that others in the family were being neglected, prompted them to think about their own needs. They identified a range of practical and psychological strategies that helped their own recovery, in addition to talking, gaining support and the service user becoming independent. Interestingly, the top two factors described as hindering their recovery were health services and professionals, often in terms of poor communication and not valuing or respecting their expertise as relatives, as well as confidentiality issues impeding their access to services.

This is a developing field that deserves further attention, and it is important for anyone involved in rehabilitation and recovery services to keep abreast of developments. The idea of self-help for carers is also being considered and an extensive manual addressing carers' own needs and their own recovery is now available (Fadden *et al*, 2012).

Conclusions

It is estimated that carers save the UK economy £119 billion each year in care costs, which is equivalent to £18 473 per year per carer (Royal College of General Practitioners, 2013). Studies of caring continue to show that the impact on those in caring roles is far-reaching and significant (Chan, 2011). Evidence-based interventions are not widely available and, in spite of guidance in this area, concerns about confidentiality frequently result in the family not getting help (Slade *et al*, 2007). There are barriers to the implementation of many healthcare interventions (Laws & D'Ambrosio, 2007; Barnett *et al*, 2011) but the area of family work is particularly difficult. It is time to develop a new relationship with families in mental health services. An interesting idea is that proposed by Rowe (2012), who suggests the development of a covenant outlining the mutual obligations between mental health services and families, as well as the obligation they both have towards the service user. Families would welcome this – the question is whether health services are ready to change.

References

Abramowitz IA, Coursey RD (1989) Impact of an educational support group on family participants who take care of their schizophrenic relatives. *Journal of Consulting and Clinical Psychology*, **57**: 232–6.

Absalom V, McGovern J, Gooding P, *et al* (2010) An assessment of patient need for family intervention in forensic services and staff skill in implementing family interventions. *Journal of Forensic Psychiatry and Psychology*, **21**: 350.

Atchinson M, Ginty M, Close J (2009) The Tuesday group: adapting family work within an inpatient child and adolescent mental health service (CAMHS) forensic service. *Meriden Family Programme Newsletter*, **3** (9): 12–14. Available at http://www.meridenfamilyprogramme.com (accessed December 2014).

Barnett J, Vasileiou K, Djemil F, *et al* (2011) Understanding innovators' experiences of barriers and facilitators in implementation and diffusion of healthcare service innovations: a qualitative study. *BMC Health Service Research*, **11**: 342.

Barrowclough C (2003) Family intervention for substance use in psychosis. In *Substance Misuse in Psychosis: A Handbook to Approaches to Treatment and Service Delivery* (eds H Graham, KT Mueser, M Birchwood, *et al*): 227–43. Wiley.

Beels C, McFarlane WR (1982) Family treatments of schizophrenia: background and state of the art. *Hospital and Community Psychiatry*, **33**: 541–50.

Berry K, Haddock G (2008) The implementation of the NICE guidelines for schizophrenia: barriers to the implementation of psychological interventions and recommendations for the future. *Psychology and Psychotherapy: Theory, Research and Practice*, **81**: 419–36.

Bird V, Premkumar P, Kendall T, *et al* (2010) Early intervention services, cognitive–behavioural therapy and family intervention in early psychosis: systematic review. *British Journal of Psychiatry*, **197**: 350–6.

Bradley E, Webster T, Baker D, *et al* (2004) Translating research into practice: speeding the adoption of innovative health care programs. *Commonwealth Fund, Issue Brief*, 1–11.

Bradstreet S, McBrierty R (2012) Recovery in Scotland: beyond service development. *International Review of Psychiatry*, **24** (1), 64–9.

Brooker C, Saul C, Robinson J, *et al* (2003) Is training in psychosocial interventions worthwhile? Report of a psychosocial intervention trainee follow-up study. *International Journal of Nursing Studies*, **40**: 731–47.

Burbach FR (2012) Family interventions: fundamental considerations when developing routine and formal family intervention services. In *Psychosis: Causes, Diagnosis and Treatment* (ed. X Anastassion-Hadjicharalambous): 207–28. Nova Science Publishers.

Bustillo JR, Lauriello J, Horan WP, *et al* (2001) The psychological treatment of schizophrenia: an update. *American Journal of Psychiatry*, **158**: 163–75.

Chaffin M, Friedrich B (2004) Evidence-based treatments in child abuse and neglect. *Children and Youth Services Review*, **26**: 1097–113.

Chan SW (2011) Global perspective of burden of family caregivers for persons with schizophrenia. *Archives of Psychiatric Nursing*, **25**: 339–49.

Chandler C, Bradstreet S, Hayward M (2013) *Voicing Caregiver Experiences: Wellbeing and Recovery Narratives for Caregivers*. Fairhall & Bryant.

Cohen AN, Glynn SM, Murray-Swank AB, *et al* (2008) The family forum: directions for the implementation of family psychoeducation for severe mental illness. *Psychiatric Services*, **59**: 40–8.

Cohen AN, Drapalski AL, Glynn SM, *et al* (2013) Preferences for family involvement in care among consumers with serious mental illness. *Psychiatric Services*, **64**: 257–63.

Department of Health (1995) *Carers (Recognition and Services) Act: Policy Guidance*. Department of Health.

Department of Health (1999) *National Service Framework for Mental Health*. Department of Health.

Department of Health (2000) *Carers and Disabled Children Act: Policy Guidance*. Department of Health.

Department of Health (2002) *Developing Services for Carers and Families of People with Mental Illness*. Department of Health.

Dixon LB, Dickerson F, Bellack AS, *et al* (2010) The 2009 Schizophrenia PORT psychosocial treatment recommendations and summary statements. *Schizophrenia Bulletin*, **36**: 48–70.

Dixon LB, Lucksted A, Medoff DR, *et al* (2011) Outcomes of a randomized study of a peer-taught family-to-family education program for mental illness. *Psychiatric Services*, **62**: 591–7.

Fadden G (1997) Implementation of family interventions in routine clinical practice: a major cause for concern. *Journal of Mental Health*, **6**: 599–612.

Fadden G (2006a) Family interventions. In *Enabling Recovery: The Principles and Practice of Rehabilitation Psychiatry* (eds G Roberts, S Davenport, F Holloway, *et al*): 158–69. Gaskell.

Fadden G (2006*b*) Training and disseminating family interventions for schizophrenia: developing family intervention skills with multi-disciplinary groups. *Journal of Family Therapy*, **28**: 23–38.

Fadden G (2009) Overcoming barriers to staff offering interventions in the NHS. In *A Casebook of Family Interventions for Psychosis* (eds F Lobban, C Barrowclough): 309–35. Wiley.

Fadden G, Birchwood M (2002) British models for expanding family psychoeducation in routine practice. In *Family Interventions in Mental Illness: International Perspectives* (eds HP Lefley, DL Johnson): 25–41. Praeger.

Fadden G, Heelis R (2011) The Meriden West Midlands Family Programme: lessons learned over ten years. *Journal of Mental Health*, **20**: 79–88.

Fadden G, Birchwood M, Jackson C, *et al* (2004) Psychological therapies: implementation in early intervention services. In *Psychological Interventions in Early Psychosis: A Practical Treatment Handbook* (eds P McGorry, J Gleeson): 261–79. Wiley.

Fadden G, Heelis B, Bisnauth R (2010) Training mental health care professionals in behavioural family therapy: an audit of trainers' experiences in the West Midlands. *Journal of Mental Health, Training, Education and Practice*, **5** (2): 27–35.

Fadden G, James C, Pinfold V (2012) *Caring for Yourself – Self-help for Families and Friends Supporting People with Mental Health Problems*. Rethink Mental Illness and Meriden Family Programme. At http://www.meridenfamilyprogramme.com (accessed December 2014).

Falkov A (2013) *The Family Model Handbook: An Integrated Approach to Supporting Mentally Ill Parents and Their Children*. Pavilion Publishing and Media.

Falloon IRH, Boyd JL, McGill CW, *et al* (1982) Family management in the prevention of exacerbations of schizophrenia: a controlled study. *New England Journal of Medicine*, **306**: 1437–40.

Farhall J, Webster B, Hocking B, *et al* (1998) Training to enhance partnerships between mental health professionals and family caregivers: a comparative study. *Psychiatric Services*, **49**: 1488–90.

French P, Smith J, Shiers D, *et al* (eds) (2010) *Promoting Recovery in Early Psychosis: A Practice Manual*. Wiley Blackwell.

Froggatt D, Fadden G, Johnson DL, *et al* (eds) (2007) *Families as Partners in Care: A Guidebook for Implementing Family Work*. World Fellowship for Schizophrenia and Allied Disorders.

Geelan S, Nickford C (1999) A survey of the use of family therapy in medium secure units in England and Wales. *Journal of Forensic Psychiatry*, **10**: 317–24.

Glynn SM, Pugh R, Rose G (1993) Benefits of attendance at a state hospital family education workshop. *Psychosocial Rehabilitation Journal*, **16**: 95–101.

Gottlieb JD, Mueser KT, Glynn SM (2012) Family therapy for schizophrenia: co-occurring psychotic and substance use disorders. *Journal of Clinical Psychology: In Session*, **68**: 490–501.

Johnson DL (2007) Models of family intervention. In *Families as Partners in Care: A Guidebook for Implementing Family Work* (eds D Froggatt, G Fadden, DL Johnson, *et al*): 10–21. World Fellowship for Schizophrenia and Allied Disorders.

Kelly M, Newstead L (2004) Family intervention in routine practice: it is possible! *Journal of Psychiatric and Mental Health Nursing*, **11**: 64–72.

Kuipers E (2011) Cognitive behavioural therapy and family intervention for psychosis – evidence-based but unavailable? The next steps. *Psychoanalytic Psychotherapy*, **25**: 69–74.

Laws KE, D'Ambrosio R (2007) *What Will It Take to Implement Evidence-Based Practices Statewide? Adolescent Substance Abuse Treatment Statewide Coordination Project*. RMC Research Corporation.

Leff J, Kuipers L, Berkowitz R, *et al* (1982) A controlled trial of social intervention of the families of schizophrenic patients. *British Journal of Psychiatry*, **141**: 121–34.

Lester H, Marshall M, Jones P, *et al* (2011) Views of young people in early intervention services for first-episode psychosis in England. *Psychiatric Services*, **62**: 882–7.

Lewis C, Buffham K, Evenson E (2012) The implementation of the psychological recommendations in the NICE guideline for schizophrenia (2009) across two CMHTs: a service evaluation. *Clinical Psychology Forum*, **237**: 31–5.

Lobban F, Barrowclough C (eds) (2009) *A Casebook of Family Interventions for Psychosis*. Wiley.

Lowens I, Bowe SE, Barrowclough C (2009) Family intervention for complex cases: substance use and psychosis. In *A Casebook of Family Interventions for Psychosis* (eds F Lobban, C Barrowclough): 93–116. Wiley.

Machin K, Repper J (2013) *Implementing Recovery Through Organisational Change*. Recovery: A Carer's Perspective, Centre for Mental Health & Mental Health Network NHS Federation.

MacInnes D (2000) Relatives and informal caregivers. In *Forensic Mental Health Nursing: Current Approaches* (eds C Chaloner, M Coffey): 208–31. Blackwell.

McFarlane WR (2002) *Multifamily Groups in the Treatment of Severe Psychiatric Disorders*. Guilford Press.

National Institute for Health and Clinical Excellence (2006) *Bipolar Disorder: The Management of Bipolar Disorder in Adults, Children and Adolescents, in Primary and Secondary Care*. National Collaborating Centre for Mental Health.

National Institute for Health and Clinical Excellence (2009) *Schizophrenia: Core Interventions in the Treatment and Management of Schizophrenia in Primary and Secondary Care*. NICE.

Onwumere J, Smith B, Kuipers E (2009) Family interventions with ethnically and culturally diverse groups. In *A Casebook of Family Interventions for Psychosis* (eds F Lobban, C Barrowclough): 211–31. John Wiley.

Peddie C (2009) Rowanbank clinic embraces behavioural family therapy within the new forensic medium secure setting. *Meriden Family Programme Newsletter*, 4–6. Available at http://www.meridenfamilyprogramme.com (accessed December 2014).

Pfammatter M, Junghan UM, Brenner HD (2006) Efficacy of psychological therapy in schizophrenia: conclusions from meta-analyses. *Schizophrenia Bulletin*, **32** (suppl 1): 64–80.

Pharoah F, Mari JJ, Rathbone J, *et al* (2010) Family intervention for schizophrenia. *Cochrane Database of Systematic Reviews*, **12**: CD000088.

Pilling S, Bebbington P, Kuipers E, *et al* (2002) Psychological treatments in schizophrenia. I: Meta-analysis of family intervention and cognitive behaviour therapy. *Psychological Medicine*, **3**: 763–82.

Pitschel-Walz G, Leucht S, Bäuml J, *et al* (2001) The effect of family interventions on relapse and rehospitalisation in schizophrenia – a meta-analysis. *Schizophrenia Bulletin*, **27**: 73–92.

Prytys M, Garety PA, Jolley S, *et al* (2011) Implementing the NICE guideline for schizophrenia recommendations for psychological therapies: a qualitative analysis of the attitudes of CMHT staff. *Clinical Psychology and Psychotherapy*, **18**: 48–59.

Richards M, Doyle M, Cook P (2009) A literature review of family interventions for dual diagnosis: implications for forensic mental health services. *British Journal of Forensic Practice*, **11**: 4.

Rosenfarb IS, Bellack AS, Aziz N (2006) Family interactions and the course of schizophrenia in African American and White patients. *Journal of Abnormal Psychology*, **115**: 112–20.

Rossberg JI, Johannessen JO, Klungsoyr O, *et al* (2010) Are multi-family groups appropriate for patients with first episode psychosis? A 5-year naturalistic follow-up study. *Acta Psychiatrica Scandinavica*, **122**: 384–94.

Roth AD, Pilling S (2013) *A Competence Framework for Psychological Interventions with People with Psychosis and Bipolar Disorder*. Research Department of Clinical, Educational and Health Psychology, UCL. Available at http://www.ucl.ac.uk/clinical-psychology/CORE/competence_mentalillness_psychosisandbipolar.html (accessed December 2014).

Rowe J (2012) A covenant between mental health services and family carers. *Mental Health Practice*, **16** (2): 22–3.

Royal College of General Practitioners (2013) *Commissioning for Carers*. Royal College of General Practitioners. Available at http://www.rcgp.org.uk/carers (accessed 5 November 2013).

Royal College of Psychiatrists (2002) *Patients as Parents: Addressing the Needs, Including the Safety, of Children Whose Parents Have Mental Illness* (CR 1105). Royal College of Psychiatrists.

Royal College of Psychiatrists (2011) *Patients as Parents: Supporting the Needs of Patients Who Are Parents and Their Children* (Council Report CR 164). Royal College of Psychiatrists.

Rummel-Kluge C, Kissling W (2008) Psychoeducation for patients with schizophrenia and their families. *Expert Review of Neurotherapeutics*, **8**: 1067–77.

Sin J, Moone N, Harris P, *et al* (2012) Understanding the experiences and service needs of siblings of individuals with first-episode psychosis: a phenomenological study. *Early Intervention in Psychiatry*, **6**: 53–9.

Sin J, Henderson C, Pinfold V, *et al* (2013) The E Sibling Project – exploratory randomised controlled trial of an online multi-component psychoeducational intervention for siblings of individuals with first episode psychosis. *BMC Psychiatry*, **13**: 123.

Slade M, Pinfold V, Rapaport J, *et al* (2007) Best practice when service users do not consent to sharing information with carers. *British Journal of Psychiatry*, **190**: 148–55.

Smeerdijk M, Linszen D, Kuipers T, *et al* (2009) Family motivational interviewing in early psychosis and cannabis misuse. In *A Casebook of Family Interventions for Psychosis* (eds F Lobban, C Barrowclough): 117–38. Wiley.

Smith G, Velleman R (2002) Maintaining a family work for psychosis service by recognising and addressing the barriers to implementation. *Journal of Mental Health*, **11**: 471–9.

Smith J, Fadden G, O'Shea M (2009) Interventions with siblings. In *A Casebook of Family Interventions for Psychosis* (eds F Lobban, C Barrowclough): 185–210. Wiley.

Smith J, Fadden G, Taylor L (2010) The needs of siblings in first episode psychosis. In *Promoting Recovery in Early Psychosis* (eds P French, M Read, J Smith, *et al*): 235–44. Blackwell.

Social Care Institute for Excellence (2011) *Think Child, Think Parent, Think Family: A Guide to Parental Mental Health and Child Welfare*. SCIE. Available at http://www.scie.org.uk/publications/guides/guide30/index.asp (accessed November 2013).

Stanbridge RI, Burbach FR (2007) Developing family inclusive mainstream mental health services. *Journal of Family Therapy*, **29**: 21–43.

Tarrier M, Barrowclough C, Vaughn C, *et al* (1988) The community management of schizophrenia: a controlled trial of behavioural intervention with families to reduce relapse. *British Journal of Psychiatry*, **153**: 532–42.

Topor A, Borg M, Mezzina R, *et al* (2006) Others: the role of family, friends and professionals in the recovery process. *American Journal of Psychiatric Rehabilitation*, **9**: 17–37.

Worthington A, Rooney P, Hannan P (2013) *The Triangle of Care, Carers Included: A Guide to Best Practice in Mental Health Care in England* (2nd edn). Carers Trust. Available at http://static.carers.org/files/the-triangle-of-care-carers-included-final-6748.pdf (accessed December 2014).

CHAPTER 11

Working with challenging behaviour

Shawn Mitchell and Sanjith Kamath

Introduction

'Challenging behaviour' is a phrase that has gained much currency within mental health services since it was first introduced in the 1980s. The initial usage of the term was confined to descriptions of problematic behaviour in younger individuals with intellectual disabilities but it has since been generalised to similar behaviours across the spectrum of psychiatric diagnoses and irrespective of age. Despite its acceptance in everyday psychiatric parlance, the precise meaning and definition of 'challenging behaviour' is often unclear and the phrase has been used as a substitute for a diagnosis or as a pejorative term to encompass those aspects of the behavioural manifestations of mental disorder that are less well understood and consequently difficult to manage.

It is likely that all clinicians working with behaviourally disordered patients will be familiar with the term 'challenging behaviour', and while most will have a notion of what they mean when using the phrase, a precise definition is hard to articulate. Emerson (1995) defined it as follows:

> culturally abnormal behaviour of such an intensity, frequency or duration that the physical safety of the person or others is likely to be placed in serious jeopardy, or behaviour which is likely to seriously limit use of, or result in the person being denied access to, ordinary community facilities.

It is of significance that a diagnosis of a mental disorder or illness is not a prerequisite to classify an individual's behaviour as challenging if it meets the above broad criteria. It is therefore important for mental health practitioners to understand that challenging behaviour is not a diagnosis and can be observed in individuals with no mental disorder. It is most usefully conceptualised as a social construct that describes behaviours that fall well outside the usually accepted ideas of 'normal'.

Types or categories of challenging behaviour

Classifying challenging behaviour allows clinicians and sometimes the patient to identify the processes involved in the expression and consequences of the behaviour. Challenging behaviours can be divided into those that are likely to cause harm to the person and those that might lead to harm to others. Each of these can be further subdivided into direct and indirect behaviours.

Types of behaviour likely to lead to harm to self

The typical example of this type of challenging behaviour is repetitive self-injurious behaviour, such as cutting of skin, tying of ligatures and inserting objects. Less commonly, patients can present with behaviours such as poor interpersonal skills provoking other patients, repetitive swearing or instigating of other patients, which can lead to the patient being the subject of assaults. These are examples of challenging behaviour leading indirectly to harm to self.

Types of behaviour likely to lead to harm to others

Easily recognised examples of challenging behaviour directly leading to harm to others include physical assaults, aggression and fire-setting, either deliberate or accidental. However, some patients, typically with dissocial personality disorder or traits, may harm others through collusion or incitement of others, which can lead to harm to others indirectly. This type of challenging behaviour, particularly in a forensic population, can be as dangerous as, if not more so than, behaviours directly leading to harm.

Levels of severity of behaviour

Challenging behaviours can also be graded according to their severity. The grading of the severity of challenging behaviour is arbitrary and is probably best decided by the teams managing each clinical area according to the level of professional intervention required to manage the behaviour. The vignette in Case example 11.1, relating to a fictional Ms B, gives an example of how challenging behaviour can be graded and illustrates how one patient can present with a number of challenging behaviours.

Understanding challenging behaviour

Challenging behaviour as a form of communication

Some challenging behaviours serve as a means of communication. Individuals with borderline personality disorder who engage in acts of self-harm may do so to communicate distress that they find difficult to verbalise.

Psychological mechanisms underlying challenging behaviour

There are a number of psychological mechanisms useful in understanding both the evolution of and the management of challenging behaviour that

Case example 11.1 Grading levels of challenging behaviour

Ms B is a 35-year-old woman with an emotionally unstable personality disorder. She has a long history of abusive relationships and repeated admissions to psychiatric hospitals. Her current admission to a secure unit occurred after a violent assault.

Her stay on the ward has been characterised by disengagement from the therapeutic programme, episodes of self-harm through superficial cuts to her arms, tying ligatures, and head-banging as well as outbursts of verbal abuse and physical aggression to staff and other patients. She has broken pieces of furniture on occasion. At times she will pace the corridors of the ward in an agitated manner and repeatedly knock on the door of the nursing office demanding cigarettes, even though the ward has set smoking times.

At times, some of her actions, particularly the repetitive swearing, can upset other patients, to the extent that she has been the subject of assaults. On other occasions she has been known to befriend patients, typically new admissions to the ward, and try to incite them to attack persons who have assaulted her.

In attempting to understand Ms B's challenging behaviours and to plan interventions to address them, they can be usefully graded as:

- Mild – repeatedly knocking on the door demanding cigarettes; disengagement from therapy, verbal abuse and agitation
- Moderate – property damage, superficial self-harm, inciting others
- Severe – tying ligatures, head-banging, physical aggression.

derive from classical learning theory. These include positive and negative reinforcement, extinction and punishment.

Positive reinforcement occurs when a behaviour (appropriate or challenging) results in a reward for the individual. An example would be when engagement in therapy is taken as an indication of the patient maintaining safety and consequently the patient is granted increased leave in the hope that this will encourage even more engagement. However, inappropriate behaviour can be maintained in a similar manner. If a patient who wanted to change wards assaulted someone on that ward and was indeed transferred to a different ward, the patient might then form the view that violence to others is a means of achieving further transfers (for example if faced with challenging psychotherapeutic work).

Classical learning theory holds that an individual is likely to engage in desirable behaviour if it results in the cessation of unpleasant consequences. This is negative reinforcement. An example is a patient not acting on thoughts of self-harm when experiencing such urges, owing to the likely negative consequences of doing so.

Extinction occurs when a behaviour eventually stops because the factor that reinforced it is removed. Returning to the above example, a patient who is aggressive in order to move ward would be expected to cease such behaviour if the aggressive episodes did not lead to a transfer. An important practice issue is that if a behaviour is intermittently positively reinforced, extinction is delayed, so consistency of response by the staff team is vital for effective behavioural management.

All of us are familiar with the concept of punishment, where an undesirable behaviour results in a perceived negative consequence for the individual. The theory is that an individual will stop engaging in a particular behaviour to avoid the negative consequence. A simple example of this is giving errant children more homework if they have been talkative in class or the imposing of points on a driving licence of someone caught speeding. In a clinical setting, punishment is seen as punitive, inhumane and counter-therapeutic, and the evidence does not support the use of punishment in eradicating challenging behaviour.

Physiological mechanisms underlying challenging behaviour

Physiological mechanisms can also lead to challenging behaviour. Some patients have abnormalities of arousal, which is often a common factor behind many forms of challenging behaviour. It is thought that early childhood trauma, including abuse as well as neglect, may lead to a state of hyperarousal, leading in turn to later mental health difficulties, possibly through pathway abnormalities in the hypothalamic–pituitary–adrenal axis, and parasympathetic and catecholamine responses (Glaser, 2000).

Assessing challenging behaviour

Often patients can be said to present with challenging behaviour without detailed thought being given to the specific nature of the behaviour. Sometimes the term is used by staff to describe a patient they find difficult to work with. Therefore, even before attempts are made to understand and plan interventions for the behaviour, it is important for individual clinicians and the clinical team to reflect on possible reasons why the patient is considered to present with challenging behaviour.

The starting point of addressing challenging behaviour is to attempt to understand the behaviour in a context, which could be the patient's mental illness, personality structure, upbringing and life experiences, and the possible purposes that the challenging behaviours serve for the patient. To understand behaviours that occur in the context of a mental disorder, it is important to assess all aspects of the individual's history, including developmental, psychosexual, family, social, medical, forensic, educational and occupational, and psychiatric aspects, as well as the patient's personality and alcohol and substance use. Some challenging behaviours are clearly related to symptoms of a mental disorder. For example, agitated repetition is frequently seen in patients with a generalised anxiety disorder, and severe self-neglect can be seen in patients with chronic schizophrenia. Early childhood neglect or abuse can play a significant role in adult mental health problems, most significantly emotionally unstable personality disorder, as well as schizophrenia and affective disorders, and can lead to adult sexual difficulties, which in themselves can lead to challenging behaviours in a person with a severe and complex mental illness. A detailed developmental history is important in assessing for intellectual disability and autistic spectrum disorder, but can also be helpful in the assessment of personality disorder and schizophrenia.

It is important to ensure that the information used for an assessment is correct. Often these patients have had contact with many services, which can lead to incorrect or incomplete information being passed on. Copies of previous records may need to be requested.

A detailed assessment of the patient's mental state is also important. Consideration needs to be given to using assessment schedules to assist in this process, for example the Brief Psychiatric Rating Scale (Overall & Gorham, 1962) or Beck Depression Inventory (Beck *et al*, 1996) for mental state, the International Personality Disorder Examination (Loranger *et al*, 1997) for personality and the Autism Diagnostic Observation Schedule (Western Psychological Services, 2012) if autism is suspected.

Assessing and planning interventions to address challenging behaviour must be done in a systematic way. This involves: (1) identifying the target behaviour(s); (2) assessing or reassessing the patient; (3) measuring the behaviour(s) of concern; (4) developing a formulation, which leads to the generation of hypotheses (medical, psychological and social) about the possible causes and maintenance of the behaviour; (5) delivery of interventions based on the formulation, ensuring that this is done in a single sequential way, to ensure that the effect of the intervention is not contaminated by other interventions; (6) allowing sufficient time for the intervention to work; and (7) evaluating the effectiveness of the intervention. If the intervention is not successful it will be necessary to reformulate and repeat the cycle.

Measuring the behaviour

A behavioural assessment template can allow clinicians to record and communicate details of the behaviour (see Box 11.1). Assessing the challenging behaviours that a patient presents is an important part of understanding the behaviour. The first step is to define the problematic behaviour, its frequency, duration and intensity. It is also important to identify possible internal factors, such as mental state, physical health, sleeping, eating and other habits, and external factors, such as daily routines, shift patterns of support staff, and contact with friends or family, which may influence the behaviour. It can be useful to record the behaviour over a period of time, the length depending on its frequency, in order to establish a baseline and to identify if there are any patterns to the

---

Box 11.1 Behavioural assessment template

1 What exactly is the behaviour?
2 Frequency of behaviour
3 Duration of behaviour
4 Intensity of behaviour
5 Where the behaviour takes place
6 What personal factors are relevant?
7 Is there a relationship with environmental variables:
   • staff
   • other patients
   • carers
   • setting?
8 Is there a relationship with:
   • diurnal variables
   • psychiatric disorder
   • medical disorder
   • sleep cycle
   • drugs (including prescription medication)
   • alcohol
   • eating routines?
9 What are the consequences of the behaviour:
   • for the patient
   • for others?

---

behaviour. Recording significant events can be helpful to identify whether there are any antecedents to the behaviour or behaviours. The behaviour or behaviours can then be further assessed by the use of an ABC chart, which identifies possible antecedents, the behaviours themselves and the consequences of the behaviour. There are many examples of such charts, with minor variations. Fig. 11.1 gives a simple example.

For patients who present primarily with aggression, the Modified Overt Aggression Scale (Alderman *et al*, 1997) can be used to monitor their behaviour in more detail. The tool is subdivided into verbal aggression, aggression against property, auto-aggression and physical aggression. In dialectical behavioural therapy, behavioural chain analysis (Dimeff &

Name:			
Date	Behaviour	Antecedants (what happened before the behaviour)	Consequences (what happened as a result of the behaviour)

Fig. 11.1 A simple ABC chart

Koerner, 2007) is a structured analysis patients can use to understand their cognitions as well as their behaviours, focusing on the sequential events that form the behaviour chain, in order to identify more adaptive ways in which they could have dealt with a difficult situation. Patients describe the problem behaviours, analyse the precipitating events, vulnerability factors, consequences, alternative solutions, prevention plans and repair.

Formulation

Formulation can be key in trying to understand a patient's difficulties. The formulation will inform planning treatment and therapeutic interventions, as well as risk management and assessment. Formulation can be described as an organisational framework for producing a narrative that explains the underlying mechanism and proposes hypotheses regarding action to facilitate change. Formulation begins with describing the problem and then identifies: predisposing factors (social, biological and environmental), motivating factors, precipitating factors (including immediate triggers), longer-term factors (e.g. stress, deterioration of mental health), disinhibiting factors, perpetuating factors, protective factors (including internal strengths) and external factors (e.g. social support).

When there are differences within a clinical team, formulation meetings can be used to arrive at a shared understanding. Recovery-oriented services would ensure that the patient is integral to this process, in order that there is transparency (Ayub *et al*, 2013). However, when there is splitting within the team, exposing these differences to the patient can be counter-therapeutic, for a number of reasons, including distressing the patient, or the patient seeing vulnerabilities in the team and playing on these. Therefore, before involving the patient, the team needs to ensure that they have arrived at a shared understanding (see Case example 11.2).

The vignette in Case example 11.2 illustrates a number of the issues that arise in a patient who is seen as presenting with challenging behaviour, including comorbidity, treatment resistance, differences within the clinical team as to formulation, and staff feelings of clinical failure, manifest in attitudes that the patient was deliberately behaving in a challenging manner, which is then ascribed to personality disorder.

Interventions

Establishing a therapeutic relationship

Therapeutic relationships are reliable predictors of patient outcomes (McCabe & Priebe, 2004). Establishing a therapeutic relationship when a service user presents with challenging behaviour is a vital first step in reducing behaviours that cause difficulties for the patient or others. Patients who present with such behaviours invariably have had experience of difficult relationships, both personal and with professionals. They will

Case example 11.2 Patient involvement in the formulation

Mary, a 48-year-old single woman, was diagnosed with schizophrenia in her late teens. Her father also had a diagnosis of schizophrenia and she reports that she was sexually abused as a child; she did tell her mother but nothing was ever done about it. In her early 20s she had a son, whom she cared for on her own for 6 months, but found this increasingly difficult and so went to live with her mother, who took over caring for her son. Thereafter Mary moved frequently between admissions, usually under the Mental Health Act, precipitated by aggression to members of the mental health team, or neighbours, and on two occasions she attempted suicide. In the community she was poorly adherent with medication and misused alcohol and illicit substances, often in the company of friends, who would take her benefits and on one occasion started living with her. Her current admission was precipitated by her setting a fire, for which she was charged and convicted and placed on section 37/41. She said she set the fire because she felt she was not receiving sufficient support from the community mental health team.

In hospital she continued to experience intermittent psychotic symptoms, with fluctuating insight. On a regular basis she was irritable, which would lead to aggression to staff and fellow service users. Sometimes her irritability appeared to be due to psychotic symptoms, but at other times this was not apparent. She also had a significant affective component to her illness and at times she expressed feelings of hopelessness and suicidal ideation. Within the team there was discussion as to whether she had a concurrent depressive disorder; however, some members of the team were of the opinion that her behaviour was as a result of personality difficulties, and therefore Mary was choosing to behave in this way. She had been unable to tolerate clozapine and risperidone, so was placed back on zuclopenthixol decanoate, and the dose increased owing to her ongoing psychotic symptoms. It was agreed to treat Mary for depression and so she was commenced on sertraline.

On discussion with her, she disclosed that she often felt extremely anxious on waking in the morning, and so was commenced on regular diazepam. Her goal was to achieve unescorted leave, but she found it difficult to sustain at least 3 weeks of no aggression to others. She reported that she found it helpful to have daily feedback on her progress, to help her achieve this goal, and following further discussion she started receiving feedback from staff twice a day, which she recorded as a visual indicator of her progress. She also started recording her mood, and identified ways of dealing with her irritability, the main one being to go to her room to avoid conflict. This combination of pharmacological and low-level psychosocial intervention resulted in her achieving her goal, which led to her being able to progress from a low secure to an open unit.

often have been treated in a number of facilities, and at each one have had to establish new therapeutic relationships. Agreeing shared goals can help to foster therapeutic relationships in which patients feel that their wishes and hopes and plans are acknowledged, rather than being dismissed, which is often their experience. This can be facilitated by using the framework of the Care Programme Approach (Department of Health, 2008), identifying the patient's needs, and developing a care package around these needs. My Shared Pathway, developed for secure services in England by the National Mental Health Development Unit, focuses on shared goals, jointly identified by the patient and involved professionals. However, it is important that when using these frameworks the focus remains on patients, identifying their goals and needs, rather than the framework being diverted to meet the needs of professionals and commissioning and regulatory organisations.

Knowing the patient

Some patients are difficult to engage in addressing challenging behaviour collaboratively. This may be due to resistance on their part, an unwillingness or inability to accept that some of their behaviour is problematic for themselves or for others. Some may not be able to engage in such discussion due to severe thought disorder or cognitive deficits. In such circumstances, in order to minimise risk, it is important to use the care staff's knowledge of the patient to be able to identify:

- when the challenging behaviours are more likely to occur
- what circumstances are likely to trigger the challenging behaviours
- what the warning signs are, exhibited by the patient
- what interventions avoid an escalation to challenging behaviour, such as distraction
- how to respond to challenging behaviour.

Psychological interventions

In planning behavioural interventions it is first necessary to have clearly identified the target behaviours, the interventions planned and how the outcome will be measured. A wide range of psychological interventions may be employed (see Box 11.2). It is important that the multidisciplinary team has the resources to deliver them, and that the team and the individuals delivering the interventions are supported in the process, to ensure consistency.

Box 11.2 Psychological interventions in challenging behaviour

- Behavioural interventions
- Cognitive therapy
- Family therapy
- Psychodynamic and systemic therapy
- Family therapy
- Dialectical behavioural therapy
- Eye movement desensitisation and reprocessing
- Motivational interviewing

Behavioural interventions

Pure behavioural approaches are not commonly used, although there can be a role for positive reinforcement. This can be delivered through a simple mechanism such as a chart recording positive or appropriate behaviour, thereby reinforcing such behaviour, and possibly linked to a reward.

This approach is systematised in the RAID approach (Davies, 2005). RAID is a whole-ward system described as a 'relentlessly positive approach to working with extreme behaviour'. The underlying principle is the development of appropriate behaviours, which will overwhelm challenging behaviour, while the latter is consistently played down where it is safe to do so (hence the acronym Reinforce Appropriate Implode Disruptive). The uniqueness of the RAID approach is the shift from the clinical instinct to focus on disruptive behaviour to reinforcing appropriate behaviours. This change in focus allows staff to identify and support positive behaviour and promotes positive interactions between staff and patients while improving therapeutic relationships. Patients realise that appropriate behaviour is reinforced through explicit reward systems such as incentive programmes or implicitly through positive interactions, and they are therefore less likely to engage in disruptive or challenging behaviour. Staff are required to be trained to identify, record and reinforce these appropriate or 'green' behaviours and to provide as many opportunities as possible for these behaviours to occur.

Cognitive therapies

There are a variety of models of cognitive approaches. There is an extensive evidence base for the use of cognitive–behavioural therapy in treatment-resistant schizophrenia and depression (see Chapter 9, 'Cognitive approaches'). Schema therapy is sometimes used for patients with personality disorder. It focuses on maladaptive schemas, which are self-defeating, core themes or patterns that people keep repeating through their lives, often related to specific emotional needs that were not met in early childhood or adolescence, and the person's response to these, either surrendering to them or finding ways of blocking or avoiding emotional pain, or fighting back and overcompensating. In adulthood, schema modes, which are the moment-to-moment emotional states and coping responses, can be triggered by life events, leading to over-reaction to situations, or acting in damaging ways (Young *et al*, 2003).

Family therapy

For patients with schizophrenia there is evidence that family therapy reduces the rate of relapse (National Collaborating Centre for Mental Health, 2010; see also Chapter 10, 'Family interventions'), and therefore this should be considered for service users with a primary diagnosis of schizophrenia, and who live with, or have close contact with, family and other main carers. Sometimes professional carers may interact with patients in a similar manner as family members and therefore, arguably, the same principles and interventions could be used.

Psychodynamic and systemic therapies

There is a limited evidence base in the use of psychodynamic psychotherapy in challenging behaviour. NICE guidelines for schizophrenia report no clear evidence to support the use of psychodynamic and psychoanalytic therapies (National Collaborating Centre for Mental Health, 2010). However, they do suggest that psychodynamic and psychoanalytic principles and theories can help healthcare professionals to understand the experiences of people with schizophrenia and their interpersonal relationships. These principles can also be used in helping understand and arrive at a formulation for people with challenging behaviour, irrespective of their diagnosis, as well as helping healthcare professionals to examine and understand some of their own reactions to patients who present with challenging behaviour.

Dialectical behaviour therapy

Dialectical behaviour therapy (DBT) is a comprehensive cognitive–behavioural treatment for patients with complex and difficult-to-treat mental disorders, which was originally developed for chronically suicidal patients but since has been extended to use for all patients with a diagnosis of borderline personality disorder (Dimeff & Koerner, 2007). This is based on the view that patients with borderline personality disorder lack interpersonal, self-regulation (including emotional regulation) and distress tolerance skills and that there are personal and environmental factors that block or at least inhibit the use of behavioural skills and thereby reinforce dysfunctional behaviour.

In DBT, skills training is delivered in groups. The role of the therapist is to validate and accept patients as they are while simultaneously helping them to change (the dialect). Mindfulness is a key element in the acceptance procedures. Important in DBT is therapist support through regular consultation meetings. There are aspects of DBT that can be used in patients with variety of mental health difficulties and therefore in patients who present with challenging behaviour. Mindfulness can be used in a variety of mental health settings, and emotional skills training, as well as interpersonal skills training, can help patients with a variety of psychiatric diagnoses. Interpersonal skills and emotional regulation skills can be beneficial to patients irrespective of their diagnosis.

Eye movement desensitisation and reprocessing

Eye movement desensitisation and reprocessing is a therapy developed primarily for patients who have experienced severe trauma that remains unresolved, based of the hypothesis that when a traumatic or distressing experience occurs, it may overwhelm normal cognitive and neurological coping mechanisms (Shapiro, 1989). It was primarily developed for patients with post-traumatic stress disorder, but is also used in other conditions.

Motivational interviewing

Motivational interviewing is a type of patient-centred counselling with the aim of helping the patients explore and resolve their ambivalence about behaviour change. It is discussed in detail in Chapter 8, 'Rehabilitation at the coalface'. Its key components are focused reflective listening, undertaken with warmth and empathy. A strong principle of motivational interviewing is that conflict is unhelpful and the focus is on a collaborative relationship between therapist and patient, in which they tackle the problem together, with the aim of the patient rather than the therapist identifying the benefits and costs involved. The therapist elaborates a discrepancy between the patient's most deeply held values and current behaviour. Resistance is sidestepped by responding with warmth and empathy, rather than confrontation. The patient's self-efficacy is developed by building up the patient's confidence that change is possible (Treasure, 2004).

Compliance therapy

Compliance therapy uses motivational interviewing with particular application to medication adherence, focusing on symptoms and side-effects, exploring patients' ambivalence about their medication and discrepancies between actions and beliefs and finally considering that drugs are a freely chosen strategy to enhance quality of life, thereby reducing the stigma of medication. Metaphors such as 'protective layer' and 'insurance policy' are used to reinforce this (Kemp et al, 1996).

Medication

As discussed earlier, patients who present with challenging behaviour have a variety of diagnoses, and often more than one. In those patients who have more than one diagnosis, it is important to ensure that there is a systematic approach to pharmacological treatment following the relevant condition guidelines, such as those produced by the National Institute for Health and Care Excellence. The Maudsley Prescribing Guidelines in Psychiatry (Taylor et al, 2012) provides useful comprehensive guidance to prescribing for mental disorders for which there is an evidence base for pharmacological treatment. In patients with schizophrenia, mood disturbance should be adequately treated, with antidepressants or mood stabilisers. It is important prior to commencing any medication to identify what measures will be used to review the response to treatment, in order to avoid potential incremental polypharmacy.

Increased arousal appears to be a factor behind much challenging behaviour. It is not always possible to identify the cause of this arousal. There is evidence that clozapine has greater beneficial effect on aggressive behaviour than other antipsychotic medication. There is also limited

Table 11.1 Side-effects of medication potentially contributing to challenging behaviours

Side-effect	Symptoms of side-effect	Medications likely to cause side-effect	Interventions
Akathisia	Unpleasant sensations of inner restlessness; can be experienced as agitation	Antipsychotics – droperidol, pimozide, trifluoperazine, amisulpride, risperidone, aripiprazole	Change to an antipsychotic less likely to cause akathisia
		Antidepressants – fluoxetine, paroxetine, venlafaxine, tricyclics, trazodone	Change antidepressant treatments – propranolol, anticholinergics, such as procyclidine, benzotropine
Tachycardia	Can be interpreted as anxiety	Some antipsychotics, most significantly clozapine, most tricyclic antidepressants; non-selective monoamine oxidase inhibitors (MAOIs); and all anti-Parkinsonian anticholinergics	Changing clozapine to olanzapine
Sexual side-effects	Loss of sexual interest Erectile dysfunction Drug-induced priapism Delayed or inhibition of ejaculation	Antipsychotics – typical and atypical Antidepressants	Changing to a different group of antipsychotic medication, particularly a group that does not cause elevated prolactin levels Changing to a different group and antidepressants, particularly selective serotonin reuptake inhibitors to mirtazapine

evidence that clozapine can have a beneficial effect in patients with borderline personality disorder (Frogley *et al*, 2013), probably due to clozapine decreasing arousal. In patients with autism spectrum disorder there is limited evidence to suggest that risperidone, usually 0.5 mg, can have a beneficial effect (Barnard *et al*, 2002).

Once the appropriate prescribing guidelines have been followed and in situations where patients have more than one diagnosis, the approach to pharmacological treatment can become more challenging, with pharmacological treatment often based on symptoms rather than diagnosis, particularly when it is difficult to ascribe specific symptoms to a specific diagnosis.

Side-effects of medication

Side-effects of medication can be factors contributing to challenging behaviour, and therefore need to be considered when assessing the patient's behaviour. This may in turn necessitate a review of medication. Table 11.1 lists common and important side-effects.

Staff factors

Feelings of failure

Feelings of failure on the part of some members of the team, added to the behaviours of the patient, can lead to 'malignant alienation' of the patient from the service, which has been associated with suicide (Watts & Morgan, 1994). In psychiatry, a professional's main therapeutic tool is the therapeutic relationship. This is largely dependent on personality and therefore professionals' capacity to heal can be linked to their feelings of self-worth. A patient not responding to the professional's attempts at healing, or even worse, rejecting the staff member's attempts to heal, can be interpreted by the staff member as rejection, which in turn can lead to the staff member rejecting the patient, described psychodynamically as countertransference.

This can be mitigated through individual supervision, in which staff can:

- be able to appreciate challenging behaviour as an inability to seek help in other ways, and acknowledgement of the patient's possible inner distress
- develop insight into and understanding of their own vulnerabilities and expectations in providing care (such self-awareness is vital in those who have a need to develop special close relationships with certain patients and who encourage close dependency).

Reflective practice groups for staff can also be helpful for addressing these issues through promoting a ward environment in which any negative feelings among staff members can be acknowledged openly and be supported

Ward factors

The ward environment and ward milieu can be a significant factor, increasing or decreasing challenging behaviour. Challenging behaviour can often result in restrictive behaviours, such as restrictions on leave, move to a more secure environment, enhanced support, seclusion, physical interventions and even seclusion or other forms of isolation. The 'Safewards' model (Bowers *et al*, 2014), which focuses on reducing restrictive practices, can be helpful in understanding and analysing the ward factors and identifying any that can increase safety of patients and staff on the ward. There are six domains within the Safewards model:

- patient characteristics – individual patients' symptoms, including paranoia, irritability, low mood; demographics, such as age, gender, alcohol and drug use
- patient community – patient interactions, including contagion effects, as well as discord

- regulatory framework – national and local policies, processes related to the Mental Health Act
- staff team – efficiency, ideology, rules and routine, custom and practice
- physical environments – quality, security, complexity, layout, quiet rooms
- outside hospital – visitors, friends and family, dependency and institutionalisation, demands and home.

Exploring these factors in detail and identifying any that might reduce potential conflict may have a beneficial effect on challenging behaviour.

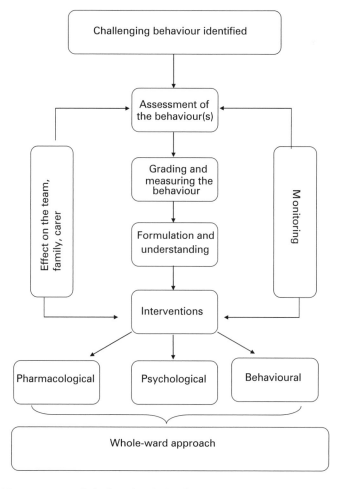

Fig. 11.2 Management of challenging behaviour

Conclusions

Patients with challenging behaviour not only provide a challenge for healthcare professionals as a result of their behaviour, but there are additional challenges in trying to find research and clinical guidelines to help with understanding the behaviour as well as planning clinical interventions. Patients with multiple diagnoses and other comorbid factors are often excluded from research projects, and if included may be difficult to keep engaged in such research. We have presented a systematic approach to the assessment and management of challenging behaviours. The approach is summarised diagrammatically in Fig. 11.2.

It is important for the healthcare professional to approach the challenges in a multidisciplinary way, with additional outside support if needed. The challenging behaviour needs to be systematically assessed and interventions planned in a staged way, with monitoring of outcomes. Staff need to be supported in understanding their own reactions to the challenging behaviour to ensure that they remain objective in their approaches, rather than relying on subjective feelings, which may adversely affect their responses.

References

Alderman N, Knight C, Morgan C (1997) Use of a modified version of the Overt Aggression Scale in the measurement and assessment of aggressive behaviours following brain injury. *Brain Injury*, **11**: 503–23.

Ayub R, Callaghan I, Haque Q, *et al* (2013) Increasing patient involvement in care pathways. *Health Service Journal*, 3 June.

Barnard L, Young AH, Pearson J, *et al* (2002) A systematic review of the use of atypical antipsychotics in autism. *Journal of Psychopharmacology*, **16**: 93–101.

Beck AT, Steer RA, Brown GK (1996) *Manual for the Beck Depression Inventory – II*. Psychological Corporation.

Bowers L, Alexander J, Bilgin H, *et al* (2014) Safewards: a new mode of conflict and containment on psychiatric ward. *Journal of Psychiatric and Mental Health Nursing*, **21**: 499–508.

Davies W (2005) *The RAID Manual: A Relentlessly Positive Approach to Working with Extreme Behaviour, to Minimise It At Source*. APT Press.

Department of Health (2008) *Refocusing the Care Programme Approach. Policy and Positive Practice Guidance*. Department of Health.

Dimeff L, Koerner K (eds) (2007) *Dialectical Behavior Therapy in Practice. Application Across Disorders and Settings*. Guilford Press.

Emerson E (1995) *Challenging Behaviour: Analysis and Intervention in People with Learning Difficulties*. Cambridge University Press.

Frogley C, Anagonstakis K, Mitchell S, *et al* (2013) A case series of clozapine for borderline personality disorder. *Annals of Clinical Psychiatry*, **25**: 125–34.

Glaser D (2000) Child abuse and neglect and the brain – a review. *Journal of Child Psychology and Psychiatry*, **41**: 97–116.

Kemp R, Hayward P, Applewhaite G, *et al* (1996) Compliance therapy in psychotic patients: randomised controlled trial. *BMJ*, **312**: 345–9.

Loranger A, Janca A, Sartorius N (eds) (1997) *Assessment and Diagnosis of Personality Disorders. The ICD-10 International Personality Disorder Examination (IPDE)*. Cambridge University Press.

McCabe R, Priebe S (2004) The therapeutic relationship in the treatment of severe mental illness: a review of methods and findings. *International Journal of Social Psychiatry*, **50**: 115–28.

National Collaborating Centre for Mental Health (2010) *Schizophrenia. The NICE Guidelines on Core Interventions in the Treatment and Management of Schizophrenia in Adults in Primary and Secondary Care* (National Clinical Guideline Number 82). British Psychological Society & Royal College of Psychiatrists.

Overall JE, Gorham DR (1962) The Brief Psychiatric Rating Scale. *Psychological Reports*, **10**: 799–812.

Shapiro F (1989) Efficacy of the eye movement desensitization procedure in the treatment of traumatic memories. *Journal of Traumatic Stress*, **2**: 199–223.

Taylor D, Paton C, Kapur S (eds) (2012) *Maudsley Prescribing Guidelines in Psychiatry* (11th edn). Wiley–Blackwell.

Treasure J (2004) Motivational interviewing. *Advances in Psychiatric Therapy*, **10**: 331–7.

Watts D, Morgan G (1994) Malignant alienation: dangers for patients who are hard to like. *British Journal of Psychiatry*, **164**: 11–15.

Western Psychological Services (2012) *Autism Diagnostic Observation Schedule* (2nd edn). Western Psychological Services.

Young JE, Klosko JS, Weishaar M (2003) *Schema Therapy: A Practitioner's Guide*. Guilford Press.

CHAPTER 12

Working with coexisting substance misuse

Cheryl Kipping

Workers need to recognise that people with multiple complex problems (dual diagnosis) can, and do, recover. Seeing opportunities for change and believing that these can be achieved makes a big difference. Leroy Simpson (service user) (Kipping & Simpson, 2010)

Introduction: a challenging context

Dual diagnosis, in this context the coexistence of substance misuse and severe mental illness, has been officially identified as 'the most challenging clinical problem that we face' (Department of Health, 2004: p. 1). Despite prevalence studies drawing on different samples, measures and time frames, a consistent finding is that at least a third of people with schizophrenia or other psychotic disorders also have problems with substances (Regier *et al*, 1990; Menezes *et al*, 1996; Weaver *et al*, 2002; Kavanagh *et al*, 2004; Carra *et al*, 2012). Alcohol and cannabis are the substances most frequently used and polysubstance use is common (Weaver *et al*, 2002; Kavanagh *et al*, 2004; Barrowclough *et al*, 2010).

The challenges of working with 'dual diagnosis'

Service user factors

'Dual diagnosis' implies just two areas of need, yet people with coexisting mental health and substance misuse problems usually have multiple needs. They may have more than one mental health diagnosis (e.g. psychosis and anxiety, depression or personality disorder), be misusing more than one substance, have physical health problems (often triggered or exacerbated by substance misuse) and have a range of social difficulties.

When compared with people with mental illness alone, people with dual diagnosis have higher rates of suicidal and violent behaviour, homelessness, hepatitis and HIV infection, more contact with the criminal justice system, worse psychiatric symptoms, poorer adherence with medication, make greater use of institutional services, and have longer hospital admissions (Banerjee *et al*, 2002; Department of Health, 2002; NICE, 2011*a*). Nevertheless, people enjoy using substances. Some find them helpful in managing mental health symptoms and many are not ready to stop (Barrowclough *et al*, 2010). Even if people do want to modify their use, change can be difficult and relapse is common.

Workforce deficits and separation of services

Regardless of discipline, the extent to which professional training equips staff to work with dual diagnosis is limited. This has been compounded by addiction being seen as a specialist area. Mental health clinicians therefore often lack knowledge and confidence in working with substance misuse.

Organisationally, at national and local level, in high-income countries mental health and substance misuse are conceptualised as separate entities. In the UK they have different policies and funding streams, and services are often delivered by different providers and even when delivered by the same provider are organisationally separate.

Mental health and substance misuse services also have different ways of working. If necessary, mental health services can enforce treatment against the person's will (in England and Wales under the Mental Health Act 1983). Substance misuse services usually expect the person to be motivated for change and to approach services for help. The separation of services promotes the view that mental health and substance misuse can be treated separately. In reality, each is likely to impact on the other, so considering one in isolation from the other is unlikely to be effective.

Together, the separation of services and deficits in staff knowledge have often resulted in mental health clinicians referring people to substance misuse services regardless of whether or not the clients themselves have identified such needs. Unsurprisingly, many do not follow through and this can result in substance misuse remaining an unmet need. Sometimes, even if the person wants to access substance misuse treatment, the way in which services operate can make this difficult. For example, some services are largely based on group work, which can be challenging for people with mental health problems (e.g. social anxiety, paranoia, auditory hallucinations). Also, substance misuse services are generally not commissioned to engage assertively with potential clients.

Lack of evidence regarding 'what works'

Although research on dual diagnosis is increasing, studies are often methodologically weak. There is a lack of robust evidence regarding the most effective treatment models and interventions (psychosocial and pharmacological) (NICE, 2011*a*, 2012; Hunt *et al*, 2013). Clinical practice in the field of dual diagnosis is therefore guided by weaker levels of evidence than are available in the management of mental illness or substance misuse as single problems.

Use of substances on wards and in residential facilities

Many people continue to use substances in hospital and other residential facilities (Phillips & Johnson, 2003) or use substances off site and return in an intoxicated state. Strategies for minimising and managing use can place staff in a 'policing' or controlling role, for example searching people and their property, using drug detection dogs and testing urine for drugs. Such roles appear at odds with the concept of a caring professional; relationships between service users and staff can become strained.

Dual diagnosis: tackling the challenges

Given this background, it is not surprising that working with people with dual diagnosis can be experienced as frustrating and demoralising. A sense of hopelessness and pessimism about a person's ability to make and sustain change is, however, counter to the principles of recovery, which focus on people's strengths (what they can do, rather than what they can't), people gaining control over their lives, and maintaining hope and optimism (Shepherd *et al*, 2008).

The remainder of this chapter draws on the available evidence and guidance, and provides suggestions on how mental health staff from all disciplines and backgrounds can work with people with dual diagnosis to support their recovery. As suggested, an integration of principles from mental health and substance misuse is required (Drake *et al*, 2001; Department of Health, 2002; Graham, 2004). For pragmatic reasons, the focus in this chapter is on substance misuse assessment and interventions, but these cannot be seen in isolation from mental health assessment and interventions. Both are crucial in promoting dual diagnosis recovery.

Recovery is defined as living a satisfying, meaningful and purposeful life within the limitations imposed by illness (Anthony, 1993). It is noteworthy that in the substance misuse field there is now an emphasis on recovery being 'getting off drugs for good' (Home Office, 2010). These contrasting conceptualisations may provide further challenges for services working with people with dual diagnosis.

The next section considers service delivery models, before attention is given to assessment and interventions. Finally, consideration is given to accommodation and working with families and carers. This structure is informed by the processes and language that guide mental health services. Service users may not view their contact with services in such ways. Wherever possible, service users and their needs should be the focus, despite the barriers that organisational processes and service requirements may present.

Service delivery models

Traditionally, treatment of 'dual diagnosis' in the UK has been based either on the *serial* model, where the person is required to address one problem before the other can be considered, or the *parallel* model, where mental health services address mental health needs and quite separately substance misuse services the substance misuse needs.

Recognising the high prevalence of coexisting mental health and substance misuse disorders, and that many service users are not ready to stop using substances, dual diagnosis work is now seen as a core component of mental healthcare (Department of Health, 2002; Appleby *et al*, 2006; Care Services Improvement Partnership, 2008) and an *integrated treatment* model is advocated. Within this model, mental health and substance misuse problems are treated at the same time, in one setting, by one team (Department of Health, 2002). Substance misuse services are expected to provide specialist advice to mental health teams (Department of Health, 2002; NICE, 2011*a*). In some areas, dual diagnosis roles and teams have also been developed to support the delivery of integrated treatment (Department of Health, 2002; Turning Point, 2007).

Although integrated treatment will be appropriate for most people, there are circumstances when the parallel model is helpful, such as when the person is physically dependent on substances and requires specialist prescribing (particularly for opiate dependence) or when the person is ready to address the substance misuse and can utilise specialist substance misuse services (NICE, 2011*a*). Parallel care and treatment require robust liaison and information-sharing to promote a consistent and coordinated approach. Service users may need support to negotiate the two treatment systems.

Assessment and review

Central to assessment is identification of the person's recovery goals – what does she or he want in terms of care and treatment? Although substance misuse may be a major concern for the mental health team, it may not be for the person. Nevertheless, to work effectively with people with dual diagnosis a good overview is needed of current substance use (what the person is using, the quantity, frequency of use, route of administration and length of time use has been at the current level), the interrelationship between the person's mental health and substance misuse, and the impact use has on physical health and social circumstances (e.g. relationships, accommodation, education/employment, finance, criminal activity, ability to care for children). Understanding the part substances play in a person's life, the reasons for using substances and readiness for change are also important for care and treatment planning (NICE, 2011*a*).

Most organisations have a template for collating information about current substance use as part of their patient record. The National Institute for Health and Care Excellence (NICE, 2010*a*, 2011*b*) recommends use of standardised assessment tools, including the Alcohol Use Disorders Identification Test (AUDIT; Babor *et al*, 1989), the Severity of Alcohol Dependence Questionnaire (SADQ; Stockwell *et al*, 1983) and the Leeds Dependency Questionnaire (LDQ; Raistrick *et al*, 1994). A substance misuse history can also be helpful: understanding why substance use was initiated, how it developed, the impact on health and social circumstances over time, whether abstinence has ever been achieved and if so how, and how the person's life was different during that period. The full guideline for psychosis with coexisting substance misuse includes details on comprehensive assessment for this group (NICE, 2011*a*). The National Institute for Health and Care Excellence provides guidance on alcohol assessment (2011*b*) and on drug assessment (2007*a*, 2007*b*; see also Department of Health (England) and The Devolved Administrations, 2007).

Good engagement is a prerequisite for good assessment. A non-judgemental approach is essential: negative attitudes and a confrontational approach can be barriers. Assessment tools that promote a closed question–answer approach can inhibit dialogue. Assessment is an ongoing process that requires pragmatism, flexibility and persistence. Collateral information from family, friends and other services should be sought. Home visits may also be useful, as they may reveal empty alcohol cans or drug-using paraphernalia. In-patient admissions for mental health relapse provide an opportunity to assess the person (relatively) substance-free and determine the extent to which symptoms are related to mental disorder or substance misuse.

If service users are willing to openly discuss their substance use, several other tools can help develop a greater understanding and highlight areas for intervention (for both the healthcare team and the person). Asking about a typical day, for example, can provide information about the type and pattern of substance use, people's relationships, diet, and how they structure their time.

Drink or drug diaries (see Fig. 12.1) provide information about the amount of substance(s) being used as well as insights into the context, motivations and consequences of use. Decision matrices, which explore the good and not so good things about using and reducing or stopping use, provide insights into reasons for use and possible motivators for change (see Fig. 12.2). Constructing a timeline that draws together information about life events, mental health and substance misuse can highlight relationships between these and enhance insight (Fig. 12.3).

Tools should be adapted to meet individual needs. For example, some people can complete a detailed diary as 'homework' between sessions, whereas a chaotic lifestyle or poor literacy skills may preclude this for others. Tools can be simplified, expanded or serve solely as a framework to guide conversation. Martino & Moyers (2008) suggest ways in which

Day	Amount and type of alcohol/ drugs	Time started– ended	Who with	Where	No. of units of alcohol	Cost (£s)	Thoughts, feelings, consequences
Mon.	2 cans strong lager 2 spliffs	16.00– 22.00	Alone	Home	9	4	Feeling rough from heavy session with Joe on Sunday. Didn't wake up until 14.00. No money left – got 2 cans on tick from shop
Tues.	2 spliffs	21.00– 22.00	Alone	Home			Mum came round. Went shopping and out for meal. No money for drink. Bit anxious and agitated
Wed.	4 spliffs	10.00– 22.00	Alone	Home			Stayed in all day. Shop won't give me more tick. Bored. Restless. Want a drink
Thurs.	6 cans strong lager 4 spliffs 2 rocks crack	12.00– 24.00	With mates	Joe's flat	27	12 30 40	Got money today. Joe called. Went round there. Can't really remember much. Think I forgot to take my meds. Bought £40 skunk
Fri.	6 cans strong lager 4 spliffs	12.00– 22.00	Joe	Home	27	12	Voices bad today. Drank to take edge off and Joe came round

Fig. 12.1 Example section from a drink and drug diary

Continuing to drink alcohol	
Advantages/pros	*Disadvantages/cons*
Like drinking and socialising with friends Like being drunk Helps me relax Takes edge of voices Something to do – helps boredom	Spending more than I can afford, getting into debt – threat of electric being cut off Getting into rows with sister – she won't let me see nephew when I've been drinking Might be having a bad effect on my liver
Stopping drinking alcohol	
Disadvantages/cons	*Advantages/pros*
Will get stressed and anxious Voices might get really out of control Boredom – what will I do if I'm not out drinking?	Won't need to worry about bills Will have money for new clothes Less rows Could think about starting a course

Fig. 12.2 Example of a decision matrix: continuing to drink alcohol

Life events	Mental health	Substance use
Age 12. Parents separated. Lived with mother, infrequent contact with father. Started missing school	Feeling low in mood and anxious at times	Started drinking, initially cider at weekends, then with peers during week, 3–4 times a week
Relationship with mother difficult – lots of rows in part due to drinking and drug use	Episodes of low mood and anxiety continue	Age 14. Continued alcohol use (cider and beer – standard strength). Some occasional cannabis use
Left school at 16, no qualifications	Occasional suspiciousness/ paranoia	Increasing cannabis use. By 16 using most days. Heavy alcohol use at weekends
		Episodes of threatening behaviour to mother when drunk
Age 17. First girlfriend. Got 'cash in hand' job, labouring	More positive about life. Mood & anxiety still present but not such a problem. No paranoia	Reduced alcohol and cannabis to mainly weekends (girlfriend not drug user – 'social drinker')
Age 18. Relationship breaks down Lost job due to drinking	Low mood and anxiety more severe again. Episodes of paranoia return	Drinking escalates to daily to cope with relationship breakdown and anxiety and depression. 6–8 cans strong beer. Cannabis use most days
Mother remarries, sells house and moves away	1st admission	Starts using amphetamine with friends – alcohol and cannabis continue
Re-established contact with some old school friends	Suicide attempt – jumped from bridge when intoxicated with alcohol, anxious and paranoid	

Fig. 12.3 Example section from a parallel timeline

some motivational tools can be adapted to meet the needs of people with severe mental illness.

Assessment, if conducted skilfully, can also be an intervention, promoting reflection and a decision for change. In England, assessment is important for allocation to a care cluster for payment and pricing. Cluster 16 ('dual diagnosis') is for people with psychosis and substance misuse (Department of Health, 2013).

Monitoring and review of substance misuse should be integral to ongoing care/treatment. Care Programme Approach (CPA) reviews provide an opportunity for more formally updating information and monitoring outcomes. AUDIT, SADQ and the LDQ can all be used as outcome measures. Other measures specifically developed for people with severe mental illness and substance misuse include the Clinicians Drug Use Scale and Clinicians Alcohol Use Scale (Mueser *et al*, 2003) and the Substance Abuse Treatment Scale (McHugo *et al*, 1995). Discussion of the results with the service user can provide an opportunity for reflection and review of recovery goals as well as providing a measure that may be useful for services.

Risk assessment and management

People with dual diagnosis have been identified as a particularly risky group (Appelby *et al*, 2006; Royal College of Psychiatrists, 2008). They may pose risks to themselves and others (family/carers, children, staff, the wider community). They may also be vulnerable to abuse and exploitation by others. Although simplistic, one way of conceptualising the risks is considering those associated with mental health/illness, those associated with substance misuse, and social risks. Inevitably there is overlap. Risks traditionally considered mental health risks include self-harm, suicide and violence. These are strongly associated with comorbid substance misuse (Fazel *et al*, 2009; National Confidential Inquiry into Suicide and Homicide by People with Mental Illness, 2014).

Substance misuse may damage physical health. Problems can be a direct consequence of use, such as: lung damage from smoking drugs; cardiac arrhythmia from using stimulant drugs; liver disease due to alcohol use; local and systemic infections from injecting; the effects of withdrawal (e.g. seizures, delirium tremens); falls when intoxicated; and accidental overdose. They may also be indirect consequences of use, such as: sexual health problems from engaging in sex work to fund use; or general poor health due to inadequate diet and self-neglect.

Social risks are often linked to the chaotic lifestyle that can be associated with substance misuse. They include involvement with the criminal justice system (to fund or as a consequence of use), debt, vulnerability to violence (particularly associated with debts to drug dealers), relationship breakdown, homelessness and exploitation (drug users taking over a property, being coerced into holding or buying drugs for others).

Staff need to be alert to child safeguarding issues (including unborn children), particularly the 'toxic trio' of mental illness, substance misuse and domestic violence (Brandon *et al*, 2010). Consideration also needs to be given to whether the person may pose a risk to a vulnerable adult, or may be a vulnerable adult themselves. Appropriate safeguarding procedures should be initiated.

195

The potentially dangerous interactions of substances and prescribed medication (particularly combinations of central nervous system depressants) and the potential for substances to impact on the effectiveness of medication need to be considered (NICE, 2011a; Taylor *et al*, 2012).

It is beyond the scope of this chapter to provide a comprehensive review of risks associated with dual diagnosis. The Department of Health (2011) provides a helpful overview of physical and mental health harms associated with drugs and alcohol. Risk needs to be regularly reviewed – at each contact and more formally at each CPA.

Rowchowdury (2011) suggests that the paradigm and values underlying recovery and risk are seemingly opposite (this apparent tension is discussed further in Chapter 26, 'Risk management in rehabilitation practice'). Service users should be active participants in identifying and developing plans to manage risk. Healthcare professionals need to accept that people with capacity have a right to make what professionals might view as 'bad' decisions (detrimental to their health and well-being). There will, however, be times when the risks associated with dual diagnosis will result in professionals taking actions that prioritise safety and limit service user self-determination. Advanced directives or care plans can enable the person to retain some control, even at times of restricted choices.

Interventions

Dual diagnosis interventions need to be staged according to the person's readiness for change (Drake *et al*, 2001; Mueser & Drake, 2003; Graham, 2004). A framework for identifying appropriate interventions has been developed by drawing on the 'cycle of change' (Prochaska & DiClemente, 1986) and Osher & Kofoed's (1989) four-stage treatment model. The 'cycle of change' conceptualises the person as moving from *pre-contemplation*, where the behaviour is not seen as problematic and change is therefore not considered, through *contemplation*, where there is some acknowledgement of difficulties and the possibility of change, on to *preparation/determination*, where a decision to change is made and change plans are developed, and then *action*, when changes are implemented. *Maintenance* concerns sustaining change. People are often unable to maintain change and so *relapse*. Osher & Kofoed's (1989) staged treatment model maps onto the cycle of change and provides pointers to interventions appropriate for different positions on the cycle: engagement, building motivation (persuasion), active treatment and relapse prevention (see Fig. 12.4 and Table 12.1).

Movement back and forth around the cycle several times is usually required before change is sustained. A long-term perspective is therefore required. Drake *et al* (2006) found evidence of change at 10-year follow-up: control of schizophrenia symptoms, remission from substance misuse, independent living and employment. The following sections describe in more detail interventions for each stage.

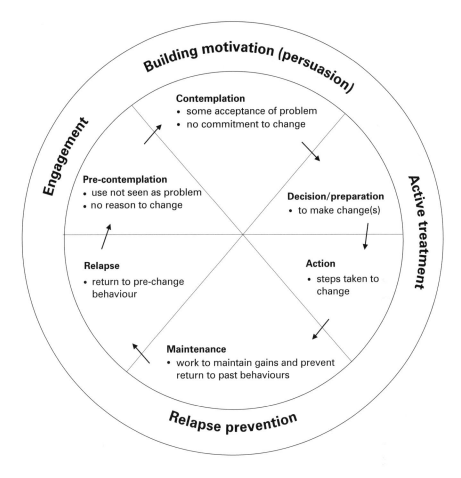

Fig. 12.4 Cycle of change and four-stage treatment model

Pre-contemplation – engagement

When the person does not view the substance misuse as problematic (pre-contemplation) interventions focus on engaging the person and building a positive relationship. The National Institute for Health and Care Excellence (2011a) highlighted the importance of being respectful, trusting, non-judgemental, hopeful and optimistic, and suggested that sensitivity, flexibility, persistence and a motivational approach are required. The 'spirit of motivational interviewing' has been identified as essential for engagement (Miller & Rollnick, 2013). It comprises four elements:

*   working collaboratively as experts – mental health practitioners have expertise in working with mental health problems, service users are experts on themselves

Table 12.1 Cycle of change, four-stage treatment model and treatment approaches/interventions

Cycle of change	Four-stage model	Treatment approaches/interventions
Pre-contemplation	Engagement	Building relationships Motivational interviewing ('spirit') Assertive outreach Flexible working practices Identifying needs Address practical issues e.g. housing, benefits Pharmacotherapy – for stabilisation of psychiatric symptoms Harm minimisation Offering information Assessment of carers' needs Obtain initial information to begin building comprehensive assessment
Contemplation	Building motivation ('persuasion')	Continue building relationship Motivational interviewing Comprehensive assessment Diaries Time lines Decision matrices Pharmacotherapy – for psychiatric symptoms Offer of information Importance and confidence rulers
Decision/ preparation Action	Active treatment	Motivational interviewing Formulating change plan Goal setting and planning Diaries Development of new skills and lifestyle changes e.g. budgeting, building social networks, enhancing social skills, developing leisure interests, developing vocational skills Activity scheduling Cognitive–behavioural therapy for psychosis Family interventions Pharmacotherapy– for psychiatric symptoms – for detoxification from substances Adjunctive therapy to address specific problems e.g. bereavement issues, childhood sexual abuse Self-help/mutual aid groups (e.g. Alcoholics Anonymous, SMART Recovery)
Maintenance	Relapse prevention	Pharmacotherapy – for psychiatric symptoms – for substance misuse relapse prevention Relapse prevention – mental health and substance misuse Day programmes, residential programmes Consolidation of skills and lifestyle changes Self-help/mutual aid groups

- acceptance – valuing the person, understanding the person's perspective, respecting choices and acknowledging strengths
- evocation – drawing out the person's own perspectives, values, ideas, strengths, resources and motivations for change
- compassion.

The 'righting reflex' – the professional's desire to set the person on the right course – inhibits collaborative working (Miller & Rollnick, 2013). Too often professionals try to direct service users into doing what they think is best. This creates tensions and closes down opportunities for honest conversations and the possibility of change.

Alongside relationship-building, practical action is needed. Offering help with benefit claims and housing, for example, can strengthen the therapeutic relationship, as well as supporting the person with their needs. Meeting clients at a location and time that best suits them (e.g. at home, in a café) can further enhance engagement (Drake *et al*, 2001; Mueser & Drake, 2003).

At this stage there may be little focus on substance misuse. The priority is retaining contact and building a collaborative relationship. Clinicians need to be attuned to opportunities that arise for discussing and obtaining information about substance use and maximise these.

Contemplation – building motivation (persuasion)

'Contemplation' is characterised by ambivalence – being in two minds. Typically, people have conflicting feelings about their substance use, with reasons for and against making changes (e.g. spending more money than they can afford, use affecting health, getting into rows with family, yet they like the feeling of being intoxicated, it is the norm in their social group, it helps take the 'edge' off voices and deals with boredom). 'Persuasion', Osher & Kofoed's term for describing interventions for this stage, has largely been replaced by 'building motivation'. The clinician should not be persuading the person to change; people need to talk themselves into change. Motivational interviewing has been defined as 'a collaborative conversation style for strengthening a person's own motivation and commitment to change' (Miller & Rollnick, 2013: p. 12). Understanding people's values and goals, the part substances play in their life, and eliciting and exploring any reasons they have for changing will be a focus. Discrepancy between the person's values and goals and the reality of the situation can be a powerful motivator for change. Reflecting 'change talk' – any talk that suggests the person wants to change (e.g. 'I'm fed up of getting into trouble with the police', 'I'm worried about my health', 'I could be a better mum if I stopped', 'I'd like to get a job') can help develop discrepancy and promote a decision for change.

At this stage tools such as diaries, timelines and decision matrices can be useful.

To help people make informed choices about their substance use, verbal and written information about the potential effects of substances on physical and mental health should be offered and the person's perceptions of this explored (NICE, 2011a). Several websites provide alcohol and drug information (e.g. http://www.talktofrank.com, http://www.drugscope.org.uk/resources/drugsearch).

Although the person may not be ready to make changes to the substance use, he or she may be ready for change in other areas: taking medication, engaging in daytime activities, improving budgeting, developing vocational skills. Everyone is motivated by something. Working with people's own priorities may produce changes that can subsequently equip them to progress in other areas. For example, deciding to develop vocational skills by attending a computing course may promote time structuring, strengthen social networks and enhance self-confidence, all of which could be beneficial if or when the person decides to modify the substance use.

Verbalising reasons for change, while characteristic of the contemplation phase, may not mean that the person is ready for change. Clinicians need to be wary of jumping ahead of the service user. Pushing for change when the person is not ready can promote discord and damage engagement. The importance and confidence rulers – scaling tools that ask people to rate how important it is for them to make a particular change (0–10 scale), and how confident they feel in their ability to achieve it (0–10 scale) – can indicate where further work is required. For example, a high level of importance but low confidence suggests that interventions are needed to boost confidence. If ratings on both scales are high, it is reasonable to assume that the person is ready to plan for change (Miller & Rollnick, 2013).

Decision/preparation, action – active treatment

Although some people will decide to stop using substances, others may choose to reduce or use in a less harmful way. A polysubstance user may decide to modify use of one substance but not another. Harm minimisation acknowledges that some people are unwilling, or unable, to stop using substances, and aims instead to reduce the physical, mental, social and economic harms of use (see the website of the UK Harm Reduction Alliance, http://www.ukhra.org/harm_reduction_definition.html). It can be a first step towards recovery (Department of Health, 2002, 2006).

Once the person has identified goals, in keeping with the 'evocative' element of motivational interviewing, the clinician should elicit ideas about how these can be attained, and provide information and suggestions when asked, or with permission (maintaining a collaborative approach). Plans might incorporate pharmacological and psychosocial approaches and include cognitive, behavioural and lifestyle components. Fig. 12.5 gives an example of a change plan.

Given that accessing substance misuse services may be an option, clinicians need a working knowledge of these. Having a colleague in the substance misuse service who can coordinate referrals from mental health teams can be invaluable. In addition, or as an alternative to formal substance misuse services, service users may benefit from self-help or mutual aid groups such as Alcoholics Anonymous, Marijuana Anonymous, Dual Recovery Anonymous, SMART Recovery (Self-Management And Recovery Training) (NICE, 2007*b*, 2011*b*). All have websites with information about their approach and details of local meetings.

In some cases substance misuse services are not suitable: the person may be vulnerable to exploitation by hardened drug users or the demands of the programme may be too challenging. Mental health clinicians have transferable skills and can include substance misuse in their ongoing work, in line with the integrated model.

An in-patient admission is likely to be a suitable treatment option for people who are physically dependent and want detoxification (from alcohol, opioids, benzodiazepines, GHB/GBL) (NICE, 2007*a*, 2011*b*). Specialist substance misuse services may be the best option but are often not equipped to provide high-level mental healthcare, so a planned psychiatric admission may be necessary. Inevitably, some people admitted to psychiatric wards because of a mental health relapse will be dependent on substances, so detoxification or substitute prescribing will be required to maintain their safety. Regardless of the pathway, substance misuse services

Change goal	Reduce cannabis use to £20 a week
Reasons for goal	Concerned about effect on lungs Spending more than I can afford/getting into debt Mental health team say it's bad for my mental health (I'm not sure)
How goal can be achieved	Don't start smoking until after 3pm Start doing other things – find out about college courses, find out about gym membership Go to Mum's (she won't let me use at her house) Keep away from Martin
People that can provide support	Mum Sister Care coordinator
How I will know plan is working	If I've kept to budget
Possible barriers and how I can overcome them	Leroy gives me cannabis (no money needed) Martin comes round – he's always got plenty (bad influence) Boredom May be phone Mum, sister or care coordinator Remind myself about things I want to buy if I can save money Keep to plan to do new things

Fig. 12.5 Example of a change plan for harm minimisation

should provide expert advice. Pharmacological interventions for substance misuse should be implemented in line with best-practice guidance (e.g. Department of Health (England) and The Devolved Administrations, 2007; NICE, 2007a, 2007c, 2010b, 2010c, 2011b; Taylor et al, 2012).

Although some people may benefit from residential substance misuse rehabilitation, few services are equipped for working with people with severe mental illness. Local social services' substance misuse care management teams can advise.

Several other services and people are likely to be working with service users to achieve their recovery goals, such as families/carers, housing workers, primary care, children and families social services. Being clear about the contribution of each and, with the permission of the service user, sharing information between services on a regular basis is important for developing a coherent and consistent plan.

Relapse prevention

Relapse in mental health and substance misuse are often closely related, relapse in one triggering relapse in the other. A cognitive–behavioural approach to preventing and managing substance misuse relapse has been developed by Marlatt and colleagues (Marlatt & Gordon, 1985; Wanigaratne et al, 1990; Marlatt & Donovan, 2005). High-risk situations and triggers for use (e.g. boredom, anxiety, being with particular people, craving) are identified and strategies to manage them developed. Some of the tools described above can be useful for identifying triggers (e.g. diaries, decision matrices).

An important aspect of preventing relapse is differentiating a lapse (using on one or two occasions) from a relapse (returning to previous regular use). The 'abstinence violation effect' is the thinking pattern that can occur following use after a period of abstinence: 'I've blown it. I'm back to square one. I knew I couldn't do it.' Reframing the experience as a lapse, from which learning is possible, can enable the person to refocus and resume progress. For example: 'I've had a slip and can get back on track. I have been able to change. I've made a mistake and can keep on trying.'

Identifying a relapse signature by mapping out the chain of events that led to a (re)lapse can help the person identify warning signs (linked to mental health and substance misuse) and consider where and how things could have happened differently. A relapse drill, strategies to manage situations differently, can then be developed to prevent future relapse (Birchwood et al, 2000).

Work needs to continue on building cognitive, behavioural and life skills, to promote continued change. Lifestyle changes are also essential if change is to be sustained. Pharmacological interventions for preventing substance misuse relapse may be helpful: acamprosate, naltrexone and disulfiram to prevent alcohol relapse (NICE, 2011b) and naltrexone for opioids (NICE, 2007d).

Accommodation

Regardless of where the person is in relation to the cycle of change, safe accommodation is usually a prerequisite for recovery. For service users unable to live independently, finding staffed accommodation that provides support with mental health and substance misuse can be difficult. Some residential projects will not accept people who have problems with alcohol and/or drugs. Chaotic substance misuse can also create difficulties for other residents (particularly those trying to remain abstinent).

Regular meetings between the service user, accommodation provider and mental health team care coordinator can help identify difficulties and develop shared plans for addressing them. Service users need to understand that they are responsible for, and have to deal with the consequences of, their actions. This may result in police involvement and losing a placement. For the mental health team the challenge of finding another placement is a common outcome.

Many of the staff running supported accommodation are unqualified and have little training for working with dual diagnosis. Statutory sector professionals can play a supporting role, for example providing advice on maintaining a substance-free environment and safe management of people who are intoxicated.

Family/carers

Although some people with dual diagnosis are not in contact with their families (Barrowclough *et al*, 2010), others are. Families, carers and friends (hereafter referred to as carers, for convenience) can be important partners in the care team, contributing their expert knowledge of the person (Worthington *et al*, 2013). Like service users, they need to be engaged in a collaborative relationship with clinicians.

Carer assessments provide an opportunity to build relationships and learn more of the carers' circumstances and perspectives. Some carers will, for the best of intentions, act in ways that promote continued use, for example by financing the person's substance use, paying bills, providing accommodation and food. People may have no need to change if carers support them in such ways. Some carers may be at risk from the service user, as a victim of theft (possessions being sold for money for drugs or money itself being stolen) or by being coerced into giving money by threats of, or actual, violence. Some carers will be exasperated by the substance use and argue with the person to try to get him or her to stop. Such confrontation can increase distress (for service users and carers) and may contribute to relapse of the mental disorder. Carers may also feel frustrated that mental health services are not doing enough to 'make' the person stop using. Barrowclough *et al* (2001) suggest that to enable carers to be effective in helping their relative they need to learn an approach consistent with the stages-of-change model and motivational interviewing approach.

Some carers will think that substance use is acceptable and may use alcohol or drugs themselves (possibly in a problematic way). This can be challenging and, where possible, it will be important to work with the carer, offering information and reviewing the experience of the service user with them, with a view to challenging perceptions and enlisting their support.

Mental health professionals can play an important role in providing carers with information about the person's illness, the effects of substances on mental health and the interactions of substances with prescribed medications. Information about carer support organisations should also be offered (NICE, 2011a). Dual diagnosis carers' groups are rare. There are national organisations and local groups specifically for the carers of people with substance misuse problems (e.g. Al-Anon, Families Anonymous).

Conclusions

People with dual diagnosis are often viewed as particularly challenging for services. Service configurations and workforce deficits, along with a lack of robust evidence regarding treatment options, can militate against effective support of people in their recovery. Change can be difficult for anyone, but for people with dual diagnosis it can be particularly challenging. Nevertheless, people with psychosis and substance misuse can and do change. Gains are often small: not deteriorating, or extending the period between hospital admissions, may be an achievement. Over time, many people are able to make significant changes, including living a drug-free life, stabilising mental health symptoms and gaining paid employment. Greater awareness of transformational stories such as that of Mark (2010) help promote the optimism and hope that are essential for service users and staff if positive change is to be achieved.

References

Anthony W (1993) Recovery from mental illness: the guiding vision of the mental health service system in the 1990s. *Psychosocial Rehabilitation Journal*, 16: 11–23.

Appleby L, Kapur N, Shaw J, *et al* (2006) *Avoidable Deaths: Five Year Report of the National Confidential Inquiry into Suicide and Homicide by People with Mental Illness*. National Confidential Inquiry into Suicide and Homicide by People with Mental Illness, University of Manchester.

Babor T, de la Fuente J, Saunders J, *et al* (1989) *AUDIT. The Alcohol Use Disorders Identification Test: Guidelines for Use in Primary Care*. World Health Organization.

Banerjee S, Clancy C, Crome I (eds) (2002) *Co-existing Problems of Mental Disorder and Substance Misuse (Dual Diagnosis): An Information Manual*. Research Unit, Royal College of Psychiatrists.

Barrowclough C, Haddock G, Tarrier N, *et al* (2001) Randomised control trial of motivational interviewing, cognitive behaviour therapy, and family interventions for patients with co-morbid schizophrenia and substance use disorders. *American Journal of Psychiatry*, **158**: 1706–13.

Barrowclough, C, Haddock G, Wykes T, *et al* (2010) Integrated motivational interviewing and cognitive behavioural therapy for people with psychosis and comorbid substance misuse: randomized control trial. *BMJ*, **341**: c6325.

Birchwood M, Spencer E, McGovern D (2000) Schizophrenia: early warning signs. *Advances in Psychiatric Treatment*, **6**: 93–101.

Brandon M, Bailey S, Belderson P (2010) *Building on the Learning from Serious Case Reviews: A Two-Year Analysis of Child Protection Database Notifications 2007–2009*. Department for Education, University of East Anglia.

Care Services Improvement Partnership (2008) *Mental Health NSF Autumn Assessment 2007 – Dual Diagnosis Themed Review*. CSIP.

Carra G, Johnson S, Bebbington P, *et al* (2012) The lifetime and past-year prevalence of dual diagnosis in people with schizophrenia across Europe: findings from the European Schizophrenia Cohort (EuroSC). *European Archives of Psychiatry and Clinical Neuroscience*, **262**: 607–16.

Department of Health (2002) *Mental Health Policy Implementation Guide: Dual Diagnosis Good Practice Guide*. Department of Health.

Department of Health (2004) *The National Service Framework for Mental Health – Five Years On*. Department of Health.

Department of Health (2006) *Dual Diagnosis in Mental Health Inpatient and Day Hospital Settings*. Department of Health.

Department of Health (2011) *A Summary of the Health Harms of Drugs*. Department of Health.

Department of Health (2013) *Mental Health Clustering Booklet* (v3.0). At http://webarchive.nationalarchives.gov.uk/20130507000015/https://www.gov.uk/government/uploads/system/uploads/attachment_data/file/127287/Draft-2013-14-Mental-Health-Clustering-Booklet.pdf.pdf (accessed June 2013).

Department of Health (England) and The Devolved Administrations (2007) *Drug Misuse and Dependence: UK Guidelines on Clinical Management*. Department of Health (England), Scottish Government, Welsh Assembly Government and Northern Ireland Executive.

Drake R, Essock S, Shaner A, *et al* (2001) Implementing dual diagnosis services for clients with severe mental illness. *Psychiatric Services*, **52**: 469–76.

Drake R, McHugo G, Xie H, *et al* (2006) Ten-year recovery outcomes for clients with co-occurring schizophrenia and substance use disorders. *Schizophrenia Bulletin*, **32**: 464–73.

Fazel S, Gulati G, Linsell L, *et al* (2009) Schizophrenia and violence: systematic review and meta-analysis. *PLoS Med*, **6** (8): e1000120.doi:10.1371/journal.pmed.1000120.

Graham H (2004) *Cognitive–Behavioural Integrated Treatment (C-BIT): A Treatment Manual for Substance Misuse in People with Severe Mental Health Problems*. Wiley.

Home Office (2010) *Drug Strategy 2010 Reducing Demand, Restricting Supply, Building Recovery: Supporting People to Live a Drug Free Life*. At http://www.homeoffice.gov.uk/publications/alcohol-drugs/drugs/drug-strategy/drug-strategy-2010 (accessed June 2013).

Hunt GE, Siegfried N, Morley K, *et al* (2013) Psychosocial interventions for people with both severe mental illness and substance misuse (review). *The Cochrane Library*, **10**: CD001088.pub3.

Kavanagh DJ, Waghorn G, Jenner L, *et al* (2004) Demographic and clinical correlates of comorbid substance use disorders in psychosis: multivariate analyses from an epidemiological sample. *Schizophrenia Research*, **66**: 115–24.

Kipping C, Simpson L (2010) Contrasting maintenance and recovery approaches to the care of people with dual diagnosis. *Advances in Dual Diagnosis*, **1** (3): 15–18.

Mark B (2010) Good dual diagnosis practice promotes real recovery. *Advances in Dual Diagnosis*, **3**: 19–22.

Marlatt GA, Donovan DM (2005) *Relapse Prevention: Maintenance Strategies in the Treatment of Addictive Behaviours* (2nd edn). Guilford Press.

Marlatt GA, Gordon JR (1985) *Relapse Prevention: Maintenance Strategies in the Treatment of Addictive Behaviours*. Guilford Press.

Martino S, Moyers T (2008) Motivational interviewing with dually diagnosed patients. In *Motivational Interviewing in the Treatment of Psychological Problems* (eds H Arkowitz, HA Weston, WR Miller, S Rollnick): 277–303. Guilford Press.

McHugo G, Drake R, Burton H, *et al* (1995) A scale for assessing the stage of substance abuse treatment in persons with severe mental illness. *Journal of Nervous and Mental Disease*, **183**: 762–7.

Menezes P, Johnson S, Thornicroft G, *et al* (1996) Drug and alcohol problems among people with severe mental illness in south London. *British Journal of Psychiatry*, **168**: 612–19.

Miller W, Rollnick S (2013) *Motivational Interviewing: Helping People Change* (3rd edn). Guilford Press.

Mueser K, Drake R (2003) Integrated dual disorder treatment in New Hampshire. In *Substance Misuse in Psychosis: Approaches to Treatment and Service Delivery* (eds HL Graham, A Copello, MJ Birchwood, *et al*): 93–105. Wiley.

Mueser KT, Noordsy DL, Drake RE, *et al* (2003) *Integrated Treatment for Dual Disorders: A Guide to Effective Practice*. Guilford Press.

National Confidential Inquiry into Suicide and Homicide by People with Mental Illness (2014) *Annual Report 2014: England, Northern Ireland, Scotland and Wales*. University of Manchester (http://www.bbmh.manchester.ac.uk/cmhr/centreforsuicideprevention/nci/reports/Annualreport2014.pdf).

National Institute for Health and Clinical Excellence (2007a) *Drug Misuse: Opiate Detoxification* (NICE Clinical Guideline 52). NICE.

National Institute for Health and Clinical Excellence (2007b) *Drug Misuse: Psychosocial Interventions* (NICE Clinical Guideline 51). NICE.

National Institute for Health and Clinical Excellence (2007c) *Methadone and Buprenorphine for the Management of Opioid Dependence* (NICE Technology Appraisal 114). NICE.

National Institute for Health and Clinical Excellence (2007d) *Naltrexone for the Management of Opioid Dependence* (NICE Technology Appraisal 115). NICE.

National Institute for Health and Clinical Excellence (2010a) *Alcohol Use Disorders: Preventing Harmful Drinking* (Public Health Guidance 24). NICE.

National Institute for Health and Clinical Excellence (2010b) *Alcohol Use Disorders: Sample Chlordiazepoxide Dosing Regimens for Use in Managing Alcohol Withdrawal*. NICE.

National Institute for Health and Clinical Excellence (2010c) *Alcohol Use Disorders: Diagnosis and Clinical Management of Alcohol-Related Physical Complications* (Clinical Guideline 100). NICE.

National Institute for Health and Clinical Excellence (2011a) *Psychosis with Coexisting Substance Misuse* (Clinical Guideline 120, full guideline). British Psychological Society & Royal College of Psychiatrists. Quick reference guide version available at: http://guidance.nice.org.uk/CG120/QuickRefGuide/pdf/English (accessed June 2013)

National Institute for Health and Clinical Excellence (2011b) *Alcohol Use Disorders: Diagnosis, Assessment and Management of Harmful Drinking and Alcohol Dependence* (Clinical Guideline 115). NICE.

National Institute for Health and Clinical Excellence (2012) *Psychosis with Coexisting Substance Misuse* (Evidence Update 26). NICE.

Osher F, Kofoed L (1989) Treatment of patients with psychiatric and psychoactive substance abuse disorders. *Hospital and Community Psychiatry*, **40**: 1025–30.

Phillips P, Johnson S (2003) Drug and alcohol use among in-patients with psychotic illnesses in three inner-London psychiatric units. *Psychiatric Bulletin*, **27**: 217–20.

Prochaska J, DiClemente C (1986) Towards a comprehensive model of change. In *Treating Addictive Behaviours: Processes of Change* (eds W Miller, N Heather): 3–27. Plenum.

Raistrick D, Bradshaw J, Tober G, *et al* (1994) Development of the Leeds Dependency Questionnaire (LDQ): a questionnaire to measure alcohol and opiate dependence in the context of a treatment evaluation package. *Addiction*, **89**: 563–72.

Regier D, Farmer M, Rae D, *et al* (1990) Comorbidity of mental disorders with alcohol and other substances: results from the Epidemiological Catchment Area Study. *JAMA*, **264**: 2511–18.

Rowchowdury A (2011) Bridging the gaps between risk and recovery: a human needs approach. *The Psychiatrist*, **35**: 68–73.

Royal College of Psychiatrists (2008) *Rethinking Risk to Others in Mental Health Services* (College Report CR150). Royal College of Psychiatrists.

Shepherd G, Boardman J, Slade M (2008) *Making Recovery a Reality*. Sainsbury Centre for Mental Health.

Stockwell T, Murphy D, Hodgson R (1983) The Severity of Alcohol Dependence Questionnaire: its use, reliability and validity. *British Journal of Addiction*, **78**: 145–55.

Taylor D, Paton C, Kapur S (2012) *The Maudsley Prescribing Guidelines in Psychiatry* (11th edn). Wiley–Blackwell.

Turning Point (2007) *Dual Diagnosis: Good Practice Handbook*. Turning Point.

Wanigaratne S, Wallace W, Pullin J, *et al* (1990) *Relapse Prevention for Addictive Behaviours*. Blackwell.

Weaver T, Charles V, Madden P, *et al* (2002) *Co-morbidity of Substance Misuse and Mental Illness Collaborative Study (COSMIC): A Study of the Prevalence and Management of Co-morbidity Amongst Adult Substance Misuse and Mental Health Treatment Populations*. National Treatment Agency, Department of Health.

Worthington A, Rooney P, Hannen R (2013) *The Triangle of Care – Carers Included: A Guide to Best Practice in Mental Health Care in England* (2nd edn). Carers Trust.

CHAPTER 13

Creative therapies and creativity

Frank Röhricht, Stuart Webster and Simon Procter

Introduction

Creative therapies, also referred to under umbrella terms such as art therapies or non-verbal therapies, have over many years been discreetly introduced into the portfolio of psychological therapies in many mental health services in the UK. This is despite the fact that it is only relatively recently that an evidence base has been developed, to the extent that the National Institute for Health and Care Excellence (NICE, 2009: pp. 251–257) recommended arts therapies as the only effective treatment of negative symptoms in schizophrenia.

There are a number of reasons why creative therapies have always been attractive to both service users and healthcare providers. Most importantly, these therapies offer a very different way of expressing thoughts and feelings and new ways of communicating with each other. They can help service users who otherwise struggle to engage with or respond to treatment and who have profound difficulty verbalising their feelings, thoughts and life experiences. This is particularly relevant for those service users who have severe, complex and often enduring mental disorders. Creative therapies foster the development of empathy and social interaction, thereby introducing hard-to-engage patients to psychological work in a less direct way.

Rehabilitation psychiatrists have always aimed to work in a holistic way, incorporating the biopsychosocial model. Living well is the aim, not necessarily a complete cure, which for people with longer-term, severe mental illness may not always be achievable. 'The recovery model' has further shifted the focus to subjective quality of life and individual psychosocial functioning. While this carries the risk of accepting a degree of ongoing pathology too easily, there are some features at the core of the recovery model that seem more unambiguous: self-empowerment and a clinical strategy that aims to nurture individual skills and capabilities.

Warner (2010) addressed the question of the scientific evidence supporting the recovery model. He emphasised an important additional aspect: 'The conclusion we may draw from this body of research is that the empowerment of people with mental illness and helping them reduce their internalised sense of stigma are as important as helping them find insight into their illnesses'. Creative therapies lend themselves strongly to this set of objectives, as they require individuals to view things in new ways or from a different perspective, including generating new possibilities or alternatives.

Art therapies or creative therapies are commonly (although not exclusively) delivered in groups. They can be used in multicultural settings in which many service users speak little English. The therapies include art therapy, drama therapy, music therapy and dance movement psychotherapy. The last has roots in two different categories of psychological therapy, namely the arts therapies (the dance therapy element) and body psychotherapy (the movement therapy element). All creative therapies have non-verbal activities at the core of their approach, although they frequently also use verbal communication, which may be opened and expanded through non-verbal activities. Therapy sessions usually end with time to reflect on the shared experience and to make links between actions, feelings and thoughts, with acknowledgement of the similarities and differences between one another.

Arts therapists and creative therapists can be found working across various types of setting, including in-patient units and community services. There is, however, a significant geographical inequity in the provision of these services, ranging from large arts therapies departments that include therapists from different modalities to little such provision or (frequently) none at all. Another model is where services operate from outside mental health institutions and provide an in-reach service as well as a social enterprise environment (see examples at the end of this chapter).

Artists and arts therapists and creative therapists seek to link service users into other forms of (non-psychiatric) provision, creating pathways that intersect with more general care pathways. Likewise, within a particular place, therapists may seek not only to work with particular clients but also more broadly to 'musicalise' the institution, creating a culture within which engagement is made available to all in a variety of ways. This necessitates being prepared to work 'out of the room' for at least some of the time. An example of this form of practice is 'community music therapy' (e.g. Pavlicevic & Ansdell, 2004; Stige & Aarø, 2011). The term indicates not simply the likely location of such work but its understanding of the value of the communal dimension. The impact of art and creativity as a therapeutic tool is far-reaching: it enables a coming together, a sharing of positive experiences, working in partnership through difficulties and performing jointly in public. This approach can remove common power imbalances in healthcare settings and so creates a culture of trust and mutual support.

209

The different modalities: models and examples of practice in recovery services

Art therapy

Art therapy is generally defined as a form of expressive therapy that uses art materials as its primary mode of communication. The therapy combines psychotherapeutic theories and techniques with an understanding of the psychological aspects of the creative process. The International Art Therapy Organization (IATO) characterises the specific work in art therapy as follows:

> When words are not enough, we turn to images and symbols to tell our stories. And in telling our stories through art, we can find a path to health and wellness, emotional reparation, recovery, and ultimately, transformation. (http://www.internationalarttherapy.org)

Another definition, from the Art Therapy Alliance, emphasises the specific areas in which art therapy can be helpful, including fostering self-expression, enhancing coping skills, managing stress and strengthening a sense of self. Art therapy is, of course, mediated through the visual:

> art therapists are trained to recognize the nonverbal symbols and metaphors that are communicated within the creative process, symbols and metaphors which might be difficult to express in words or in other modalities. Art making is seen as an opportunity to express oneself imaginatively, authentically, and spontaneously, an experience that, over time, can lead to personal fulfillment, emotional reparation, and transformation. (http://www.internationalarttherapy.org)

Typically, an art therapy session will involve access to a range of art materials, carefully selected for their visual and tactile variety, and the opportunity to make use of them and engage in art-making processes, such as drawing, painting, sculpture and collage. This 'making' period of connecting with the art materials is followed by a period of 'looking' – of reflecting and exploring the visual images made, together with a trained art therapist. Within these processes of visual and tactile expression, Woodcock (2003) says, are the 'features that make art therapy so powerful ... its facility as a non-verbal therapy, its ability to work with unconscious processes, and its capability of bringing together domains of experience'.

The overall psychotherapeutic aim of art therapy is to enhance the emotional capacity of people who, for whatever reason, find it difficult to express themselves in words alone. This form of therapy can enable them to accept and understand emotions that may emerge during their involvement in the sensorimotor, perceptual, cognitive, physical, interpersonal and, for some, spiritual aspects of art therapy.

A particular contribution of art psychotherapy is working with people who have experienced trauma, where this cannot be expressed with words because it cannot be thought about in the first place, and the capacity for making meaningful links is seriously disturbed. Through the art psychotherapist's empathic attunement, and by facilitating pre-verbal symbol formation, the visual artwork contains and gives meaning to individual experience. The therapy can be used as a bridge to verbal dialogue, restoring links and attachments to the individual's own thoughts, feelings and personal narrative. With direct eye contact experienced by many service users as abusive and traumatic, art therapy enables the intimacy of looking and interpersonal relating to be rerouted in a creative and constructive way, which enables being seen by others to be more tolerable. The process of 'looking' is central and amplified in art therapy. It aims to create a visual containing environment – akin to the 'listening' in a talking therapy. The opportunity for insight and change, and developing new ways of being with, and of relating to self and others, offers unique possibilities to service users for their recovery process. The client is at the centre of art therapy and involved in the whole therapeutic process.

Recovery of optimism and hope through art therapy has been expressed by users of services in the following ways: 'Art de-frags my brain, like a computer rearranging the files into different places.' 'I learnt to face my feelings and my thoughts on paper in disarray just like my mind. I also found that it became a mirror image of my feelings. It has helped me face reality.' 'It was good meeting people and seeing things from other people's point of view.' 'Kind of gives you time to think things through in a group. The art therapy helps and gives me something to work with; it will be a part of my future.'

Drama therapy

Drama therapy incorporates a range of techniques and approaches, such as the use of culturally diverse stories, role-play, improvisation and structured story-making. The British Association of Dramatherapists defines the approach on its website:

> Dramatherapy is a form of psychological therapy in which all of the performance arts are utilised within the therapeutic relationship.... The therapy gives equal validity to body and mind within the dramatic context; stories, myths, play texts, puppetry, masks and improvisation are examples of the range of artistic interventions a Dramatherapist may employ. These will enable the client to explore difficult and painful life experiences through an indirect approach. (https://badth.org.uk/)

The approach aims to use the notion of 'dramatic distance' in order to promote a sense of safety in the exploratory psychological work with clients, while also remaining mindful of the personal elements that are likely to emerge in the process. Participants are not expected to have prior acting experience.

Sessions will start with a range of warm-up activities. Once a main theme or topic has emerged, the therapist, in negotiation with the group, leads an exploration of this. This can be through the use of either projected play (with objects) or personal play (embodied). After the main theme has been explored creatively, the therapeutic process aims to connect the scenes of 'enactment' and the 'here and now' of participants' realities. The therapist thereby encourages the group members to reflect upon and share their experiences, focusing on conflict resolution and problem-solving. Drama therapy encourages participants to learn or rediscover 'playfulness', which helps promote self-expression, develop self-confidence and increase self-esteem. It can help to develop spontaneity and flexibility of thinking and to contain difficult feelings. It addresses basic developmental deficits such as issues relating to lack of basic trust, autonomy and initiative and a range of emotional problems. It encourages social interaction and helps increase mutual understanding of forming and maintaining relationships.

In rehabilitation and recovery services, drama therapy can make significant contributions to the overall multidisciplinary care plan. One of the many ways in which drama therapy is intrinsically linked to the recovery model is the explicit work with patients' stories (in terms of enacted narratives). Multidisciplinary teams benefit from feedback regarding a different dimension to the patient's profile, such as unknown aspects of his or her personal 'story', or 'shadow' gestures and other non-verbal expressions indicating unconscious disturbance. As a patient-centred approach, drama therapy facilitates and encourages active engagement with the creative work and engagement with the immediate (peers) and wider community. Taking responsibility and making a commitment to the format of interactive role-play in the drama therapy group provide an experiential field for preparing for other commitments in the community, such as going to work. Close links with community-based arts projects can be cultivated by joint working between organisations and by helping individuals to take a lead in participating in this process.

Music therapy

The term 'music therapy' may be applied to different practices in different parts of the world. There is generally a major distinction between 'receptive' music therapy (where recordings of music are listened to as a form of therapy) and 'active', improvisational music therapy. Music therapy as practised in the UK is usually described as 'active': both therapist and client(s) are actively engaged in the making of music together. While clients need have no prior experience of playing music, therapists need to be not only skilled in using their instrument(s) but also able to use their musicianship to engage clients, support them musically and lead them into new experiences of self and of self in relation to other(s). Contrary to the popularly held assumption that music therapy is a means of soothing, calming or relaxing people, music therapists often work with the full range of music's expressivity.

Music therapists employ a range of theoretical constructs when describing their work. Some make use of psychodynamic or psychoanalytic theory (as used in psychotherapy) and may indeed consider their work a form of psychotherapy, emphasising the role of verbal reflection on the music-making. Others conceive of their work as having to do with the social (and hence interpersonal) affordances of music itself, describing their work as 'music centred'. They place emphasis on the musical relating that happens moment by moment. Nevertheless, common theoretical ground lies in the notion of 'communicative musicality' (Trevarthen & Malloch, 2000). This suggests that people are born hard-wired for and predisposed to musical interaction. From birth we use musical features improvisationally to develop communication and relationship with our primary carers and hence, ultimately, a sense of self.

Music therapists typically have a room full of different types of instruments available to their clients (as well as to themselves) to play. The music in music therapy is usually improvised, since this enables the therapist to be led very much by the client's musical self-presentation. Unlike in speech, in musical interaction it is possible to give people a sense of being supported, responded to or even offered new experiences of self while they are themselves producing continuously; there is no prerequisite for turn-taking. To take a crude example, someone who is drumming continually can be accompanied with a matching tempo, but the strategic use by the music therapist of other musical features in addition, such as harmony or melody or idiomatic style, can dramatically recontextualise that person's experience of his or her own playing. This may ultimately lead to shifts in tempo too. Likewise, people whose playing is sparse and unconnected can be given an experience of 'joined-up-ness' and being drawn into greater commitment to participation and relating by the accompanying therapist. People whose presentation is chaotic can find themselves being 'organised' by clear musical structure. Clients often report surprise at the extent to which they feel listened to or accompanied, or invited into new ways of interacting. Music therapy may equally make use of familiar musical material – for example, songs known to and valued by the client. It may also involve the writing of songs or other forms of music, the development of musical skills, and lead to performance.

Dance movement psychotherapy

'The dance' has always been important in human society because of its essentially transformative ability, for example in wedding rituals, religious ceremonies and harvest celebrations. It provides a medium through which body and psyche are brought together, allowing for the expression of thoughts and feelings. Movement therapy developed out of natural health movements, reformist gymnastics and health pedagogies. Its aim is to improve well-being through creative techniques that allow individuals to use their natural and liberated breathing and movement pattern. From the mid-20th century, the use of movement and dance has become more formalised in healthcare settings, both clinically and also in respect of general health promotion.

The professional body, the Association for Dance Movement Psychotherapy UK (ADMP UK), defines dance movement psychotherapy (DMP) as follows:

> DMP is the psychotherapeutic use of movement and dance through which a person can engage creatively in a process to further their emotional, cognitive, physical and social integration. It is founded on the principle that movement reflects an individual's patterns of thinking and feeling. Through acknowledging and supporting clients' movements the therapist encourages development and integration of new adaptive movement patterns together with the emotional experiences that accompany such changes. Dance Movement Psychotherapy is practised as both individual and group therapy in health, education and social service settings and in private practice. (http://www.admt.org.uk)

It adheres to the same general psychotherapeutic principles as other forms of psychotherapy, including creating a consistent, safe, therapeutic space, maintaining appropriate therapeutic boundaries, and being mindful of transference and countertransference issues. In addition, in group work, DMP attends to the stages of development of the group and to the complex psychological dynamics, projections and relationships that may emerge between group members. DMP has a unique position within creative therapies, straddling the body psychotherapy approaches in its use of the body and movement and the arts psychotherapy approaches in its use of dance as a creative medium, and offering the opportunity for expressive symbolic movement work.

Body psychotherapy (BPT) is deeply rooted within depth psychology frameworks and, in its modern version, BPT can be provided as a form of embodied relational psychotherapy (e.g. Hartley, 2009), while sharing some historic roots with DMP in respect of influences from reformist gymnastics and health pedagogies (Geuter, 2006). Both BPT and DMP utilise the creative potential of the 'body in motion' as a means of identifying psychological processes and habitual patterns of responses to adversity or conflict, and also in respect of emotional expressiveness, communication and solution-focused work. Given this overlap and for the purpose of this overview, the authors include both DMP and BPT under the umbrella term 'body-oriented psychological therapies'.

The evidence base

The emerging evidence base from clinical trials points towards disorder-specific areas of effectiveness for creative, arts, non-verbal therapies. The approaches require clear training and supervision strategies to ensure adherence to the fidelity of the particular model being employed and cost-effective delivery. This overview is focused on clinical trials and systematic (e.g. Cochrane) reviews and randomised control trials (RCTs). Clinical, naturalistic and case-based outcome studies are reported elsewhere (e.g. Röhricht, 2000, 2009; Gilroy, 2006; Hartley, 2009; Stige & Aarø, 2011).

Schizophrenia

Negative symptoms can be long-standing and may seriously affect a service user's social inclusion, hence hampering recovery. The best evidence base is currently available for music therapy (eight studies) and body-oriented psychological therapy (three RCTs and a multicentre trial under way).

The findings from the MATISSE trial (Crawford *et al*, 2012) have brought into question outcomes from earlier art therapy trials (Green *et al*, 1987; Richardson *et al*, 2007) considered by the schizophrenia update from the National Institute for Clinical Excellence (2009). There are case studies pointing towards good effects of art therapy in individual therapy settings and as an adjunct for in-patient treatment, enabling patients with an acute psychosis to use the art medium in order to express themselves and illustrate their difficult-to-verbalise experiences (e.g. Killick, 1991, 1997, 2000).

A Cochrane review on music therapy (Mössler *et al*, 2013) concluded that 'Music therapy as an addition to standard care helps people with schizophrenia to improve their global state, mental state (including negative symptoms) and social functioning if a sufficient number of music therapy sessions are provided by qualified music therapists'. It includes an exploratory RCT by Talwar *et al* (2006), which is unusual in that it examines fairly typical UK music therapy practice in in-patient settings. Crawford & Patterson (2007) identify music therapy as the arts therapy for which there is most evidence as an intervention for people with schizophrenia.

Randomised control trials of BPT in chronic schizophrenia (Nitsun *et al*, 1974; Röhricht & Priebe, 2006) found that patients receiving BPT had significantly lower scores for negative symptoms after treatment. Another clinical trial has since been published (Röhricht *et al*, 2011) and the results of this naturalistic study are consistent with findings from previous RCTs, indicating that BPT is associated with reduced negative symptoms.

A Cochrane review on drama therapy in schizophrenia (Ruddy & Dent-Brown, 2008) identified five studies that met the inclusion criteria, but owing to significant methodological problems the authors were unable to reach conclusive findings.

Two more RCT studies have been completed recently utilising the same manual (Röhricht, 2000) for chronic schizophrenia, but at the time of writing their results are not yet published. Whereas one study conducted at the University of Heidelberg in Germany replicated the positive findings and demonstrated similar benefits (S. Koch, personal communication, 2015), a multicentre trial across four sites in the UK did not; the trial showed that patients' expressive behaviour significantly improved post-treatment (as compared with patient groups receiving Pilates), but PANSS-measured negative symptoms did not change (further details available from the authors). This has important implications for future research aiming to identify predictors for treatment response, investigating whether longer-term treatments (i.e. 40 sessions instead of short treatments with 10–20 sessions) are required for patients with very chronic severe conditions to achieve effects on negative symptoms for most patients (allowing improvements in range of expressive behaviour to translate into more substantial, clinically significant improvements).

Depression

There are a number of effective, evidence-based treatments provided for depressive disorders, mainly cognitive–behavioural therapy, interpersonal psychotherapy and psychodynamic psychotherapy. However, about 20% of patients do not recover within 2 years and at least 10% of patients have chronic depression. The effectiveness of arts psychotherapy among patients with severe (and chronic) depression has so far been insufficiently addressed in research. Clinical cohort studies point towards positive effects of dance/movement psychotherapy and BPT on depressive and anxiety symptoms (e.g. Brooks & Stark, 1989; Weber *et al*, 1994; Koemeda-Lutz *et al*, 2006; Koch *et al*, 2007). Stewart *et al* (2004) carried out a study (randomised single-case experimental design) on movement therapy in a sample of in-patients with depression and found that the therapy had a positive effect on mood. In an RCT pilot study, Röhricht *et al* (2013) demonstrated good efficacy for BPT on core depressive symptoms and improved self-esteem despite the participants having treatment-refractory conditions.

A Cochrane review on music therapy in depression (Maratos *et al*, 2008) identified five studies for evaluation that met the inclusion criteria; despite methodological shortcomings it concluded that music therapy is accepted by patients with depression and that the therapy is associated with improvements in mood. Erkkilä *et al* (2011) conducted another successful RCT on individual music therapy for depression.

Post-traumatic stress disorder and other stress disorders

Several outcome studies (predominantly case studies – e.g. Grigsby, 1987; Morgan & Johnson, 1995; Gantt & Tinnin, 2007; Greenwood, 2011) suggest the effectiveness of short-term group and individual art therapy for patients with post-traumatic stress disorder (PTSD) and other stress disorders. The main effects are a decrease in anxiety and depression and symptoms of PTSD, and improvements in self-esteem (Gilroy, 2006). One exploratory RCT of music therapy in a group of patients with persistent PTSD (Carr *et al*, 2012) demonstrated good feasibility and effectiveness for those who had not sufficiently responded to cognitive–behavioural therapy. There is only preliminary evidence for BPT in this patient group. A pilot RCT with a small sample of patients who had experienced childhood sexual abuse confirmed the results from an earlier study (Mattsson *et al*, 1998) and suggested that body-oriented therapy is efficacious as an adjunct to psychotherapy in sexual abuse recovery and for patients with PTSD (Price, 2006; Price *et al*, 2007).

Personality disorder

Studies indicate that art therapy can improve the management of highly charged emotional experiences, ameliorating destructive tendencies. Initial reports suggest the use of body-oriented psychological therapy in specific personality disorders such as borderline disorder (Gottschalk & Boekholt, 2004); for those disorders the focus in BPT is directed towards stabilising experiences, fostering coherent self-experiences across the domains of movement (action), perception and affect and the containing elements in BPT with regard to a holding therapeutic relationship. Discussing BPT for borderline personality disorders, Röhricht (2015) emphasised the importance of 'BPT strategies that seek to foster ego-maturation processes retrospectively, with non-verbal communication/interaction/empathy at its heart...sometimes the therapist will provide functions of an auxiliary ego' (p. 62).

Autism spectrum disorder

The results from a Cochrane review (Gold *et al*, 2010) indicate that music therapy may help children with autistic spectrum disorder improve their communicative skills. According to Gilroy (2006), individual art therapy is effective in promoting cognitive and emotional development, enabling relationships and lessening destructive behaviour.

Examples of good practice – bridging the gap

The cultural and well-being service 'blueSCI' in Trafford

The not-for-profit mental health arts, cultural and well-being service 'blueSCI' was founded in Trafford in 2004 by Stuart Webster, a professional contemporary artist, and Alicia Clare, a registered mental health nurse and modern matron of the local mental health in-patient unit (Clare *et al*, 2007). The concept for blueSCI emerged as a natural response from their work on an acute mental health in-patient unit, where they commissioned professional contemporary artists, who used a variety of art forms, including video, music, dance, drama, stone-carving and interior design. All the art activities were accessible and designed to engage with the in-patient community, viewing staff, patients and visitors as equal members of that community. This approach resulted in patients working alongside staff at all levels, including consultant psychiatrists, domestic staff and nurses. Together, they commenced a creative journey as willing participants. The approach was so successful in engaging patients in a meaningful way that patients discharged from the unit did not want to leave because they had not finished their artwork. This resulted in the discharged patients providing peer support to those still on the ward when they returned for a time to complete their artwork. blueSCI was created to meet this identified

Box 13.1 The music group at blueSCI

In response to requests 'blueSCI' commissioned a professional musician and recording artist to run a weekly music activity. The music sessions (as in all blueSCI activities) had a low entry level, i.e. an interest in music was sufficient to join. Members attending helped shape the direction of the weekly sessions which allowed it to grow, bottom up. Members set up a community bank account and were provided with support to apply for grants. This funded a recording studio in a space identified in the blueSCI building. The Seed Studio was designed by a respected musician and producer, who continue providing an advisory role to the studio, giving it credibility as a professional community music studio. This attracted professional musicians who have since recorded at the studio and who run free workshops. Members at the studio have performed in public. The studio has become recognised in its own right and receives contracts for services which provide opportunities for members to be commissioned along with other artists to deliver programmes of work. Alongside the high-level arts activity taking place, the studio has not lost sight of its fundamental purpose and membership remains open only for people who currently, or have previously, accessed the blueSCI service. The studio members engage with musicians, who use the studio and reciprocate by sharing their skills with others.

Box 13.2 The Seymour Poets at blueSCI

Seymour Poets is an informal poetry group that was formed by individuals coming together through a shared interest in spoken and written poetry and creative writing. The group is supported by volunteers who have an interest in poetry. blueSCI provides the group with free meeting space and has assisted them in applying for funding for projects. One such project brought together a visual arts group, the poetry group and two artists (a visual artist and a poet). The arts group provided artworks to illustrate a book of personal recovery stories and poems produced by Seymour Poets. The poems and stories were performed at a public launch, which included performances of new personal recordings by Seed Studio members. The book is available for purchase with money raised going back to support the group. The group continues to meet beyond the funded projects and individuals can join or leave at any point, the focus of common interest being the arts activity.

need, providing patients on discharge with an opportunity to participate continuously in high-quality arts and cultural engagement. It provided an opportunity to achieve, to recognise ability, to improve self-esteem and to create positive social networks and sustainable partnerships with mainstream cultural organisations.

blueSCI was established as a community service positioned in the third sector and this allows the service to be modelled to the context of life recovery principles (as opposed to a medical or clinical recovery approach; Collier, 2010). The approach removes the requirement to identify with a medical diagnosis in order to access the service. The service enables individuals to work towards their chosen goals, for example the wish to recover the skills to ride a bike, or to recover confidence to undertake cultural creative activities (Box 13.1 and Box 13.2). The service functions as a support to access the wider community rather than as an escape from it. This is underpinned with active engagement with mainstream partners as opposed to mental health partners, taking a 'critical friend' approach to influence, challenge and support.

blueSCI promotes ethics and values of respect, individual rights, freedom from discrimination and social capital. It is important to ensure that the positive emotional environment is reflected in the physical environment. This was achieved by refurbishing a council community building. It was converted into a high-quality cultural centre that includes an internet café and an artist-designed backlit reception area; solid oak is used throughout the café area to avoid the tired chipped laminate look often seen in day service environments. The building provides a positive first impression to negate any feeling of 'I'm not welcome here'.

The delivery approach of blueSCI is fundamentally a creative process that is able to respond and adapt to the influences of its partners, the community context and people who access the service. The true value of the people who access the service is recognised and they are encouraged to share their skills, knowledge and experience by delivering the service through volunteering, commissioned work or paid work (Webber, 2012). The 'Connecting People study' of social capital highlights the importance of this way of working in order to engage local people and local solutions that influence the service (Webber, 2012). This 'can do' culture is underpinned by professional contemporary arts practice, with blueSCI providing a well-being infrastructure for a number of arts organisations.

The professional artists commissioned by blueSCI do not have a clinical background or badge themselves as 'arts in health' practitioners; they are recognised artists within their field who have good communication skills and a passion for what they do. This demonstrates an equality to these dynamic relationships in that they are based on shared interest and mutual respect that each chooses to share about themselves. This is in contrast to traditional services, where relationships are more commonly based on the 'health professional' holding more personal knowledge and in turn power, thus creating the potential for a power struggle.

The key ways of working that support the arts and cultural practice at blueSCI are as follows.

- This way of working is based upon the natural way in which people form relationships. It is not forced or prescribed.
- The culture of the blueSCI team incorporates everyone.
- Access to the service is immediate because it does not rely on 'staff assessing what you need', but rather is best described as a 'if you think the service is for you then it is' approach.

- Having a 'can do' culture means that people talk openly about their ideas, dreams and aspirations and work collectively to overcome barriers and find solutions. There is no 'ask the staff', because who are the staff?
- People own the service and its assets (background, skills, knowledge, networks and resources) and enhance it by sharing their own assets.

People genuinely identify that 'giving' (one of the five ways to well-being) – accessing the service and in turn delivering the service – is a main factor in improving their well-being and ability to cope with life's difficulties. People who attend the service have a sense of purpose.

'Core Arts', promoting mental health service in East London

This service was developed in 1992 by the artist Paul Monks, using vacant space in the old Hackney Hospital in East London. The website highlights the background for this initiative:

> His studio became a haven for artistic expression, as curious patients seeking refuge from the monotony of life on the psychiatric ward immersed themselves in a world of paint. (http://www.corearts.co.uk)

As a registered charity, Core Arts is promoting the artistic and creative abilities of people who experience severe and enduring mental health problems. The service offers a range of artistic activities in classes, courses and workshops, spanning art, music, creative writing and multimedia activities. Core Arts is accessible for service users with identified mental health problems who are resident in the Borough of Hackney. Following a recovery-oriented ethos, the programme is provided by professional artists and focuses on 'what people can achieve, supporting them to increase their capacity for innovation and learning, problem-solving, confidence and leadership skills'. The service also offers open-access activities, a gardening and horticultural service, and organises events in which participants can perform in public.

'Thinking about Looking', Newham, London

'Thinking about Looking' is a partnership between Newham Centre for Mental Health and Tate Modern, initiated by Sheila Grandison (head of arts therapy in Newham). With an active commitment to social justice, this partnership bridges hospital and gallery and brings together the cultural policy and mental health agendas of access and inclusion.

The London Borough of Newham is one of the most culturally diverse and socioeconomically deprived areas in England. Recognising the cultural diversity of East London and how contemporary visual art practice can be integrated into ways of exploring identity and cultural diversity is central to the partnership. In the 'Thinking about Looking' programme, culturally diverse adults, at different points of their recovery, including during their acute admissions, come together and engage with the national resource of modern and contemporary art. Users of mental health services work alongside their professional and family carers in group study days in the busy, high-profile public gallery spaces at Tate Modern. Almost all participants are first-time gallery visitors, and for user participants the group study days are destigmatising. They provide the opportunity for shared learning in a public space as equal members of the public. All participants have the opportunity to join wider gallery networks and peer-led projects. Feedback regarding what was experienced as satisfying in the group study days at the Tate include: 'It opens your mind to other possibilities', 'Standing up and talking about art you like to the group', 'Being with everybody in the energy room', 'When you are at Tate Modern you feel free', 'I found the experience very good by concentrating and found that I enjoyed every minute', 'Can I come to the Tate again?'

Acknowledgements

The authors would like to thank colleagues who contributed descriptions of good practice across a wide range of settings, which helped to shape the core of this text. We are particularly grateful for contributions regarding the modality-specific information to Sheila Grandison (art therapy), Aleka Loutsis (drama therapy) and Nina Papadopoulos (dance movement psychotherapy).

References

Brooks D, Stark A (1989) The effect of dance/movement therapy on affect: a pilot study. *American Journal of Dance Therapy*, **11**: 101–11.

Carr C, d'Ardenne P, Sloboda A, *et al* (2012) Group music therapy for patients with persistent post-traumatic stress disorder – an exploratory randomized controlled trial with mixed methods evaluation. *Psychology and Psychotherapy*, **85**: 179–202.

Clare A, Collier E, Higgin S (2007) Enabling mental health through social and cultural inclusion. *A Life in the Day*, **11**: 22–6.

Collier E (2010) Confusion of recovery: one solution. *International Journal of Mental Health Nursing*, **19**: 16–21.

Crawford M, Patterson S (2007) Arts therapies for people with schizophrenia: an emerging evidence base. *Evidence Based Mental Health*, **10**: 69–70.

Crawford M, Killaspy H, Barnes TR, *et al* (2012) Group art therapy as an adjunctive treatment for people with schizophrenia: multicentre pragmatic randomised trial. *BMJ*, **344**: e846.

Erkkilä J, Punkanen M, Fachner J, *et al* (2011) Individual music therapy for depression: randomised controlled trial. *British Journal of Psychiatry*, **199**: 132–9.

Gantt L, Tinnin LW (2007) Intensive trauma therapy of PTSD and dissociation: an outcome study. *The Arts in Psychotherapy*, **34**: 68–80.

Geuter U (2006) Geschichte der Körperpsychotherapie. [History of body psychotherapy.] In *Handbuch der Körperpsychotherapie* [*Handbook of Body Psychotherapy*] (eds G Marlock, H Weiss): 17–32. Schattauer.

Gilroy A (2006) *Art Therapy: Research and Evidence-based Practice*. Sage.

Gold C, Wigram T, Elefant C (2010) Music therapy for autistic spectrum disorder. *Cochrane Database of Systematic Reviews*, **19**: CD004381.

Gottschalk G, Boekholt C (2004) Body-therapeutic work with borderline patients. *Persönlichkeitsstörungen Theorie und Therapie*, **8**: 154–60.

Green BL, Wehling C, Talsky GJ (1987) Group art therapy as an adjunct to treatment for chronic outpatients. *Hospital and Community Psychiatry*, **38**: 988–91.

Greenwood H (2011) Long term individual art psychotherapy. Art for art's sake: The effect of early relational trauma. *International Journal of Art Therapy*, **16**: 41–51.

Grigsby JP (1987) Single case study: the use of imagery in the treatment of posttraumatic stress disorder. *Journal of Nervous and Mental Disease*, **175**: 55–9.

Hartley E (ed) (2009) *Contemporary Body Psychotherapy: The Chiron Approach*. Routledge.

Killick K (1991) The practice of art therapy with patients in acute psychotic states. *Inscape*, winter: 2–6.

Killick K (1997) Unintegration and containment in acute psychosis. In *Art, Psychotherapy and Psychosis* (eds K Killick, J Schaverien): 38–51. Routledge.

Killick K (2000) The art room as container in analytical art psychotherapy with patients in psychotic states. In *The Changing Shape of Art Therapy* (eds A Gilroy, G McNeilly): 99–114. Jessica Kingsley.

Koch SC, Morlinghaus K, Fuchs T (2007) The joy dance. *Specific effects of a single dance intervention on psychiatric patients with depression. The Arts in Psychotherapy*, **34**: 340–9.

Koemeda-Lutz M, Kaschke M, Revenstorf D, *et al* (2006) Evaluation der Wirksamkeit von ambulanten Körperpsychotherapien – EWAK. Eine Multizenterstudie in Deutschland und der Schweiz [Evaluation of the efficacy of outpatient psychotherapies body – EWAK. A multicenter study in Germany and Switzerland]. *Psychotherapie Psychosomatik medizinische Psychologie*, **56**: 1–8.

Maratos AS, Gold C, Wang X, *et al* (2008) Music therapy for depression. *Cochrane Database of Systematic Reviews* 1: CD004517.pub2.

Mattsson M, Wikman M, Dahlgren L, *et al* (1998) Body awareness therapy with sexually abused women. Part 2: Evaluation of body awareness in a group setting. *Journal of Bodywork and Movement Therapies*, **2**: 38–45.

Morgan C, Johnson D (1995) Use of a drawing task in the treatment of nightmares in combat-related post-traumatic stress disorder. *Art Therapy Journal of the American Association of Art Therapists*, **12**: 244–7.

Mössler K, Chen X, Heldal TO, *et al* (2013) Music therapy for people with schizophrenia and schizophrenia-like disorders. *Cochrane Database of Systematic Reviews*, **12**: CD004025.pub3.

National Institute for Clinical Excellence (2009) *Schizophrenia: Core Interventions in the Treatment and Management of Schizophrenia in Adults in Primary and Secondary Care*. NICE.

Nitsun M, Stapleton JH, Bender MP (1974) Movement and drama therapy with long-stay schizophrenics. *British Journal of Medical Psychology*, **47**: 101–19.

Pavlicevic M, Ansdell G (eds) (2004) *Community Music Therapy*. Jessica Kingsley.

Price CJ (2006) Body-oriented therapy in sexual abuse recovery: a pilot-test comparison. *Journal of Bodywork and Movement Therapies*, **10**: 58–64.

Price CJ, McBride B, Hyerle L, *et al* (2007) Mindful awareness in body-oriented therapy for female veterans with post-traumatic stress disorder taking prescription analgesics for chronic pain: a feasibility study. *Alternative Therapies in Health and Medicine*, **13**: 32–40.

Richardson P, Jones K, Evans C, *et al* (2007) Exploratory RCT of art therapy as an adjunctive treatment in schizophrenia. *Journal of Mental Health*, **16**: 483–91.

Röhricht F (2000) *Die körperorientierte Psychotherapie psychischer Störungen. Ein Leitfaden für Forschung und Praxis. [Body-Oriented Psychotherapy in Mental Illness. A Manual for Research and Practice.]* Hogrefe.

Röhricht F (2009) Body oriented psychotherapy – the state of the art in empirical research and evidence based practice: a clinical perspective. *Body, Movement and Dance in Psychotherapy. An International Journal for Theory, Research and Practice*, **4**: 135–56.

Röhricht F (2015) Body psychotherapy for the treatment of severe mental disorders – an overview. *Body, Movement and Dance in Psychotherapy: An International Journal for Theory, Research and Practice*, **10**: 51–67.

Röhricht F, Priebe S (2006) Effect of body oriented psychological therapy on negative symptoms in schizophrenia: a randomised controlled trial. *Psychological Medicine*, **36**: 669–78.

Röhricht F, Papadopoulos N, Holden S, *et al* (2011) Clinical effectiveness and therapeutic processes of body psychotherapy in chronic schizophrenia – an open clinical trial. *Arts in Psychotherapy*, **38**: 196–203.

Röhricht F, Papadopoulos N, Priebe S (2013) An exploratory randomized controlled trial of body psychotherapy for patients with chronic depression. *Journal of Affective Disorders*, **151**: 85–91.

Ruddy R, Dent-Brown K (2008) Drama therapy for schizophrenia or schizophrenia-like illnesses (Review). *Cochrane Database of Systematic Reviews*, **1**: CD005378.pub2.

Stewart NJ, McMullen LM, Rubin LD (2004) Movement therapy with depressed inpatients: a randomized multiple single case design. *Archives of Psychiatric Nursing*, **8**: 22–9.

Stige B, Aarø LE (2011) *Invitation to Community Music Therapy*. Routledge.

Talwar N, Crawford MJ, Maratos A, *et al* (2006) Music therapy for in-patients with schizophrenia. Exploratory randomised controlled trial. *British Journal of Psychiatry*, **189**: 405–9.

Trevarthen C, Malloch SN (2000) The dance of well-being: defining the musical therapeutic effect. *Nordic Journal of Music Therapy*, **9**: 3–17.

Warner R (2010) Does the scientific evidence support the recovery model? *The Psychiatrist*, **34**: 3–5.

Webber M (2012) *The Role of the Third Sector in Social Capital Enhancement and Mobilisation: Evidence from an Ethnographic Study*. King's College London.

Weber C, Haltenhof H, Combecher J, *et al* (1994) Bewegungstherapie bei Patienten mit psychischen Störungen: Eine Verlaufsstudie. [Exercise therapy in patients with mental disorders: a longitudinal study.] In *Salutogenese: ein neues Konzept in der Psychosomatik? [Salutogenesis: a new concept in psychosomatic?]* (eds F Lamprecht, R Johnen): 536–43. Verlag für Akademische Schriften.

Woodcock J (2003) Comment – art therapy and family therapy'. *Journal of Family Therapy*, **25**: 233–5.

CHAPTER 14

Management of medication when treatment is failing

Georgina Boon, Melinda Sweeting and James MacCabe

Introduction

Pharmacological treatment plays an essential role in the treatment, care and support of people experiencing major mental illnesses. In this chapter we discuss how to assess and then optimise medication management for people with schizophrenia and schizoaffective disorder, the most common conditions resulting in referral to psychiatric rehabilitation services, from the perspective of the clinician taking over responsibility for treatment. We focus on people who are identified as 'treatment resistant', that is, remain significantly symptomatic despite standard care, and the practicalities of prescribing clozapine. We have constructed this chapter to address five key issues in medication management: establishing treatment resistance, managing treatment resistance, maximising adherence, managing adverse effects and adhering to the schizophrenia guidelines from the National Institute for Health and Care Excellence (NICE) (2014).

Establishing treatment resistance

The NICE schizophrenia guidelines define treatment-resistant schizophrenia as a lack of satisfactory clinical improvement despite the sequential use of the recommended doses for 4–6 weeks of at least two antipsychotics, at least one of which is a second-generation antipsychotic. Before one can conclude that an individual is treatment resistant, it is important to review thoroughly key aspects of previous and current medication (see Box 14.1).

The clinician should review the patient's history at this stage, which enables a critical evaluation of the diagnosis(es). It is important to consider comorbid or primary disorders that might have been missed, such as an organic mental disorder (e.g. temporal lobe epilepsy) or autism spectrum disorder. Equally, one should review the current symptoms to ensure that treatment is effectively targeting those that are distressing the patient and carers. Reviewing the medication history is important: what worked in the past might be effective again now. Similarly, it is important to assess previous adherence to treatment, drug levels where available and, finally, to evaluate side-effects.

Box 14.1 Approaches to the assessment of the patient whose symptoms persist

Review the patient's history
- Is the diagnosis correct?
- Have organic mental illnesses been excluded?
- Are there any unaddressed perpetuating factors?
- Have psychosocial difficulties been addressed?
- What are the views of the patient and carer and how might these be affecting symptoms or adherence?

Review patient's current symptoms
- Are the psychotic symptoms primary?
- Does the patient have affective symptoms and are they being treated?
- Does the patient have anxiety symptoms and are they being treated?

Review medication history, current use and patient's knowledge
- What has been tried before?
- What worked and what didn't (including doses, levels, evidence of adherence, adverse effects)?
- If there are other family members with the illness, what treatment did they have and was it successful?
- What medication is the patient taking now? And how was it chosen? (By the patient, carer and/or professional?)

Is the patient adhering to the medication regimen?
- Have blood medication levels been assessed? Simple blood tests to determine levels have been found to be useful for clozapine, olanzapine, amisulpride, valproate, lamotrigine, lithium and some tricyclic antidepressants
- If the patient is not compliant, why not? Do they have insight? Do they have side-effects from existing medications?

Can side-effects be addressed?
- Is the patient taking as few medications as possible? Are minimum effective doses being prescribed?
- Can the patient be switched to an alternative antipsychotic to alleviate side-effects?

At this point one should be in a position to identify the best treatment options, in terms of medication and psychological and social interventions. Treatment options should be discussed in as much detail as possible with the patient and any involved carer and this discussion recorded in the case-notes (NICE, 2014). The better the patient and carer(s) understand the illness and the available treatments, including medication, the more informed their choices can be. Being given choice should increase treatment adherence and encourage patients on their way to recovery (both in the sense of decreased symptoms and, just as importantly, in gaining autonomy in the management of the illness). Active dialogue about treatment options should, of course, continue even when the individual is being treated under mental health legislation.

Managing treatment resistance

The role of clozapine

Clozapine is the treatment of choice in treatment-resistant schizophrenia and is the only antipsychotic that has robustly demonstrated effectiveness in treatment-resistant illness (Davis *et al*, 2003). Early use of clozapine is much more likely than anything else to be successful (Agid *et al*, 2011). Although not in its product licence, clozapine is also an effective antimanic agent.

The most well known of clozapine's side-effects are neutropenia and agranulocytosis, which initially resulted in its withdrawal from most markets in the world. Since its reintroduction, close haematological monitoring has been mandatory with clozapine. With haematological monitoring in place, weight gain and its consequences, impaired glucose tolerance and constipation are, in practice, more concerning. Early side-effects include sedation, hypersalivation, hypertension, hypotension, tachycardia, fever, nausea and constipation (which may become life-threatening in cases of intestinal obstruction). A combination of tachycardia and fever may indicate myocarditis. There is anecdotal evidence that clozapine may be associated with an increased risk of chest infections, which may prove fatal (Taylor *et al*, 2009). Although this has not yet been reported extensively in the medical literature, clinicians should be aware that if pneumonia occurs in a patient taking clozapine, with no other obvious risk factors, clozapine may be considered a possible cause. Nocturnal enuresis is common and distressing, and the risk of seizures increases during titration and at higher plasma levels. Other rare but serious side-effects include thromboembolism and cardiomyopathy.

General principles for commencing clozapine

The general eligibility criteria for commencing clozapine are that:

- the patient, when well, is willing to take oral medication and allow blood tests
- symptoms are resistant to at least two other antipsychotics (one of which is a second-generation drug)
- if possible, the patient gives informed consent to taking the drug and understands both the risks and potential benefits associated with it.

Although it is possible to commence clozapine on an out-patient or day-patient basis, for people who have a history of non-adherence or substance misuse, who present a risk to themselves or others, or who have physical health problems, treatment may have to be started in hospital. Before prescribing clozapine, the clinician must review the patient's medical history, checking in particular that there is no history of significant cardiac problems, seizures, agranulocytosis or active liver disease. The *Maudsley*

Prescribing Guidelines (Taylor *et al*, 2012*a*) recommend baseline measurement of full blood count, glucose, HbA$_{1c}$ (glycosylated haemoglobin, type 1c), liver function, pulse rate, blood pressure, temperature, weight, body mass index (BMI), waist circumference, lipids and electrocardiogram (ECG). These tests allow monitoring for some of the documented adverse effects of clozapine. Determination of baseline urea and electrolyte levels, fasting blood lipid levels and creatine phosphokinase level is also recommended. Consideration can also be given to monitoring plasma troponin and C-reactive protein in the first 6 weeks, especially if there is any suspicion of myocarditis. Any patient prescribed clozapine must also be registered with a clozapine monitoring service. In the UK there are currently three brands of clozapine available (Clozaril, Zaponex and Denzapine) and therefore three different monitoring services: Clozaril Patient Monitoring Service, Zaponex Treatment Access System and Denzapine Monitoring System.

The *Maudsley Prescribing Guidelines* (Taylor *et al*, 2012*a*) provide a titration regimen for in-patient and out-patient initiation of prescribing, the latter being significantly slower. The standard in-patient titration regimen results in a dose of 300 mg/day in divided doses after 15 days. If dose increases are required beyond 300 mg, they should be made in increments of 50 mg every 3 days, with the aim of achieving a trough level of 350–500 mg/L. It is recommended that blood serum levels are measured when the patient reaches a dose of 300 mg/day or earlier if the patient is elderly, of East Asian descent, female or a non-smoker, or if treatment non-adherence is suspected. Blood serum levels should also be checked following a change in smoking habit, as smoking may reduce plasma levels by up to 50% (Taylor *et al*, 2012*a*). It is recommended that an anticonvulsant (sodium valproate or lamotrigine) is considered as prophylaxis against seizures when plasma levels are above 500 mg/L (Varma *et al*, 2011).

If using the in-patient titration regimen, on initiating clozapine, blood pressure and pulse should be monitored hourly for the first 6 hours. Temperature, blood pressure and pulse should then be taken twice daily (as well as before and after the morning dose) for at least 2 weeks, or until there are no unacceptable adverse effects. Monitoring should continue daily or every other day (depending on the rate of titration) until a stable dose is reached. Thereafter, these parameters should be monitored when blood tests are taken. The *Maudsley Prescribing Guidelines* give recommendations on monitoring using the out-patient titration regimen.

With either regimen, staff should inform the prescriber if:

- the patient's temperature rises above 38°C (although it is important to note that elevated temperatures are common and clozapine does not usually need to be stopped in these situations)
- the pulse rate rises to more than 100 bpm or more than 20 bpm above baseline (which is also common, but important, as in rare cases it may be a sign of myocarditis, a severe and potentially fatal side-effect of clozapine)

- there is a postural blood pressure drop of greater than 30 mmHg
- the patient is clearly over-sedated or otherwise distressed by side-effects.

As with a number of other second-generation antipsychotics, weight gain is a major problem with clozapine and weight should be regularly monitored. The *Maudsley Prescribing Guidelines* provide additional recommendations for monitoring the metabolic and cardiac effects of clozapine and these are regularly updated as the evidence base expands. Much of the skill in using clozapine is in effectively managing its side-effects, which includes supporting the patient who is experiencing them. One of the disadvantages of clozapine is that if there is a break in treatment of over 48 hours it must be re-titrated, albeit at a faster rate than for drug-naïve patients. There is also some evidence that a rebound psychosis may occur on abrupt discontinuation of clozapine (Moncrieff, 2006).

Augmentation strategies

Full benefit from clozapine may take many months to emerge. If a patient continues to have distressing symptoms, even though clozapine is improving the illness, augmentation with other medications may be considered. Generally, a trial of at least 3 months should occur before augmentation is considered. When deciding on augmentation options, first consider whether the individual has symptoms that would suggest particular drugs. For example, for symptoms of mania consider adding a mood stabiliser, and for depression, an antidepressant. When considering the use of multiple medications, it is important to note the possibility of additional side-effects, pharmacological interactions, compliance and cost-effectiveness.

Meta-analyses (Cipriani *et al*, 2009; Taylor *et al*, 2012*b*) have concluded that there is evidence to show modest benefit in augmentation with a second antipsychotic, but it is not clear which medication is the most effective. Options include sulpiride (Shiloh *et al*, 1997), amisulpride (Munro *et al*, 2004) and risperidone (Yagcioglu *et al*, 2005; Weiner *et al*, 2010). Aripiprazole has limited evidence of therapeutic benefit when used for clozapine augmentation but can improve metabolic parameters (Fleischhacker *et al*, 2010; Muscatello *et al*, 2011).

A systematic review by Sommer *et al* (2012) also concluded that evidence for the efficacy of clozapine augmentation is scarce. Some improvement in symptom severity was seen with lamotrigine, topiramate, sulpiride, citalopram and CX516, an experimental glutamatergic agonist. However, all positive effects were either based on one outlying study or were derived from a single randomised controlled trial. It should be noted that topiramate has been reported to worsen psychosis in some patients (Dursun & Deakin, 2001; Millson *et al*, 2002.)

There are reasons to avoid olanzapine (it may increase the risk of agranulocytosis and compound metabolic adverse effects), and agents that have a documented effect on the QTc interval, for example pimozide, quetiapine and ziprasidone (the last of which is not licensed in the UK).

Many people with treatment-resistant psychosis have affective features to their illness, and there is some evidence that sodium valproate can be useful as an adjunctive treatment for these (Kando et al, 1994). It also has the advantage of being prophylactic against clozapine-induced seizures, used at the same doses and usual therapeutic range. However, sodium valproate is also commonly known to cause weight gain. Lamotrigine has been reported to be an effective augmenting agent at doses of up to 400 mg/day, with effects on both positive and negative symptoms (Tiihonen et al, 2009). Reported side-effects include hypersalivation, asthenia, rash, constipation, ejaculatory dysfunction and failing memory. One case of lamotrigine-associated agranulocytosis has been reported. Lithium has also been shown to be effective in augmentation of clozapine (Small et al, 2003) at plasma levels ≥ 0.5 mmol/L. Carbamazepine is not recommended for clozapine augmentation owing to the additive risk of agranulocytosis, neuroleptic malignant syndrome and lowering of clozapine serum levels. Phenytoin should not be used because of the risk of agranulocytosis.

Trials of augmentation with antidepressants are sparse and conflicting. Selective serotonin reuptake inhibitors may increase clozapine serum levels and should therefore be used with caution because side-effects may be exacerbated. The exception is citalopram, which has been shown to improve negative symptoms compared with placebo (Sommer et al, 2012) and is probably therefore the drug of choice in treating comorbid depression. Citalopram is associated with dose-dependent prolongation of the QT interval and should not be used in those with congenital long QT syndrome, known pre-existing QT interval prolongation, or in combination with other medicines that prolong the QT interval. Electrolyte disturbances should be corrected before the patient starts treatment and an ECG should be considered for patients with cardiac disease.

There have been several double-blind randomised trials of the use of omega 3 fatty acids as augmentation agents. On balance, although doubts remain about the extent of the effects, it appears that omega 3 fatty acids may be a worthwhile augmentation option, particularly as they are cheap and well tolerated (Taylor et al, 2012a).

There are some case reports of the safe use of electroconvulsive therapy (ECT) as an adjunctive agent, although a lengthening of seizures has been noted. ECT, combined with antipsychotic drugs, may be considered an option when rapid global improvement and reduction of symptoms is desired. There is some evidence to show that using ECT in combination with antipsychotic drugs results in greater improvement in mental state than with antipsychotics alone (Tharyan & Adams, 2005).

Demjaha et al (2013) have shown that treatment resistance in schizophrenia is associated with a combination of relatively normal striatal dopamine synthesis and elevated levels of glutamate in the anterior cingulate cortex. Substances acting on the glutamate system may improve symptoms when added to regular antipsychotic medication, although the evidence base is too limited to allow for firm conclusions (Tiihonen & Wahlbeck, 2006). Currently, glutaminergic drugs are not available for clinical use.

Haematological rechallenge with clozapine

Because patients requiring clozapine are by definition unresponsive to other antipsychotics, if clozapine has been stopped owing to haematological side-effects, rechallenge may be discussed by patients, families and staff, despite the risks involved.

Approximately 2.7% of patients treated with clozapine develop neutropenia. Of these, half do so within the first 18 weeks of treatment and three-quarters by the end of the first year (Munro *et al*, 1999). The risk is not dose related. Of those rechallenged, one-third will again develop a blood dyscrasia, which is likely to be more severe than the first. The risks of rechallenge vary according to the cause and nature of the blood dyscrasia.

Neutropenia can arise because of factors unrelated or indirectly related to clozapine treatment, including coexisting medical conditions, concomitant medication and benign ethnic neutropenia (BEN, a normal ethnic reduction in the baseline levels of neutrophils).

After a neutropenic episode, the patient's individual clinical circum-stances must be taken into account. Close liaison with a local haematologist is imperative when considering rechallenge of clozapine after a blood dyscrasia. For patients taking clozapine, a diagnosis of BEN is important. In people with BEN, clozapine monitoring services allow a lower level of neutrophils without the need to stop clozapine treatment, in recognition of the lowered baseline levels. If non-clozapine causes of neutropenia are identified and eliminated (e.g. infections, bone marrow disease, lupus), clozapine may reasonably be restarted, with appropriate liaison and haematological monitoring.

Where low baseline levels of white blood cells continue to preclude the initiation of clozapine, despite consideration of a diagnosis of BEN, lithium may be used to increase neutrophil and total white blood cell counts (Taylor *et al*, 2012a). It is important to note that although lithium increases white cell counts, it does not protect against clozapine-induced agranulocytosis. One case of fatal agranulocytosis (Gerson *et al*, 1991) and one of treatment resistance to granulocyte/macrophage colony-stimulating factor (GM-CSF) (Valevski *et al*, 1993) have been reported with lithium and clozapine. If using lithium to boost white blood cells, aim for the same therapeutic blood range used in bipolar disorder, and monitor for symptoms of lithium toxicity (which can occur in the absence of raised lithium levels).

In exceptional circumstances, where severe and prolonged relapse occurs on cessation of clozapine, rechallenge may be tried after clozapine-induced neutropenia or agranulocytosis (Whiskey & Taylor, 2007). This is usually done in a specialist centre and is a very high-risk strategy that requires extreme vigilance. Facilities for close and frequent monitoring are essential and concurrent granulocyte colony stimulating factor (G-CSF) may be required, although it is important to note that G-CSF does not protect against agranulocytosis.

Rechallenge with clozapine after myocarditis and cardiomyopathy

The exact incidence of myocarditis and cardiomyopathy with clozapine is not known. An Australian study estimated the incidence of myocarditis to be around 1% of those treated (Haas *et al*, 2007). As with haematological rechallenge, close liaison with local physical health colleagues is essential. A local cardiologist should be identified prior to rechallenge in order to optimise any cardiac treatments and facilitate ECG monitoring once clozapine is restarted. If myocarditis or cardiomyopathy has been suspected in the past, intensive monitoring should be carried out upon rechallenge, to aid early detection of recurrence. However, any sign of heart failure should provoke immediate cessation of clozapine and referral to the local cardiologist. The *Maudsley Prescribing Guidelines* (Taylor *et al*, 2012a) detail a suggested monitoring procedure for myocarditis (from an Australian group), including echocardiography, troponin and C-reactive protein testing.

What if clozapine cannot be used?

Some patients are unable to tolerate clozapine or do not show symptom improvement after a reasonable trial. Pharmacological options for these individuals are very limited. It is doubtful that second-generation antipsychotics in standard doses would be effective alone in treatment-resistant schizophrenia and the practice of 'mega-dosage' therapy using first-generation antipsychotics is now discredited. High-dose olanzapine (30–60 mg/day) may be effective, although there are contradictory findings in the literature and its use at such doses is outside the product licence and risks increased likelihood of severe metabolic changes.

Electroconvulsive therapy is another option. The 2005 Cochrane review (Tharyan & Adams, 2005) concluded that courses of ECT can increase global improvement for some people with schizophrenia. The authors noted that even though the beneficial effect may not last beyond the short term, there is no clear evidence to refute the use of ECT in schizophrenia.

Using a combination of non-clozapine second-generation antipsychotics to treat patients with treatment-resistant illness who are intolerant to clozapine is common, despite a very sparse evidence base. Chan & Sweeting (2007) report that combinations using olanzapine with either amisulpride or risperidone, or quetiapine with risperidone, which act in theory on different receptor profiles, show improvement in symptoms in the limited data available, have been used frequently and on balance have more data on safety. A subsequent naturalistic observation study (Quintero *et al*,

2011) suggests benefit of quetiapine and amisulpride. Although there is no evidence of improved clinical symptoms of schizophrenia when aripiprazole is combined with other second-generation antipsychotics, it has been shown to reduce hyperprolactinaemia associated with risperidone (Chen *et al*, 2009) and improve metabolic parameters with clozapine, as mentioned previously in this chapter. Owing to the lack of data on safety, caution is recommended when combining non-clozapine second-generation antipsychotics, owing to the additive metabolic side-effects; increased monitoring of ECG, weight, blood glucose and other metabolic parameters is needed.

Maximising adherence

Ongoing symptoms may reflect non-adherence to medication regimens rather than true treatment resistance. Adherence to medication is likely to be greater if patients have input into choices of drugs and are aware of the likely benefits and potential side-effects of their medication and the treatment options available to ameliorate side-effects. Dolder *et al* (2003) reviewed the literature on interventions to improve adherence to antipsychotic medication. Combinations of educational and behavioural strategies appear to be the most successful in terms of adherence and secondary outcomes (such as symptoms, relapse and admissions).

In a meta-analysis by Nosé *et al* (2003) looking at clinical interventions for treatment non-adherence in psychosis, at a median follow-up of 6 months, these had more than doubled the likelihood of adherence to psychotropic

---

Box 14.2 Principles of compliance therapy

- Symptoms or problems reported by the patient are used as treatment targets
- The therapist openly predicts common misgivings about treatment, such as fears of addiction, loss of control, loss of personality. If the patient has any untoward fears, a cognitive approach is used to address them
- Confusion between illness symptoms and side-effects is discussed
- Any other meanings attached to medication are explored
- The natural tendency to stop medication if feeling well is discussed, in combination with an exploration of the patient's views of the consequences
- Indirect benefits of medication are highlighted, such as getting on better with other people
- The therapist tries to instil a feeling that poor adherence works against the patient's long-term goals, for example sustaining work, avoiding hospital, looking after children
- Certain metaphors are introduced, like 'medication offers a protective layer', 'medication is an insurance policy'

(After Kemp *et al*, 1998)

medications and attendance at scheduled appointments. The interventions included educational sessions, psychotherapeutic approaches and telephone prompts. One well-structured approach is compliance therapy (Kemp *et al*, 1998), which uses a combination of motivational interviewing and cognitive techniques to encourage individuals to reflect on their illness and the role that psychotropic treatment might play in its management (Box 14.2), although not all studies of compliance therapy have shown it to be superior to non-specific counselling (O'Donnell *et al*, 2003). Depot administration is recommended if non-adherence is a serious concern.

The use of depot and other preparations

Medication does not work if the patient does not take it or if therapeutic levels are not established. Unfortunately, simple blood tests to determine levels of antipsychotic medication are routinely available only for some agents. Systematic reviews suggest that 40–60% of patients with schizophrenia are partially or totally non-adherent to oral antipsychotic medication (Patel *et al*, 2009). Even in supervised settings, people may avoid taking prescribed treatment. Depot medication (using long-acting injectable preparations) should be considered if there is evidence that the individual has an established pattern of non-adherence with oral medication. The advantage of depot is that it is clear whether the medication has been taken or not. There is evidence that prescription of depot antipsychotic preparations improves treatment adherence in the long term (Leucht *et al*, 2011) and leads to reduced risk of hospitalisation (Haddad *et al*, 2009). Some patients prefer depot administration since it relieves them of responsibility for taking medication daily and provides a reason for regular contact with services. The choice of drug will depend on individual patient variation and side-effect profile, a detailed discussion of which is beyond the scope of this chapter. It is important to note that the pharmacokinetic properties of depot preparations make frequent dosage alteration illogical.

Risperidone, paliperidone, aripiprazole and olanzapine are the second-generation depot preparations available at the time of writing. In a study of risperidone long-acting injection, prior use of clozapine was associated with less-favourable outcomes compared with those of people not previously exposed to clozapine (Taylor & Cornelius, 2010). If depot risperidone is planned, the patient should be established on the oral preparation, and the full oral drug dose should be maintained for 3–4 weeks after the first injection. This ensures therapeutic plasma levels, and also reduces the risk of administering a long-acting drug that causes unacceptable side-effects.

Paliperidone, the major active metabolite of risperidone, is a monthly depot, whereas risperidone is given fortnightly. Following administration of paliperidone depot, active plasma levels are seen within a day or so, negating the need for co-administration of an oral preparation. Dosing consists of two initiation doses (deltoid) followed by monthly maintenance doses (deltoid or gluteal).

Olanzapine depot may be given every 2 or every 4 weeks. Again, the patient should be established on the oral preparation prior to the depot. Post-injection syndrome occurs after 0.07% of injections and is characterised by confusion and delirium, followed by profound sedation. Because of this risk, patients must be observed for 3 hours after administration. This requirement obviously presents challenges in terms of asking out-patients to remain in clinics for observation and the resources needed to provide this level of supervision as opposed to regular depot clinics where patients simply receive their dose and leave.

Aripiprazole, olanzapine and risperidone are also available in rapidly dispersing oral preparations that may aid healthcare professionals in ensuring compliance. Unless the patient has a strong preference, there is no obvious reason to continue to prescribe these preparations if concerns about compliance are no longer present, or observation by clinicians of dose administration is no longer occurring.

Managing adverse effects

Adverse effects of medication may create significant problems for patients, affecting their attitudes to their illness, medication adherence and their relationship with staff and carers. In the past, inadequate attention was paid to the burden of adverse effects of treatment, and some side-effects were under-recognised (e.g. the effects of antipsychotics and antidepressants on sexual functioning). Side-effects are commonly related to plasma levels, and so it is important when prescribing antipsychotics to use the minimum effective dose. Standard psychopharmacology textbooks such as those by Stahl (2013) and Taylor *et al* (2012*a*) provide accounts of the side-effect profiles of medications in common use; the latter also contains an extended discussion of side-effect management.

The greatest concerns of clinicians used to relate to the extrapyramidal effects of first-generation antipsychotics and the rare but potentially fatal neuroleptic malignant syndrome. With second-generation antipsychotics now dominating the market, concern has shifted to the physical health burden from these newer antipsychotics and the impact of the metabolic syndrome. This comprises obesity, dyslipidaemia, hypertension and impaired glucose tolerance. The rare occurrence of sudden death due to antipsychotics, which is thought to be related to ventricular arrhythmia, is also a concern. More recently, concerns about hyperprolactinaemia leading to possible increase risk of breast cancer and decreased bone mineral density have led to recommendations for routine monitoring of prolactin levels.

People with schizophrenia have an increased risk of dying from cardiovascular disorders, which is significantly exacerbated by smoking and obesity (Ohlsen & Gaughran, 2011). Weight gain is particularly associated with clozapine and olanzapine and is less likely with amisulpride and aripiprazole. A small volume of literature examining behavioural interventions to reduce weight gain has shown some positive results (Werneke *et al*, 2013) and this is discussed in more depth in Chapter 15, 'Physical healthcare'. It is important that patients are warned about the risks when starting on antipsychotics, that weight is monitored regularly and that dietetic advice is available. Switching to a medication with a lower propensity for weight gain can also be beneficial, though switching obviously carries the risk of relapse. Other strategies, including adding low-dose aripiprazole to olanzapine or clozapine, have also been shown to reduce weight gain (Fleischhacker *et al*, 2010).

Owing to concern about potential cardiac and metabolic side-effects, routine monitoring of ECGs (particularly when dosages are high) and plasma glucose levels in patients taking antipsychotics over the long term is recommended. More immediately relevant to the prescriber of clozapine are the array of common but distressing adverse effects associated with its complex pharmacology, such as sialorrhoea (treated with hyoscine) and enuresis (which responds to desmopressin). Sedation is usually short-lived and may be managed by careful adjustment of the timing of doses. Constipation (often requiring treatment with laxatives) must be monitored and managed actively, as clozapine-induced intestinal obstruction can be fatal.

The NICE schizophrenia guidelines

The National Institute for Health and Care Excellence is responsible for making recommendations about the treatments to be provided within the National Health Service in England and Wales. It has published a number of documents on psychosis and its treatment, including clinical guidelines on the treatment of schizophrenia and a technology appraisal on the use of second-generation antipsychotics. These documents have been combined and fully revised as NICE Clinical Guideline 178, *Psychosis and Schizophrenia in Adults: Treatment and Management* (NICE, 2014), which makes recommendations for social, psychological and pharmacological management. All practitioners in England and Wales need to be aware of NICE recommendations and should deviate from them only if they have good reason.

The guidelines make few specific recommendations regarding choice of medication. There remains a recommendation of clozapine if two medications have failed (one of which should be a non-clozapine second-generation antipsychotic). Depot medication is suggested where adherence is suspected to be poor.

There is an increased emphasis on joint decision-making with the patient and carer if appropriate. The aim is that decisions are made by the patient as an informed choice. Information is to be provided and advance directives should be encouraged and followed. While this may not be achievable in all cases, particularly with a patient who does not acknowledge the need for medication, it represents a major and probably irreversible paradigm shift in the treatment of psychosis. It is fully in line with the overall theme of this book, which focuses on the individual with a major mental illness as an active participant in the management of the illness and his or her individual process of recovery.

Conclusions

People coming into psychiatric rehabilitation services have generally responded poorly or incompletely to pharmacological treatments for their psychotic illnesses and may experience a significant burden of side-effects. Careful attention to detail, including assessment of adherence to treatment, identifying comorbid conditions, optimising standard treatments and judicious use of adjunctive strategies can result in marked symptomatic improvement. It is important for rehabilitation practitioners to remain aware of advances in pharmacological treatment and take an evidence-based approach. It is recommended that prescribers considering prescribing medication where there is a poor evidence base for doing so seek a second opinion and expert advice.

Further reading

An exhaustive review of the pharmacological management of treatment-resistant psychosis is beyond the remit of this chapter. Readers seeking to increase their understanding of the mechanisms of drug action should consult one of the standard textbooks on psychopharmacology. Stahl (2013), for example, provides an excellent introduction. For advice on the practical aspects of prescribing, the *Maudsley Prescribing Guidelines* (Taylor *et al*, 2012*a*) is recommended.

References

Agid O, Arenovich T, Sajeev G, *et al* (2011) An algorithm-based approach to first-episode schizophrenia: response rates over 3 prospective antipsychotic trials with a retrospective data analysis. *Journal of Clinical Psychiatry*, **72**: 1439–44

Chan J, Sweeting M (2007) Combination therapy with non-clozapine atypical antipsychotic medication: a review of current evidence. *Journal of Psychopharmacology*, **21**: 657–64.

Chen JX, Su YA, Wang SL, *et al* (2009) Aripiprazole treatment of risperidone-induced hyperprolactinaemia. *Journal of Clinical Psychiatry*, **70**: 1058–9.

Cipriani A, Boso M, Barbui C (2009) Clozapine combined with different antipsychotic drugs for treatment resistant schizophrenia. *Cochrane Database of Systematic Reviews*, **8(3)**: CD006324.

Davis JM, Chen N, Glick ID (2003) A meta-analysis of the efficacy of second-generation antipsychotics. *Archives of General Psychiatry*, **60**: 553–64.

Demjaha A, Egerton A, Murray R *et al* (2013) Antipsychotic treatment resistance in schizophrenia associated with elevated glutamate levels but normal dopamine function. *Biological Psychiatry*, **75** (5): e11–13 (doi: 10.1016/j.biopsych.2013.06.011).

Dolder CR, Lacro JP, Leckband S, *et al* (2003) Interventions to improve antipsychotic medication adherence: review of recent literature. *Journal of Clinical Psychopharmacology*, **23**: 389–99.

Dursun SM, Deakin JF (2001) Augmenting antipsychotic treatment with lamotrigine or topiramate in patients with treatment-resistant schizophrenia: a naturalistic case-series outcome study. *Journal of Psychopharmacology*, **15** (4): 297–301.

Fleischhacker WW, Heikkinen ME, Olié JP, *et al* (2010) Effects of adjunctive treatment with aripiprazole on body weight and clinical efficacy in schizophrenia patients treated with clozapine: a randomized, double-blind, placebo-controlled trial. *International Journal of Neuropsychopharmacology*, **13**: 1115–25.

Gerson SL, Lieberman JA, Friedenberg WR, *et al* (1991) Polypharmacy in fatal clozapine-associated agranulocytosis. *Lancet*, **338**: 262–3.

Haas SJ, Hill R, Crum H, *et al* (2007) Clozapine-associated myocarditis: a review of 116 cases of suspected myocarditis associated with the use of clozapine in Australia during 1993–2003. *Drug Safety*, **30**: 47–50.

Haddad P, Taylor M, Niaz O (2009) First-generation antipsychotic long acting injections versus oral antipsychotics in schizophrenia: systematic review of randomised controlled trials and observational studies. *British Journal of Psychiatry*, **195** (suppl 52): S20–8.

Kando JC, Tohen M, Castillo J, *et al* (1994) Concurrent use of clozapine and valproate in affective and psychotic disorders. *Journal of Clinical Psychiatry*, **55**: 255–7.

Kemp R, Kirov G, Everitt B (1998) Randomised controlled trial of compliance therapy. 18-month follow-up. *British Journal of Psychiatry*, **172**: 413–19.

Leucht C, Heres S, Kane JM, *et al* (2011) Oral versus depot antipsychotic drugs for schizophrenia – a critical systematic review and meta-analysis of randomised long-term trials. *Schizophrenia Research*, **127**: 83–92.

Millson M, Owen J, Lorberg G, *et al* (2002) Topiramate for refractory schizophrenia. *American Journal of Psychiatry*, **159**: 675.

Moncrieff J (2006) Does antipsychotic withdrawal provoke psychosis? Review of the literature on rapid onset psychosis (supersensitivity psychosis) and withdrawal-related relapse. *Acta Psychiatrica Scandinavica*, **114**: 3–13.

Munro J, O'Sullivan D, Andrews C, *et al* (1999) Active monitoring of 12760 clozapine recipients in the UK and Ireland. *British Journal of Psychiatry*, **175**: 576–80.

Munro J, Matthiasson P, Osborne S, *et al* (2004) Amisulpride augmentation of clozapine: an open non-randomized study in patients with schizophrenia partially responsive to clozapine. *Acta Psychiatrica Scandinavica*, **110**: 292–8.

Muscatello MR, Bruno A, Pandolfo G, *et al* (2011) Effect of aripiprazole augmentation of clozapine in schizophrenia: a double-blind, placebo-controlled study. *Schizophrenia Research*, **127**: 93–9.

National Institute for Health and Care Excellence (2014) *Psychosis and Schizophrenia in Adults: Treatment and Management* (Clinical Guideline 178). NICE.

Nosé M, Barbui C, Gray R, *et al* (2003) Clinical interventions for treatment non-adherence in psychosis: meta-analysis. *British Journal of Psychiatry*, **183**: 197–206.

O'Donnell C, Donohoe G, Sharkey L, *et al* (2003) Compliance therapy: a randomised controlled trial in schizophrenia. *BMJ*, **327**: 834–6.

Ohlsen R, Gaughran F (2011) Schizophrenia: a major risk factor for cardiovascular disease. *British Journal of Cardiac Nursing*, **6** (5): 2–5.

Patel M, Taylor M, David A (2009) Antipsychotic long acting injections: mind the gap. *British Journal of Psychiatry*, **195** (suppl 52): 1–4.

Quintero J, Barbudo E, Molina JD, *et al* (2011) The effectiveness of the combination therapy of amisulpride and quetiapine for managing treatment-resistant schizophrenia: a naturalistic study. *Journal of Clinical Psychopharmacology*, **31**: 240–2.

Shiloh R, Zemishlany Z, Aizenberg D, *et al* (1997) Sulpiride augmentation in people with schizophrenia partially responsive to clozapine. A double-blind, placebo-controlled study. *British Journal of Psychiatry*, **171**: 569–3.

Small JG, Klapper MH, Malloy FW, *et al* (2003) Tolerability and efficacy of clozapine combined with lithium in schizophrenia and schizoaffective disorder. *Journal of Clinical Psychopharmacology*, **23**: 223–8.

Sommer I, Begemann MJH, Temmerman A, *et al* (2012) Pharmacological augmentation strategies for schizophrenia patients with insufficient response to clozapine: a quantitative literature review. *Schizophrenia Bulletin*, **38**: 1003–11.

Stahl SM (2013) *Essential Psychopharmacology: Neuroscientific Basis and Practical Applications*. (4th edn). Cambridge University Press.

Taylor D, Cornelius V (2010) Risperidone long-acting injection: factors associated with changes in bed stay and hospitalisation in a 3-year naturalistic follow-up. *Journal of Psychopharmacology*, **24**: 995.

Taylor D, Douglas-Hall P, Olofinjana B, *et al* (2009) Reasons for discontinuing clozapine: matched case–control comparison with risperidone long-acting injection. *British Journal of Psychiatry*, **194**: 165–7.

Taylor D, Paton C, Kapur S (2012*a*) *The Maudsley Prescribing Guidelines in Psychiatry* (11th edn). Wiley–Blackwell.

Taylor D, Smith L, Gee S, *et al* (2012*b*) Augmentation of clozapine with a second antipsychotic – a meta-analysis. *Acta Psychiatrica Scandinavica*, **125**: 15–24.

Tharyan P, Adams CE (2005) Electroconvulsive therapy for schizophrenia. *Cochrane Database of Systematic Reviews*, **18 (2)**: CD000076.

Tiihonen J, Wahlbeck K (2006) Glutamatergic drugs for schizophrenia. *Cochrane Database of Systematic Reviews*, CD003730 (DOI: 10.1002/14651858.CD003730.pub2).

Tiihonen J, Wahlbeck K, Kiviniemi V (2009) The efficacy of lamotrigine in clozapine-resistant schizophrenia: a systematic review and meta-analysis. *Schizophrenia Research*, **109**: 10–14.

Valevski A, Modai I, Labav M, *et al* (1993) Clozapine–lithium combined treatment and agranulocytosis. *International Clinical Psychopharmacology*, **8**: 63–5.

Varma S, Bishara D, Besag F, *et al* (2011) Clozapine-related EEG changes and seizures: dose and plasma-level relationships. *Therapeutic Advances in Psychopharmacology*, **1**: 47–66.

Weiner E, Conley RR, Ball MP, *et al* (2010) Adjunctive risperidone for partially responsive people with schizophrenia treated with clozapine. *Journal of Neuropsychopharmacology*, **35**: 2274–83.

Werneke U, Taylor D, Sanders T (2013) Behavioural interventions for antipsychotic-induced appetite changes. *Current Psychiatry Reports*, **15**: 347.

Whiskey E, Taylor D (2007) Restarting clozapine after neutropenia: evaluating the possibilities and practicalities. *CNS Drugs*, **1**: 25–35.

Yagcioglu AE, Akdede BB, Turgut TI, *et al* (2005) A double-blind controlled study of adjunctive treatment with risperidone in schizophrenic patients partially responsive to clozapine: efficacy and safety. *Journal of Clinical Psychiatry*, **66**: 63–72.

CHAPTER 15

Physical healthcare

Joseph Hayes and David Osborn

Introduction

There are considerable inequities in physical health outcomes between individuals with severe enduring mental illness and the general population. These include a mortality rate of up to three times that of the general population (Laursen *et al*, 2007). This mortality gap, which translates to a life expectancy shortened by 15–30 years (Vreeland, 2007), has increased in recent decades, even in high-income countries with well-regarded healthcare systems providing universal care for the entire population (Ösby *et al*, 2000).

This chapter describes the factors responsible for premature mortality and some of the common physical health problems people with severe mental illness develop. Recovery and rehabilitation services, by their very nature, care for people at the severest end of the mental illness spectrum and are likely therefore to manage individuals with more challenging physical health needs, and symptoms that are barriers to healthy living. However, the recovery model also provides an opportunity to include physical health as a central tenet of the care provided.

The interplay between mental and physical health has received significant coverage in recent years. It is at the core of the British government's mental health policy and is highlighted in reports by the Schizophrenia Commission (Schizophrenia Commission, 2012) and the Sainsbury Centre (Naylor *et al*, 2012). Within the UK, the National Health Service (NHS) has been given a clear mandate to tackle the long-standing and long-outdated disparity between mental and physical healthcare.

Mortality and morbidity statistics

Premature death in people with schizophrenia, bipolar disorder and other severe mental illnesses is a major concern. Results vary from study to study, but life expectancy could be reduced by as much as 30 years in this group. People with severe enduring mental illnesses are six to seven times more likely to die prematurely from physical illness than they are from suicide. The main cause of premature death is cardiovascular disease. People with severe mental illness under the age of 50 are three times more likely to die from a heart attack or stroke than the general population. Similarly, people aged 50–75 with a severe mental illness are twice as likely to die from cardiovascular disease (Osborn *et al*, 2007).

Why the mortality gap exists

A number of factors contribute to this increased mortality and morbidity in people with severe mental illness; these include poor access to healthcare, lifestyle factors and smoking, the effects of psychiatric treatment and factors intrinsic to particular mental disorders.

Access to healthcare

Poor access to healthcare can occur through both healthcare system failures and failure of the patient to engage 'appropriately' with the healthcare system. Psychiatrists and other doctors may regard reporting of a physical symptom as a sign of mental illness (diagnostic overshadowing). The psychiatrist may focus on the mental health issue at the expense of physical healthcare and may not possess the appropriate skills to diagnose the physical complaint. Resources for diagnosis and treatment may be lacking in a psychiatric setting. Physicians, surgeons and emergency department staff may be reluctant to treat people with severe mental illness because engagement is complicated by the mental illness, because of stigmatising attitudes or because of issues with capacity, which they may feel less well versed in.

Patients may actively avoid contact with general healthcare services, or may have poor general treatment concordance. Some may have difficulty communicating their physical health needs and problems in general, or may be unaware of physical health problems because of cognitive deficits or negative symptoms. Some patients may have difficulty undertaking tasks such as making appointments, comprehending healthcare or carrying out recommended lifestyle changes, without additional support.

Health behaviours

Individuals with severe mental illness have been shown to engage in more unhealthy and high-risk behaviours than the general population (Parks *et al*, 2006). They have been found to have poorer diets, exercise less frequently and smoke more than the general population. They are more likely to use illicit substances. They are less likely to practise safe sex. They are more at risk of coercion, exploitation and violence.

Medication effects

Antipsychotic medications, mood stabilisers and some antidepressants cause weight gain. This in turn can result in cardiovascular disease, hyperlipidaemia and diabetes. Medications also have side-effects such as sedation or Parkinsonism that can contribute to reduced physical activity.

Effects of mental illness

It has been shown that before the introduction of antipsychotic medication in the 1950s, individuals with schizophrenia were at increased risk of diabetes. This argument is further strengthened by evidence that drug-naïve patients have increased intra-abdominal fat, impaired fasting glucose tolerance and more insulin resistance than the general population (Ryan *et al*, 2003). Genes are now being identified that increase the risk of serious mental illness, and might also add incremental risk of cardiometabolic disorders.

Physical health problems

Smoking

People with mental health problems are far more likely to smoke than the general population. More than 70% of people with schizophrenia and other severe mental illnesses smoke cigarettes, a rate that is double to triple that of the general population. Explanations for the elevated prevalence of smoking among people with severe mental illness include neurological, psychological, behavioural and environmental factors. Individuals with schizophrenia often describe smoking as a way to manage symptoms such as stress, anxiety and depression; to reduce medication side-effects; to blunt distress owing to illness sequelae such as isolation, hopelessness and stigma; and to facilitate social interaction. There is also increasing evidence of a biochemical vulnerability to nicotine addiction in individuals with schizophrenia, as nicotine appears to affect sensory gating, which improves attention and filtering of aberrant stimuli (Conway, 2009).

Patients with severe mental illness also smoke more heavily than the general population, with 45–70% of smokers with schizophrenia smoking over 20 cigarettes per day. A clear connection has been shown between higher numbers of cigarettes smoked and poorer overall self-reported subjective quality of life, as well as lower satisfaction with social relationships, finances, leisure activities and health among persons with severe mental illness (Dixon *et al*, 2010).

Morbidity is increased in smokers through a number of interacting mechanisms linked to both behaviour and treatment. Smoking is a risk factor for cardiovascular, cerebrovascular and respiratory disease. Also, by way of enzyme induction in the liver, smoking reduces the available plasma levels of antipsychotics (notably olanzapine and clozapine). Therefore, it may influence the patient's behaviour and the treatment outcome. All staff and indeed the patient need to be aware that if smoking ceases, there will be reduced breakdown of antipsychotic medication and levels in the blood stream will increase, despite the oral dose remaining the same.

Obesity

Obesity is a growing health crisis worldwide. Obese individuals have shorter life spans and are at increased risk of a number of health problems. They are at three times the risk of cardiovascular disease, type 2 diabetes mellitus, hypertension, dyslipidaemia and respiratory problems, and at twice the risk of bowel cancer and hormone abnormalities (de Hert *et al*, 2011a). Obesity is classified as a body mass index (BMI) of greater than 30 kg/m^2; however, waist circumference (measuring abdominal or central adiposity) may be a more valid and reliable predictor for cardiovascular risk, type 2 diabetes and other metabolic conditions (Klein *et al*, 2007).

There is a clinically significant overlap between obesity and severe mental illness. People with severe mental illness are at increased risk of obesity, even early in their illness or without medication. People with schizophrenia are 2.8–3.5 times more likely to be obese than the general population and individuals with bipolar disorder or major depression 1.2–1.5 times (de Hert *et al*, 2011a).

As with the general population, lifestyle factors (lack of exercise, poor diet,etc.) contribute significantly to weight gain in severe mental illness. However, beyond this, treatment side-effects such as weight liability and sedation need to be considered contributors to the risk of obesity. Up to 70% of patients with schizophrenia experience weight gain during acute and maintenance treatment and there are similar effects in patients with bipolar disorder. All atypical antipsychotics have the potential to increase weight, but clozapine and olanzapine have been identified as having the greatest impact (Daumit *et al*, 2008). The majority of antidepressants and mood stabilisers have also been associated with weight gain (Zimmermann *et al*, 2003).

Diabetes

The prevalence of diabetes mellitus in people with severe mental illness is two to three times that of the general population. Again, the increased risk comes from a combination of lifestyle, genetic, disease and treatment factors (de Hert *et al*, 2009). Second-generation antipsychotics are more diabetogenic than conventional antipsychotics (relative risk 1.3). However, different second-generation antipsychotics convey different risks. Olanzapine, clozapine and to a lesser extent quetiapine and risperidone are associated with significantly increased rates of type 2 diabetes mellitus (Smith *et al*, 2008). Some studies have suggested that aripiprazole may reduce the incidence of diabetes (Kessing *et al*, 2010; Nielsen *et al*, 2010).

Antidepressants may also increase the risk of diabetes, through side-effects such as sedation, increased appetite and weight gain (Kivimäki *et al*, 2010). Many mood stabilisers, especially valproate, are associated with an elevated risk of insulin resistance, conferring a risk for diabetes. In the case of valproate, the risk is likely to be related to weight gain, fatty liver infiltration and the drug itself (Pylvänen *et al*, 2002).

Cardiovascular disease

Risk factors for cardiovascular disease include smoking, obesity, raised cholesterol levels and diabetes mellitus, as well as poor diet, physical inactivity and low economic status. People with severe mental illness have an elevated risk of cardiovascular disease and significantly higher rates of modifiable risk factors than the general population (de Hert *et al*, 2009). The risk of coronary heart disease is tripled in schizophrenia, doubled in bipolar disorder and may be as much as 4.5 times greater in major depressive disorder. The risk of cerebrovascular disease is threefold greater in schizophrenia, and double in bipolar disorder and major depression (Brown *et al*, 2000).

Antipsychotic medication appears to increase the risk of both heart disease and cerebrovascular events, probably through D_2 antagonism (García-Tornadú *et al*, 2010). Higher antipsychotic doses confer greater risk of cardiovascular disease. Both conventional and second-generation antipsychotics can increase QTc values and as such put patients at risk of sudden cardiac death (with *torsade de pointes* and ventricular arrhythmias). This relationship is also dose related (Leung *et al*, 2012).

Despite the people with severe mental illness having the highest mortality from cardiovascular disease, they continue to have lower rates of screening, appropriate drug treatment and surgical intervention (Kisely *et al*, 2007).

Cancer

Smoking, obesity and an unhealthy lifestyle are significant risks for a number of different types of cancer. It should therefore follow that people with severe mental illness have high rates of cancer. However, as it stands, studies exploring the risk of any cancer type have given conflicting results. There are reasons why an increased rate of cancer in this population may not be consistently seen. For instance, it has been shown that patients with severe mental illness are less likely than the general population to receive routine screening, that they present later, and have a higher cancer fatality than the general population. Furthermore, because of the reduced life expectancy, it may be that patients with severe mental illness die from other causes before reaching the expected age of death from cancer (de Hert *et al*, 2011*a*). It has also been hypothesised that this population may *actually* have a lower risk of developing cancer, because antipsychotic medication may have chemotherapeutic properties (Cohen *et al*, 2002) or because schizophrenia may have protective properties via a shared genetic basis (Catts & Catts, 2000).

Respiratory disease

Before 1960, respiratory diseases, including tuberculosis and pneumonia, were the main cause of death of people with severe mental illness.

Respiratory disease is still elevated in this population today. Studies consistently show higher rates of tuberculosis, pneumonia and chronic obstructive pulmonary disease (Filik *et al*, 2006). Some have found that even after adjusting for smoking status, an increased risk of chronic obstructive pulmonary disease remains (Sokal *et al*, 2004).

HIV and hepatitis

Data from the USA and Europe suggest that people with severe mental illness are at increased risk of both HIV and hepatitis C (Rosenberg *et al*, 2001; Leucht *et al*, 2007). There is a lack of information on rates of HIV and hepatitis in individuals with severe mental illness in the UK and currently national strategies around HIV prevention and sexual health do not identify them as a high-risk group. If patients have HIV or hepatitis, their needs related to this diagnosis should be assessed and addressed as part of their care plan.

It has been shown that a significant proportion of this group engage in more frequent risk behaviours (such as injecting and non-injecting substance misuse, multiple sexual partners, infrequent contraceptive use and selling sex) (Wright *et al*, 2012). Comorbidity of a severe mental illness and life-threatening viral illness incurs a worse prognosis for both conditions. Despite this, effective pharmacotherapy exists, and antipsychotics and treatments for HIV or hepatitis C can be used together successfully (Cournos *et al*, 2005). The clinical challenge is to encourage adherence to treatment and to coordinate the clinical services needed to address the diverse psychiatric and medical problems that coexist in this population. HIV or hepatitis infection can have a profound impact on individuals, their friends, family and carers, and on service provision. This may be compounded in those already suffering stigma, social exclusion and low self-esteem related to the diagnosis of severe mental illness.

Dental health

There is a higher prevalence and severity of dental disease among patients with severe mental illness. Studies suggest that the majority visit the dentist only when they have serious oral problems and less frequently attend routine checks than the general population. Again, the reasons for worse dental health are multifactorial. There is evidence that individuals with severe mental illness have poorer diets, and may also lack the motivation to adopt and maintain good oral hygiene habits. Antipsychotics, antidepressants and mood stabilisers are associated with multiple periodontal disorders (including ulcers, glossitis and caries). Symptoms can be exacerbated by the use of anticholinergic drugs, which, because of the side-effect of hyposalivation, increase the rate of caries formation. Treatment side-effects that affect orofacial muscles (such as dystonias, Parkinsonism and tardive dyskinesia) may also increase the difficulty of maintaining good oral hygiene and accessing treatment. Furthermore, there seems to be a tendency among dentists to treat psychiatric patients by extracting the teeth that cause pain instead of carrying out complex treatments of preservation or restoration (Arnaiz *et al*, 2011). This may partially be a reflection of the patients being less able, or willing, to tolerate the time and volume of appointments necessary for such dental work. In the UK, dental problems may be particularly problematic because of the reduced treatments available to NHS patients.

Recommended monitoring in severe mental illness

Worldwide, there are multiple guidelines for monitoring the physical health of people with severe mental illness. In the UK, two key guidelines are in place: the revised schizophrenia guidelines from the National Institute for Health and Care Excellence (NICE) (National Collaborating Centre for Mental Health, 2010) and the UK Quality and Outcomes Framework (QOF) for primary care (NICE, 2012). The guidelines focus on the monitoring of body mass index (BMI), blood pressure, HbA1c or glucose and the ratio of total cholesterol to high-density lipoprotein (HDL). These guidelines do not state what comprises adequate frequency of testing, but NICE suggests monitoring physical health at least once a year and states

---

Box 15.1 Physical health monitoring for people with a mental illness

Physical history and examination
- Personal physical health history
- Current medications
- Family history of physical health problems
- Smoking and physical activity history
- Physical examination
- Weight, height (and therefore BMI) and waist circumference
- Blood pressure

Physical investigations
- Fasting glucose
- Total cholesterol
- High-density lipoprotein (HDL) cholesterol (and total/HDL ratio)
- Low-density lipoprotein cholesterol
- Triglycerides
- Prolactin
- Electrocardiogram (ECG)

On commencing a new antipsychotic medication, it is recommended that all of the above be recorded at baseline and annually, with extra tests at 6 weeks and 3 months, excluding ECG. More specific recommendations exist for particular prescribing practices (e.g. clozapine, lithium).

---

that it is primary care, rather than psychiatrists, that has responsibility for this monitoring (apart from for patients who have been prescribed a high-dose antipsychotic). However, patients using rehabilitation and recovery services may have particular difficulty in engaging with general practitioners or other doctors and therefore specialist psychiatric staff are in a unique position to engage with patients and offer monitoring of their physical health.

Consensus across a number of guidelines suggests that the minimum annual monitoring should include the parameters shown in Box 15.1.

The role of psychiatric services in providing physical healthcare

As the NHS expects greater quality, and productivity, it is imperative to ensure that standards of physical healthcare retain their priority within services. Patients die on mental health wards and in the community, often without receiving adequate standards of basic screening and health interventions. Whatever the clinical, political and economic climate, routine physical assessment is part of the holistic care that modern mental health services should be providing across the board.

As our services diversify and modernise, there are elements of them that have rightly moved away from the medical model. Some services are increasingly staffed by non-clinical support workers, and clinical and medical time may be more limited. However, it is inconceivable that people using these modern services should expect inferior standards of physical healthcare. Commissioners and service managers must ensure that physical healthcare is always embedded within these new services, in terms of policy, staffing, training and availability of equipment.

Recent studies have shown that ward and community staff appreciate the need to provide patients with dietary and activity advice (Howard & Gamble, 2011). However, it is often felt that management of diabetes, smoking cessation and providing sexual health advice should be the role of doctors alone. Checking whether patients attend cancer screening and dental and optician checks was not felt to be in the work remit of many staff (Howard & Gamble, 2011; Robson *et al*, 2013), although many rehabilitation teams will undertake this work, in the knowledge that many of their patients do neglect their physical health and do not engage well with such services.

A number of tools are available for physical health assessment and screening which can be employed in recovery services. An example is the Physical Health Check Tool, which was developed by the Rethink Mental Illness charity and is freely available to download from its website (Rethink Mental Illness, 2014). The tool assists non-clinicians in enquiring about current physical problems and access to preventive healthcare (including screening for cardiovascular risk factors, cancer and oral health). It also allows clinicians to make a plan to act on any findings or omissions. With tools as straightforward and helpful as this, there is no excuse for anyone working with people with mental health problems to avoid asking about physical health, whatever their level of clinical training or confidence.

There may be additional benefits to psychiatrists and other mental health staff being involved in the physical healthcare of people with mental health problems. It is clear that a whole range of chronic health problems have a significant effect on mental state and complicate the diagnosis and treatment of both common and severe mental disorders, so identifying and treating patients physical complaints may go some way to improving their mental health. There is also the opportunity to strengthen the therapeutic alliance by addressing physical problems that the service user may feel have been neglected by other healthcare providers.

Effective physical interventions in recovery services

Most guidelines recommend advising patients and their families on physical activity and diet, encouraging smoking cessation, switching medication if necessary, treating hyperlipidaemia and diabetes, and referring to specialist services as required. We know that interventions for smoking and weight reduction can be successful in people with severe mental illness (Faulkner *et al*, 2007; Banham & Gilbody, 2010). There is good reason to be positive about addressing the physical health needs of people with long-term severe mental illnesses. Contrary to popular stereotypes, many people with mental illness rate their physical health as important. However, there is some evidence that people with psychosis are more likely to perceive the influences on their physical health as external to their own locus of control (Buhagiar *et al*, 2011). If these findings generalise to longer-stay service users, then all mental health staff can have a positive impact by routinely assessing simple physical health outcomes and motivating patients to regain a sense of agency regarding their own health. This work would fit neatly within the philosophy of recovery, by being collaborative and holistic in nature.

Box 15.2 Interventions that improve physical health

- Maintenance of an ideal body weight can reduce the risk of coronary heart disease by up to 60%
- Weight loss of 5% can eliminate the need for antihypertensive medication and halve the risk of type 2 diabetes
- A 10% drop in cholesterol can reduce heart disease by 30%
- Walking for at least 30 minutes per day can halve the risk of developing diabetes and reduce cerebrovascular events by a third
- Smoking cessation can reduce the risk of coronary heart disease by 50%

Many interventions have significant effects on physical health (de Hert *et al*, 2011*b*). These are summarised in Box 15.2. Three specific activities that can be promoted by rehabilitation and recovery services are described in more detail below: *healthy eating, exercise* and *smoking cessation.*

Healthy eating programmes

Strategies to help individuals with severe mental illness manage their weight include: external restriction of caloric intake (i.e. by in-patient ward staff or carers); pharmacological intervention; and behavioural intervention. The UK government recommends that at least five portions of fruit and vegetables be consumed each day and two portions of oily fish per week. In in-patient settings, main meals should contain less than 15 g of fat, deserts less than 10 g of sugar and daily salt intake should be less than 6 g (Department of Health, 2010). The consumption of snacks, take-away meals, confectionary and sugary drinks can significantly contribute to calorie intake.

Although restricting calorie intake in in-patient settings can be effective for weight control, it is rarely feasible in community settings. This approach is also inconsistent with the goal of recovery: designing sustainable interventions and promoting independence among persons with mental illness. Behavioural health eating programmes offer the best evidence for sustained change in this population. A recent review of healthy eating programmes for patients with severe mental illness suggests that basic approaches to caloric reduction can be as effective as more comprehensive efforts. One dietary intervention, for example, adopted a simplified approach in which participants were presented with food choices labelled by colours of traffic lights ('green – eat as much as you'd like; yellow – eat with caution; and red – stop before you eat') (Kalarchian *et al*, 2005). Another focused on multiple, complex skills, such as planning, shopping for, and preparing nutritionally complete, lower-fat meals (Centorrino *et al*, 2006), with similar results.

Exercise programmes

While structured exercise programmes ensure safe and appropriate physical activity in a supervised environment, they can be costly in terms of space, staff and equipment. Lifestyle interventions (such as walking groups) have been shown to be more effective in increasing levels of physical activity in patients with severe mental illness (Ussher *et al*, 2007). Walking, either in the form of supervised walking groups or unsupervised, is one of the easiest, safest and most inexpensive types of exercise to promote. It is also one of the most popular forms of exercise for those with and without chronic illness (Krug *et al*, 1991). Other forms of physical activity that may be low cost and popular include low-impact exercise videos and group aerobics classes. However, even low-cost programmes such as these require planning, organisation, supervision and evaluation.

Smoking cessation programmes

More than half of people with severe mental illness want to give up smoking. Recent systematic reviews confirm that treatment interventions based on behavioural support and pharmacotherapy that work in the general population are also (and approximately equally) effective in smokers with mental illness and do not appear to worsen psychiatric symptoms (Banham & Gilbody, 2010; Ratschen *et al*, 2011). Adding nicotine replacement therapy to behavioural support has been shown to increase the rate of quitting by over 50%. So there is reason to be optimistic. Guidelines, toolkits and training programmes to support appropriate treatment of smokers with mental illness are being developed. Also, the legal obligation to create smoke-free environments in mental health settings from July 2008 in England has provided a perfect opportunity to address smoking in those patients who are admitted to hospital.

When smoking cessation is being considered, clinicians must be aware of how smoking affects the course of psychiatric disorders through its profound effect on the metabolism of psychotropic drugs, and how smoking status is a contributory factor to the individual variations observed in drug responses. Nicotine metabolism is mediated primarily by cytochrome P450, therefore lowering therapeutic levels of the multiple psychiatric drugs that are also metabolised through this route (e.g. diazepam, haloperidol, olanzapine and clozapine). Smoking cessation leads to increased plasma concentrations, with increased risks of adverse effects, creating a requirement for close drug dose monitoring during smoking cessation. Conversely, antipsychotic medications may differentially affect an individual's smoking status; for example, patients with schizophrenia were found to smoke more after initiation of haloperidol treatment and less when switched from haloperidol to clozapine. Other atypical antipsychotic medications, for example olanzapine and risperidone, can also reduce cigarette consumption.

The majority of individuals using recovery services will be prescribed one or more drugs that are affected by smoking (Box 15.3).

Box 15.3 Medications affected by smoking

- Antipsychotics: clozapine, olanzapine, haloperidol, chlorpromazine, fluphenazine, thioridazine
- Anticonvulsants: phenytoin, valproate
- Hypnotics: all benzodiazepines, zolpidem
- Antidepressants: mirtazapine, duloxetine, fluvoxamine, trazodone, all tricyclic antidepressants
- Other commonly used medications: insulin, beta-blockers, warfarin, codeine, methadone

---

In-patient rehabilitation and longer-stay recovery settings should consider offering a full internal programme of smoking cessation support. These programmes should be developed and run in conjunction with local NHS Stop Smoking services, which are well placed to provide staff training, advice and resources.

Routine screening

Employment of a registered general nurse across a number of community mental health sites has been shown to significantly increase the rate of screening for cardiovascular risk factors (Osborn *et al*, 2010). However, it is unlikely that extra staffing costs will be forthcoming for physical healthcare within modern mental health services, in an era of efficiency and austerity. Staff in recovery services may be well placed to assist patients in understanding the importance of routine screening and facilitating attendance. General practitioners (GPs) will invite every patient on their severe mental illness register to annual screening for cardiovascular and diabetes risk factors. The NHS has a screening programme for a number of cancers. Women aged 25–49 are invited for screening for cervical cancer every 3 years (every 5 years for those aged 50–64) and women aged 50–70 for breast cancer screening every 5 years. There is also a biannual bowel cancer screening programme for men and women aged 60–69.

Engagement with primary care

In the UK, 97% of the population are registered with a GP. Since 2004, GPs have been incentivised to provide annual physical health checks for all patients on their severe mental illness register. This includes annually documenting BMI, blood pressure, total cholesterol/HDL ratio, blood glucose and alcohol consumption, and recording cervical screening every 5 years (NICE, 2012). In 2010/11, this information was recorded for approximately 80% of patients with a severe mental illness. However, it is clear that not all these patients are recorded on GPs' severe mental illness registers. The information collected by GPs is not automatically communicated with secondary care teams and there is no established process for mental health services to support those patients who find attending for monitoring challenging. It should be within the remit of staff working in community recovery teams to facilitate patients' engagement with GPs, by reminding them of routine screening appointments and, in special circumstances, attending with them if the patient wishes. This can be built in to the Care Programme Approach care plan in a straightforward manner. Some long-stay wards and community treatment units have had success in utilising visits by a GP to the ward on a weekly basis (Welthagen *et al*, 2004) and mental health providers may want to consider this if budgets allow.

Conclusions

There is now unequivocal evidence that people with severe mental health problems have significantly worse health outcomes than the general population. Despite the challenges of providing physical healthcare to this population, it is totally unacceptable that they receive second-rate care. Individuals cared for by recovery and rehabilitation services are at particular risk of neglecting their physical health, owing to the severity of their mental illness, difficulty engaging with services and, on occasions, long stays in psychiatric hospitals. Cardiovascular disease is the major cause of death in this population and it is likely that many of the factors that contribute to this cluster of illnesses are avoidable. Recovery and rehabilitation services are well placed to improve monitoring of physical health problems and provide simple yet effective, evidence-based interventions.

References

Arnaiz A, Zumárraga M, Díez-Altuna I, *et al* (2011) Oral health and the symptoms of schizophrenia. *Psychiatry Research*, **188**: 24–8.

Banham L, Gilbody S (2010) Smoking cessation in severe mental illness: what works? *Addiction*, **105**: 1176–89.

Brown S, Barraclough B, Inskip H (2000) Causes of the excess mortality of schizophrenia. *British Journal of Psychiatry*, **177**: 212–17.

Buhagiar K, Parsonage L, Osborn DP (2011) Physical health behaviours and health locus of control in people with schizophrenia-spectrum disorder and bipolar disorder: a cross-sectional comparative study with people with non-psychotic mental illness. *BMC Psychiatry*, **11**: 104.

Catts VS, Catts SV (2000) Apoptosis and schizophrenia: is the tumour suppressor gene, p53, a candidate susceptibility gene? *Schizophrenia Research*, **41**: 405–15.

Centorrino F, Wurtman JJ, Duca KA, *et al* (2006) Weight loss in overweight patients maintained on atypical antipsychotic agents. *International Journal of Obesity*, **30**: 1011–16.

Cohen ME, Dembling B, Schorling JB (2002) The association between schizophrenia and cancer: a population-based mortality study. *Schizophrenia Research*, **57**: 139–46.

Conway JLC (2009) Exogenous nicotine normalises sensory gating in schizophrenia; therapeutic implications. *Medical Hypotheses*, **73**: 259–62.

Cournos F, McKinnon K, Sullivan G (2005) Schizophrenia and comorbid human immunodeficiency virus or hepatitis C virus. *Journal of Clinical Psychiatry*, **66**: 27.

Daumit GL, Goff DC, Meyer JM, *et al* (2008) Antipsychotic effects on estimated 10 year coronary heart disease risk in the CATIE Schizophrenia Study. *Schizophrenia Research*, **105**: 175.

de Hert M, Dekker JM, Wood D, *et al* (2009) Cardiovascular disease and diabetes in people with severe mental illness position statement from the European Psychiatric Association (EPA), supported by the European Association for the Study of Diabetes (EASD) and the European Society of Cardiology (ESC). *European Psychiatry*, **24**: 412–24.

de Hert M, Correll CU, Bobes J, *et al* (2011a) Physical illness in patients with severe mental disorders. I. Prevalence, impact of medications and disparities in health care. *World Psychiatry*, **10**: 52.

de Hert M, Cohen D, Bobes J, *et al* (2011b) Physical illness in patients with severe mental disorders. II. Barriers to care, monitoring and treatment guidelines, plus recommendations at the system and individual level. *World Psychiatry*, **10**: 138.

Department of Health (2010) *Better Hospital Food Programme*. Department of Health.

Dixon L, Medoff DR, Wohlheiter K, *et al* (2010) Correlates of severity of smoking among persons with severe mental illness. *American Journal on Addictions*, **16**: 101–10.

Faulkner G, Taylor A, Munro S, *et al* (2007) The acceptability of physical activity programming within a smoking cessation service for individuals with severe mental illness. *Patient Education and Counselling*, **66**: 123–6.

Filik R, Sipos A, Kehoe PG, *et al* (2006) The cardiovascular and respiratory health of people with schizophrenia. *Acta Psychiatrica Scandinavica*, **113**: 298–305.

García-Tornadú I, Ornstein AM, Chamson-Reig A, *et al* (2010) Disruption of the dopamine D2 receptor impairs insulin secretion and causes glucose intolerance. *Endocrinology*, **151**: 1441–50.

Howard L, Gamble C (2011) Supporting mental health nurses to address the physical health needs of people with serious mental illness in acute inpatient care settings. *Journal of Psychiatric and Mental Health Nursing*, **18**: 105–12.

Kalarchian MA, Marcus MD, Levine MD, *et al* (2005) Behavioral treatment of obesity in patients taking antipsychotic medications. *Journal of Clinical Psychiatry*, **66**: 1058–63.

Kessing LV, Thomsen AF, Mogensen UB, *et al* (2010) Treatment with antipsychotics and the risk of diabetes in clinical practice. *British Journal of Psychiatry*, **197**: 266–71.

Kisely S, Smith M, Lawrence D, *et al* (2007) Inequitable access for mentally ill patients to some medically necessary procedures. *Canadian Medical Association Journal*, **176**: 779–84.

Kivimäki M, Hamer M, Batty GD, *et al* (2010) Antidepressant medication use, weight gain, and risk of type 2 diabetes: a population-based study. *Diabetes Care*, **33**: 2611–16.

Klein S, Allison DB, Heymsfield SB, *et al* (2007) Waist circumference and cardiometabolic risk: a consensus statement from shaping America's health: Association for Weight Management and Obesity Prevention; NAASO, the Obesity Society; the American Society for Nutrition; and the American Diabetes Association. *Obesity*, **15**: 1061–7.

Krug LM, Haire-Joshu D, Heady SA (1991) Exercise habits and exercise relapse in persons with non-insulin-dependent diabetes mellitus. *Diabetes Educator*, **17**: 185–8.

Laursen TM, Munk-Olsen T, Nordentoft M, *et al* (2007) Increased mortality among patients admitted with major psychiatric disorders: a register-based study comparing mortality in unipolar depressive disorder, bipolar affective disorder, schizoaffective disorder, and schizophrenia. *Journal of Clinical Psychiatry*, **68**: 899–907.

Leucht S, Burkard T, Henderson JH (2007) *Physical Illness and Schizophrenia. A Review of the Evidence*. Cambridge University Press.

Leung JY, Barr AM, Procyshyn RM, *et al* (2012) Cardiovascular side-effects of antipsychotic drugs: the role of the autonomic nervous system. *Pharmacology and Therapeutics*, **135**: 113–22.

National Collaborating Centre for Mental Health (2010) *Schizophrenia: Core Interventions in the Treatment and Management of Schizophrenia in Adults in Primary and Secondary Care* (Updated Edition, National Clinical Guideline Number 82). British Psychological Society & Royal College of Psychiatrists.

National Institute for Health and Clinical Excellence (2012) *Quality and Outcomes Framework for 2012/13: Guidance for PCOs and Practices*. NHS Employers.

Naylor C, Parsonage M, McDaid D, *et al* (2012) *Long-Term Conditions and Mental Health: The Cost of Co-morbidities*. King's Fund and the Centre for Mental Health.

Nielsen J, Skadhede S, Correll CU (2010) Antipsychotics associated with the development of type 2 diabetes in antipsychotic-naïve schizophrenia patients. *Neuropsychopharmacology*, **35**: 1997–2004.

Osborn DP, Levy G, Nazareth I, *et al* (2007) Relative risk of cardiovascular and cancer mortality in people with severe mental illness from the United Kingdom's General Practice Research Database. *Archives of General Psychiatry*, **64**: 242.

Osborn DP, Nazareth I, Wright CA, *et al* (2010) Impact of a nurse-led intervention to improve screening for cardiovascular risk factors in people with severe mental illnesses. Phase-two cluster randomised feasibility trial of community mental health teams. *BMC Health Services Research*, **10**: 61.

Ösby U, Correia N, Brandt L, *et al* (2000) Time trends in schizophrenia mortality in Stockholm County, Sweden: cohort study. *BMJ*, **321**: 483.

Parks J, Svendsen D, Singer P, *et al* (2006) *Morbidity and Mortality in People with Serious Mental Illness*. National Association of State Mental Health Program Directors (NASMHPD) Medical Directors Council.

Pylvänen V, Knip M, Pakarinen A, *et al* (2002) Serum insulin and leptin levels in valproate-associated obesity. *Epilepsia*, **43**: 514–17.

Ratschen E, Britton J, McNeill A (2011) The smoking culture in psychiatry: time for change. *British Journal of Psychiatry*, **198**: 6–7.

Rethink Mental Illness (2014) *My Physical Health: A Physical Health Check for People using Mental Health Services*. Rethink (http://www.rethink.org/media/1137219/Physical%20 Health%20Check%202014.pdf).

Robson D, Haddad M, Gray R, *et al* (2013) Mental health nursing and physical health care: a cross-sectional study of nurses' attitudes, practice, and perceived training needs for the physical health care of people with severe mental illness. *International Journal of Mental Health Nursing*, **22**: 409–17.

Rosenberg SD, Goodman LA, Osher FC, *et al* (2001) Prevalence of HIV, hepatitis B, and hepatitis C in people with severe mental illness. *American Journal of Public Health*, **91**: 31.

Ryan MC, Collins P, Thakore JH (2003) Impaired fasting glucose tolerance in first-episode, drug-naive patients with schizophrenia. *American Journal of Psychiatry*, **160**: 284–9.

Schizophrenia Commission (2012) *The Abandoned Illness: A Report from the Schizophrenia Commission*. Rethink Mental Illness.

Smith M, Hopkins D, Peveler RC, *et al* (2008) First- v. second-generation antipsychotics and risk for diabetes in schizophrenia: systematic review and meta-analysis. *British Journal of Psychiatry*, **192**: 406–11.

Sokal J, Messias E, Dickerson FB, *et al* (2004) Comorbidity of medical illnesses among adults with serious mental illness who are receiving community psychiatric services. *Journal of Nervous and Mental Disease*, **192**: 421–7.

Ussher M, Stanbury L, Cheeseman V, *et al* (2007) Physical activity preferences and perceived barriers to activity among persons with severe mental illness in the United Kingdom. *Psychiatric Services*, **58**: 405–8.

Vreeland B (2007) Bridging the gap between mental and physical health: a multidisciplinary approach. *Journal of Clinical Psychiatry*, **68** (suppl 4): 26–33.

Welthagen E, Talbot S, Harrison O, *et al* (2004) Providing a primary care service for psychiatric in-patients. *Psychiatric Bulletin*, **28**: 167–70.

Wright N, Akhtar A, Tosh G, *et al* (2012) *HIV Prevention Advice for People with Serious Mental Illness*. Cochrane Library, Cochrane Collaboration.

Zimmermann U, Kraus T, Himmerich H, *et al* (2003) Epidemiology, implications and mechanisms underlying drug-induced weight gain in psychiatric patients. *Journal of Psychiatric Research*, **37**: 193–220.

Part 3

Key elements of a rehabilitation service

CHAPTER 16

Key elements of a rehabilitation service: overview

Helen Killaspy, Frank Holloway, Sridevi Kalidindi and Glenn Roberts

---

Introduction

Part 3 of the book describes the main components of the 'whole system' mental health rehabilitation care pathway referred to in Chapter 2, 'What is psychiatric rehabilitation?' Patients with complex mental health needs are usually referred to rehabilitation services from acute in-patient services and secure services. They may move through a series of treatment and support environments over a number of years, with each stage providing the opportunity for them to gain the confidence and skills to manage their lives with greater independence and autonomy, building on their progress and recovery incrementally. The pathway is shown in summary in Fig. 16.1. It includes a range of in-patient mental health rehabilitation units, some of which may actually be based in a community setting rather than a hospital (see Chapter 17, 'Rehabilitation in hospital settings'), a range of supported accommodation services (see Chapter 19, 'Housing: a place to live'), vocational rehabilitation services (see Chapter 20, 'Work and employment') and peer support services (see Chapter 21, 'Peer support in mental health services'). Once out of hospital, individuals are also supported by primary care and statutory community mental health services, including community rehabilitation teams and assertive outreach teams (see Chapter 18, 'Community-based rehabilitation and recovery').

Providing a flexible pathway

The exact configuration of in-patient rehabilitation services varies in different localities according to morbidity and need, with inner-city areas tending to require more high-dependency in-patient rehabilitation units, from where service users generally move on to a community-based rehabilitation unit in preparation for more independent, but supported, community living. Most (67%) people who require in-patient rehabilitation, whether delivered in a hospital or in a community-based unit, are able to move on successfully to some form of supported accommodation within 3 years (Killaspy & Zis, 2013).

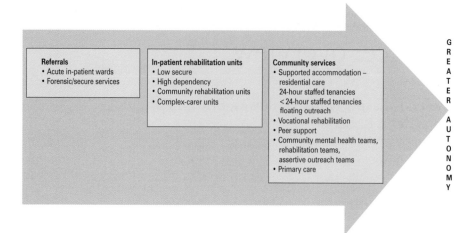

Fig. 16.1 The whole-system mental health rehabilitation care pathway (adapted from Joint Commissioning Panel for Mental Health, 2012)

Community rehabilitation services work closely with supported-accommodation services to provide comprehensive support to service users as they continue their recovery in the community. When service users are able to manage with less support they move on to less-supported accommodation. Once they are able to manage more independent living, their care is usually transferred from the rehabilitation service to a community mental health team or recovery team. However, only around 10% of service users will achieve and sustain fully independent living within 5 years of referral to rehabilitation services (Killaspy & Zis, 2013). It usually takes a number of years for individuals to move successfully through each step of the rehabilitation care pathway, owing to the severity and complexity of their mental health needs. The configuration of supported-accommodation services in many areas seems to have evolved historically and according to the interest of those commissioning these services rather than being driven by the characteristics and needs of the local population. Very little empirical evidence has been published about the effectiveness of different models of supported accommodation to guide clinicians and service planners, although this is beginning to be addressed.

While the rehabilitation care pathway appears linear, it needs to have the flexibility for people to jump stages when appropriate, to support people for as long as required at each stage, and to allow people to move back to a stage of higher support, when needed, before they progress again towards a more independent setting. Some people may need to make repeated attempts to transition successfully from a higher to a lower level of support. This flexibility requires a close and collaborative working relationship between those providing the different components of the pathway.

Productive partnerships between statutory and non-statutory services

In England, around a third of National Health Service trusts have their own low secure mental health rehabilitation unit (Mountain *et al*, 2009) and the vast majority of services provide high-dependency or community rehabilitation units; on average, each mental health trust in England has two in-patient mental health rehabilitation units (Killaspy *et al*, 2013). Many also provide a longer-term complex-care unit (Killaspy *et al*, 2005). Managing assessments and admissions to such an in-patient pathway within a single provider organisation may be fairly easily coordinated, since key clinicians (often the rehabilitation psychiatrist) and service managers will work across these units. Effective management of patient flows across the pathway is much more challenging when different components are provided by different organisations. In the UK, the majority of supported accommodation is provided by the independent and voluntary sector rather than the National Health Service. Liaison between different providers to ensure a coherent and transparent approach to the assessment process that ensures placements are agreed and prioritised according to people's needs is a key role for rehabilitation practitioners and community rehabilitation teams. However, this liaison does not only apply to the referral and assessment process. Increasingly, statutory and non-statutory services are working creatively and productively together, using their complementary skills to provide a comprehensive care pathway that supports individuals effectively and efficiently. This is described in more detail in Chapter 18, 'Community-based rehabilitation and recovery'.

Supporting social inclusion

As well as providing treatment and support directly to individuals, rehabilitation services and the wider network of services with which they work develop strong links with local community resources to facilitate service users' social inclusion. This may vary from building informal relationships with local shopkeepers to supporting people to access mainstream courses at a local college. Similarly, productive partnerships with users and carers are needed to support informal support networks. Further information about how to do this is provided in Part 2 of the book, and in particular Chapter 10, 'Family interventions'.

Supporting people with mental health problems to access meaningful occupation is important in helping to maximise their recovery and social inclusion, since occupation forms an important part of everybody's personal and social identity. A major focus for rehabilitation services is the facilitation of service users' occupation, including hobbies, leisure activities and social engagements, educational and vocational courses, and voluntary, supported and paid employment. Although employment rates for people with severe mental health problems are very low, services can help people to gain or regain work, and practical guidance on how to deliver these is given in Chapter 20, 'Work and employment'. Assisting individuals to build a programme of meaningful, enjoyable and rewarding activities takes time and requires careful, detailed care planning. It is easy to underestimate how much support a person may need to be able to achieve seemingly minor goals. Occupational therapists play a key role here in making links with local community resources (e.g. cinemas, gyms, colleges and employment organisations) and, along with nursing staff, support workers and activity workers, in supporting service users to access and engage with these. It is vital that occupational care plans are developed with service users to reflect their interests and goals and that there is recognition that not all service users are able, or wish, to work.

Peer support

Chapter 21 provides an overview of the use of peer support in mental health services, a relatively new and evolving field. Around a third of in-patient mental health rehabilitation services employ service users or ex-service users in this kind of capacity (Killaspy et al, 2013). Peer support capitalises on a person's lived experience of mental health problems by using this as a vehicle to engage service users in collaborative recovery-oriented work. Though at an early stage of evaluation, the conceptual validity and the positive experiences reported suggest it is likely to become an important addition to the rehabilitation portfolio, enhancing and quite possibly challenging more traditional ways of working.

Leadership and management

Delivering and managing such a comprehensive and complex pathway requires specialist leadership and management skills. Responding to the demands of senior managers and commissioners in a changeable economic and political context while ensuring appropriate, high-quality local services continue to be provided is a requirement of rehabilitation psychiatrists. Often they are the only people working across many components of the pathway and they thus are well placed to advise on service developments that address resource gaps in local provision. However, as mental health services adopt an increasingly business-like model of operation, they need to be equipped with the right skills and language to communicate with those commissioning and managing services. As such, Chapter 22, 'Leadership, management and service development in rehabilitation practice', is an essential read for all rehabilitation psychiatrists, especially given the recurring threats to rehabilitation services.

References

Joint Commissioning Panel for Mental Health (2012) *Guidance for Commissioners of Rehabilitation Services for People with Complex Mental Health Needs.* Royal College of Psychiatrists.

Killaspy H, Zis P (2013) Predictors of outcomes of mental health rehabilitation services: a 5-year retrospective cohort study in inner London, UK. *Social Psychiatry and Psychiatric Epidemiology,* **48**: 1005–12.

Killaspy H, Harden C, Holloway F, *et al* (2005) What do mental health rehabilitation services do and what are they for? A national survey in England. *Journal of Mental Health,* **14**: 157–66.

Killaspy H, Marston L, Omar R, *et al* (2013) Service quality and clinical outcomes: an example from mental health rehabilitation services in England. *British Journal of Psychiatry,* **202**: 28–34.

Mountain D, Killaspy H, Holloway F (2009) Mental health rehabilitation services in the UK in 2007. *Psychiatric Bulletin,* **33**: 215–18.

CHAPTER 17

Rehabilitation in hospital settings

Steffan Davies and Helen Killaspy

Introduction

In-patient services have always accounted for the bulk of expenditure on mental healthcare. Although they deal with small numbers of people, they are required to provide for all of a patient's daily needs: safety, food, accommodation, daytime activities and treatment of their mental disorders, and often wider social needs. This requires expensive buildings, 24-hour staffing and a multidisciplinary team of trained professionals. In the UK, a mental health in-patient service is defined as a unit with 'hospital beds' that provides 24-hour nursing care (NHS Confederation, 2012). It is able to care for patients detained under the Mental Health Act, with a consultant psychiatrist or other professional acting as 'responsible clinician'. This does not mean that all or even a majority of patients will be detained.

Even after decades of investment in community services, in-patient services in the UK, from acute admission wards to high-security hospitals, account for around 40% of mental health services spending by the National Health Service (NHS), with health and social care provided in other settings (including nursing and residential care homes and places funded through continuing care) accounting for a further 20%, pharmacy costs 9% and management costs 4% (Department of Health Commissioning Development, 2011). Most of this can be broadly described as being spent on rehabilitation services, that is, longer-term services aiming to improve the quality of life, independence and functional abilities of people suffering with complex mental health problems.

A comprehensive definition of UK rehabilitation is clearly relevant to many in-patient services but by virtue of their philosophy and approach rather than, necessarily, the badge on the door:

> A whole system approach to recovery from mental ill health which maximizes an individual's quality of life and social inclusion by encouraging their skills, promoting independence and autonomy in order to give them hope for the future and which leads to successful community living through appropriate support. (Killaspy *et al*, 2005: p. 163)

It is also vital to remember that in-patient services can be the opposite of rehabilitative, providing poor care, disempowering people and damaging their health (Davies, 2004), as illustrated yet again in the recent Francis report on the scandalously inadequate care provided in one physical healthcare setting in the UK (Francis, 2013).

A brief history of in-patient mental health rehabilitation services

The Retreat

The Retreat was founded in 1797 by the Society of Friends (the Quakers) in York following the death of one of their Society in the York Asylum as a result of poor care. Daniel Hack Tuke, the initial superintendent, was a coffee and tea merchant by background. He was succeeded by his son and grandson, who trained as medical practitioners before taking over leadership of The Retreat, which is still run by the Society of Friends.

The principles that the institution were run on were later termed 'moral treatment'. They are described in *The Retreat* (the best short textbook on mental health management) (Tuke, 1813) as comprising three factors:

- strengthening and assisting the patient to control the disorder
- coercion being employed only when absolutely necessary
- promoting the general comfort of the insane, including occupation and physical health.

These principles map closely onto Killaspy's definition of a modern rehabilitation service (above) with:

- strengthening and assisting in the control of the disorder being actions that encourage skills and give hope for the future
- promoting independence and autonomy being the obverse of employing coercion only where necessary
- and promoting the general comfort including occupation and physical health being things that will maximise quality of life and social inclusion.

Many features of psychiatric practice, such as meaningful occupation as an in-patient, physical healthcare and skills for employability, which have been more recent preoccupations for mental health service providers, were already recognised in the ethos of moral treatment over 200 years ago. Similarly, the following text, published in 1814, illustrates the prime importance of what today we would call 'relational security' in psychiatric settings:

> In the construction of [asylums], cure and comfort ought to be as much considered as security, and I have no hesitation in declaring that a system which, by limiting the power of the attendant, obliges him not to neglect his duty, and makes his interest to obtain the good opinion of those under

his care, provides more effectively for the safety of the keeper, as well as for the patient, than all the apparatus of chains, darkness and anodynes. (Tuke, 1814: p. 25)

The Retreat, like many reforms in psychiatry, arose out of a scandal of poor care in a large institution, in this case York Asylum. The principles set out by the Tukes have resurfaced over the years, sometimes rediscovered, sometimes (as with Killaspy's definition) synthesised anew from a national survey. The aspects of poor care have also resurfaced in physical and psychiatric healthcare settings and in other institutions such as prisons and care homes for children.

Public asylums and an end to private mad houses

A number of factors, outlined by D. G. Thompson (1914), including greater numbers of pauper lunatics, continuing abuses in private madhouses and greater public provision with the Industrial Revolution, led to Wynne's Act of 1808, which encouraged the establishment of a lunatic asylum in every county. Progress was painfully slow, with only five asylums (Nottinghamshire, Norfolk, Lancashire, Staffordshire and Yorkshire) established over the next 10 years. The 1845 Lunacy Act compelled local authorities to establish asylums and created the Lunacy Commission, the first inspectorate of in-patient mental healthcare in the UK, which had the right to enter every place in England and Wales containing insane persons, whether public asylums, workhouses, private establishments or military hospitals. The Lunacy Commission continued until replaced in 1913 by the Board of Control. Public asylums were built throughout the UK, with most English counties having city and county asylums. This system continued until 1948 and the transfer of responsibility for the asylums from local authorities to the new NHS.

Reforming the asylums and the development of therapeutic communities

By the early 1950s, many asylums contained large numbers of 'back ward' patients, many kept in locked conditions and severely institutionalised. Goffman's seminal work *Asylums: Essays on the Social Situation of Mental Patients and Other Inmates* was published in 1961. David Clark (1996) eloquently describes his experiences of taking over such an asylum (Fulbourn in Cambridgeshire). Clark was appointed as medical superintendent at the age of 33 and was one of the pioneering, reforming, medical superintendents who did a huge amount to improve these institutions in the 1950s and 1960s. The difference in therapeutic environment provided in different institutions, particularly with regard to social approaches, was illustrated in the Three Hospital Study (see Chapter 29, 'Expanding the evidence base'). Clark & Meyers (1970) advocated the 'therapeutic community approach', emphasising increased activity, freedom and responsibility. The therapeutic community approach traced its roots back to the Northfield experiments, early attempts at group therapy for the mass treatment of neurotic disorders in army personnel in the Second World War. In a time of austerity, when trained professionals were in short supply, patients were involved in their therapy, groups were used (of necessity) in preference to individual therapy, rigid hierarchies were flattened and the whole institution was thought of as therapeutic. The pioneers at Northfield went on to have major influences on the development of the therapeutic community movement proper, group therapy and group analysis (Harrison & Clark, 1992).

The improvements made in many asylums were acknowledged by Enoch Powell (1961) in his famous 'water-tower' speech, announcing the closure of the asylums and a move to psychiatric units on the sites of district general hospitals, and community services:

> This is a colossal undertaking, not so much in the new physical provision which it involves, as in the sheer inertia of mind and matter which it requires to overcome. There they stand, isolated, majestic, imperious, brooded over by the gigantic water-tower and chimney combined, rising unmistakable and daunting out of the countryside – the asylums which our forefathers built with such immense solidity to express the notions of their day. Do not for a moment underestimate their powers of resistance to our assault. Let me describe some of the defences which we have to storm.

The process of closure of the asylums in England and Wales was envisaged to be completed by the mid-1970s, but took until very recent times to achieve (a similar timescale to the building of the county Asylums took after Wynne's Act of 1808). The water-tower speech is instructive as much for the identification of obstacles to cultural change as for the practicalities of the capital programme.

Deinstitutionalisation and the virtual asylum

Over the past 50 years or so, most Western countries have closed their large mental asylums and undertaken a process of 'deinstitutionalisation'. In England and Wales this process initially involved devolving in-patient services to smaller, more local units based within the local district general hospital and developing community-based services. More recently, with the separation of mental health and physical healthcare services in different NHS organisations, there has been a regrouping of mental health in-patient services into larger, local mental health units comprising multiple wards. Alongside this, there has been major investment in specialist supported accommodation in the community for those with more long-term and complex needs (see Chapter 19, 'Housing: a place to live'). The number of NHS mental health in-patient beds in England continued to decline from around 67 000 in 1987 to around 22 000 by the late 1990s, but with the growth in independent sector provision, particularly secure and rehabilitation services, this figure is estimated to have increased again, to around 30 000 for the past decade (NHS England, 2013).

The process of deinstitutionalisation was shown to be successful, with most patients able to manage the transition from the asylum to the community without requiring readmission to hospital at 5-year follow-up (Leff & Trieman, 2000). Moreover, the majority of those with the most complex needs were able to progress to more independent supported community living (Trieman & Leff, 2002). However, the need for rehabilitation services did not disappear with the closure of the long-stay institutions and a variety of in-patient rehabilitation units are still an essential component of any comprehensive psychiatric system (Royal College of Psychiatrists, 2009). As described in Chapter 2, 'What is psychiatric rehabilitation?', these services specialise in the treatment of people with complex psychosis and other mental and physical health problems. Without them, this 'small volume, high needs' group are inadequately treated and languish on acute admission wards.

In England and Wales, the consequences of inadequate investment in mental health rehabilitation services became clear following the expansion of specialist community services as part of the National Service Framework for Mental Health (Department of Health, 1999). While this expansion was welcome, it had unforeseen consequences for those patients with the most complex needs (Killaspy & Meier, 2010). Around half of the community rehabilitation teams in existence at the time were disbanded, devolved or rebadged as assertive community treatment teams, and along with other in-patient beds, many rehabilitation wards were closed. Those with the most complex needs did not fit this new system and were not able to be discharged to the care of the new community services. There was a subsequent rapid expansion of in-patient, nursing and residential care provision within the independent sector that addressed this gap, but these services were often located many miles from the person's area of origin. These facilities have been criticised for their lack of rehabilitative ethos and the social dislocation they introduce. They are also more expensive than local provision (Killaspy & Meier, 2010). One of the largest expansions has been seen in 'low secure' in-patient provision (more recently these have been oxymoronically referred to as 'locked rehabilitation' units to differentiate them from low-secure units that form part of the 'forensic' pathway).

This process is not unique to the UK. Described by some writers as 'the virtual asylum' (Poole et al, 2002) and by others as 'reinstitutionalisation' or 'trans-institutionalisation', the expansion of independent sector provision has been reported across many deinstitutionalised countries in Europe (Priebe et al, 2005). In England, the tide appears to be turning. Policy makers have acknowledged that local in-patient rehabilitation and supported accommodation are vital components of a 'whole system' pathway for those with complex needs, and national guidance for commissioners of mental health services is now available that specifically includes mental health rehabilitation services (Joint Commissioning Panel for Mental Health, 2012).

Current definitions of in-patient mental health rehabilitation services

Killaspy *et al*'s (2005) survey of rehabilitation services showed that most NHS trusts had short-term in-patient rehabilitation services and around half also had longer-term services. Most policy documents, if they mentioned rehabilitation at all, also talked about long-term and short-term services and continuing care. These terms had their origins in the old asylums and did not accurately describe the pattern of modern services and their place in a 'whole system' of rehabilitation, particularly one fragmented between different providers.

In order to address this, the Royal College of Psychiatrists' Rehabilitation Faculty undertook a survey of its members and reviewed relevant policy in order to define better the range of services required. The survey received responses from services covering a total population of 7.5 million in the UK and the Republic of Ireland (6 million from England). The number and types of in-patient rehabilitation unit were highly variable but universally felt to be inadequate. Many units were trying to span a variety of functions described below, limiting their effectiveness for certain groups. Major service gaps were in high-dependency, low-secure rehabilitation and supported accommodation for patients to move on to.

The survey clarified that a whole-system approach to rehabilitation requires a range of different facilities that work as part of an interdependent system, a managed functional network, rather than stand-alone units. Only the largest NHS organisations could provide a full spectrum of rehabilitation services. Very specialist services, for example for people with rare comorbid conditions such as mental illness and brain injury, were viable only if provided for a large population. At the other end of the scale, shorter-term (up to 1 year) in-patient rehabilitation units, which could be hospital- or community-based and that focused on enabling users to return to independent living, were available in all but the smallest services. Between them, NHS and independent providers seemed to provide the full range of more specialist in-patient rehabilitation services at the local, regional and national level, as part of a functional network, but this was felt to have arisen piecemeal rather than through a well-organised, strategic partnership that had been built in response to the needs of the population. Nevertheless, the services were noted to provide across four main dimensions:

1   length of admission – from shorter-term assessment and treatment (of 6–12 months), through more prolonged rehabilitation (1–2 years) to longer term (over many years);
2   functional ability of residents – domestic environments concentrating on acquiring and utilising on a daily basis skills for the activities of daily living (ADL), for community living, through to high dependency with domestic services provided by the unit rather than its residents;

Box 17.1 A typology of in-patient mental health rehabilitation units

Community rehabilitation unit
- *Client group:* the many people who, while not needing an acute admission ward or intensively staffed services, need time to recover from a psychotic episode, to optimise medication and reduce side-effects to a minimum
- *Focus:* engagement with services, psychological interventions and skills in activities of daily living (ADL)
- *Recovery goal:* to develop skills and support packages, that include families and carers, for a successful return to community living with variable degrees of support
- *Site:* ideally community based, with a focus on developing practical ADL skills in a domestic environment close to a person's home
- *Length of admission:* usually up to 1 year
- *Functional ability:* domestic environments, concentrating on acquiring and utilising on a daily basis ADL skills for community living
- *Risk management:* generally low-staffed open units but may have some specialist risk assessment skills
- *Degree of specialisation:* local generic rehabilitation units predominantly for patients with treatment-resistant psychosis – should be available in all trusts serving a population of around 300 000

High-dependency rehabilitation unit
- *Client group:* highly symptomatic people, with several or severe comorbid conditions and significant risk histories; a high proportion will be detained and have 'challenging behaviours', and many will have been admitted to forensic admissions or spent periods of time in psychiatric intensive care units
- *Focus:* thorough ongoing assessment, medication, engagement, supporting clients in managing their behaviour and re-engaging with families and communities
- *Recovery goal:* usually a move on to other facilities in the rehabilitation service prior to community living or residential care
- *Site:* usually hospital based to benefit from support from other units and out-of-hours cover
- *Length of admission:* 1–3 years
- *Functional ability:* domestic services provided by the unit rather than its residents, although participation in domestic activities with support encouraged as part of a therapeutic programme
- *Risk management:* higher-staffed (often locked/lockable) units able to manage behavioural disturbance
- *Degree of specialisation:* should be available in all trusts serving a population of around 600 000–1 000 000; has a major role in returning patients from secure services and out-of-area placements

Longer-term complex-care unit
- *Client group:* usually patients with high levels of disability from complex comorbid conditions, with limited potential for future change and associated with significant risk to their own health and safety or those of others; comorbidity with serious physical health problems will be common
- *Focus:* ongoing monitoring and treatment in addition to mental health issues
- *Recovery goal:* other rehabilitation options will usually have been explored; while disability and risk issues remain, a more domestic but highly supported

setting is practical; the emphasis is on promoting personal recovery and improving social and interpersonal functioning

- *Site:* usually community based, sometimes on a hospital campus
- *Length of admission:* several years
- *Functional ability:* domestic services provided by the unit rather than its residents, although participation in domestic activities with support encouraged as part of a therapeutic programme
- *Risk management:* higher-staffed units but with emphasis on unqualified support staff; risk management based on relational skills and environmental management (e.g. low expressed emotion)
- *Degree of specialisation:* should be available in all trusts serving a population of around 600 000–1 000 000

Secure rehabilitation unit

- *Client group:* a group with diverse needs, all of whom have been involved in offending behaviour and detained under the Mental Health Act, the majority under Part III, with levels of security determined by Ministry of Justice requirements
- *Focus:* accurate assessment and management of risk; residents will have varying levels of functional skills and are likely to require therapeutic programmes tailored to their offending behaviour in addition to their mental disorders
- *Recovery goal:* to leave hospital, probably with close supervision by a local community forensic team or assertive outreach team
- *Site:* usually a hospital campus
- *Length of admission:* 2 years or more, depending on the nature of the offending behaviour and psychopathology
- *Functional ability:* domestic services provided by the unit rather than its residents, although participation in domestic activities with support encouraged as part of a therapeutic programme
- *Risk management:* higher-staffed units able to manage behavioural disturbance with full range of physical, procedural and relational security and specialist risk assessment and management skills
- *Degree of specialisation:* low secure for populations of 1 million or more, to high secure for populations of around 15 million

Highly specialist rehabilitation unit

- *Client group:* people with very particular needs such as acquired brain damage, severe personality disorder, comorbid autism spectrum disorder
- *Focus:* psychological approaches to treatment and management, with very active liaison with referrers; often, nearby step-down units will be required that allow people to move on but maintain contact with the specialist expertise they require
- *Recovery goal:* for patients to move on to more independent settings, often with complex care packages developed with the advice of the specialist service
- *Site:* within hospital complexes or in stand-alone units
- *Length of admission:* 1–3 years but highly variable, depending on the nature of the conditions and specialist treatment programmes
- *Functional ability:* variable but should cover a range from full domestic services to high levels of patient participation in ADL activities
- *Risk management:* varies with risk profile and treatment needs
- *Degree of specialisation:* highly specialist facilities for people with specific conditions and comorbidities, requiring specialist treatment programmes for populations of several million

3   risk management – including risks to self, others and health, through the provision of open, low-staffed community units through local higher-staffed (often locked/lockable) units able to manage behavioural disturbance, to secure rehabilitation;

4   specialisation – from local generic rehabilitation units predominantly for patients with treatment-resistant psychosis (these should be available in all trusts serving a population of around 300 000) through to highly specialist facilities for people with specific conditions or comorbidities (specialist treatment programmes for populations of several million).

Incorporating these dimensions and information from the survey, a new typology of in-patient rehabilitation units was devised that reflected contemporary provision more accurately. Cowan *et al* (2012) applied the definitions to existing services and client groups and found they accurately captured community rehabilitation, high-dependency and long-term complex care. The different types of in-patient rehabilitation unit are listed in Box 17.1.

Measuring the therapeutic environments: a cultural barometer?

Psychiatry and indeed medicine as a discipline are often referred to as using a biopsychosocial model of care. The biological aspect has received great attention (and research funding) over recent decades, offering advances in drug treatments for many mental health problems. With the exception of clozapine, these benefits have been limited for people with more complex and severe psychoses. Psychological interventions have also seen great advances, most notably with an increasing evidence base for cognitive–behavioural therapy (CBT) for a variety of conditions, including depression and psychosis, and other manualised treatments such as dialectical behavioural therapy (DBT) for borderline personality disorder. While these developments are welcome, there has been less of a focus on social interventions in recent years. In part, this may have been owing to an increasing preoccupation with shorter admissions in acute mental health services and the fragmentation of some longer-term services (the 'virtual asylum' referred to earlier). The effect of the social environment or therapeutic milieu is a key component of in-patient treatment and needs to be considered and managed in the same way as any other aspect of treatment.

While much has been written about therapeutic environments, often from a psychodynamic or therapeutic community perspective, the evidence base in scientific terms has been limited. This is partly because of the difficulties of reliably measuring the social aspect of therapeutic environments; attempts to do so date back to the 1960s, when Rudolph Moos and colleagues developed the Ward Atmosphere Scale (WAS) for use in large US institutions (see Timko & Moos, 2004). While this was used intermittently at times in the UK, it was laborious to administer, particularly for patients with high levels of disability, and took persistence to score and interpret. Over recent years, other measures have been developed in Europe and adopted in the UK. The Good Milieu Index (GMI) was developed in Norway in the 1980s. It is a short instrument (five items, scored on a five-point scale) and is very easy to complete, analyse and use repeatedly. It includes questions such as 'In general, how satisfied are you with the unit?', 'Does what you do on the unit help you have confidence in yourself?' This measure was employed in the national programme of research into mental health in-patient rehabilitation units in England (the REAL study, detailed in Chapter 29, 'Expanding the evidence base') and was found to be positively associated with other measures of the quality of these units (Killaspy *et al*, 2013). The GMI forms part of the AIMS-Rehab accreditation process run by the Royal College of Psychiatrists Centre for Quality Improvement, described in more detail below (see also Cresswell *et al*, 2012). Another instrument, the Essen Climate Evaluation Scale (EssenCES), was developed in German forensic psychiatric units in the late 1990s and validated in UK settings in the 2000s (Howells *et al*, 2009). This measure was adopted by secure-services commissioning groups as part of the contractual Commissioning for Quality and Innovation (CQUIN) payment framework for medium- and low-secure psychiatric units in England and Wales.

Measures to rate therapeutic environments have therefore progressed from somewhat unwieldy rather esoteric measures (although the WAS is still widely used in the USA) to much more 'user-friendly' measures that have been widely adopted by quality networks and commissioners, and have an expanding evidence base in forensic and rehabilitation services.

Quality in mental health in-patient rehabilitation services

Concerns about how to maintain quality and standards of care in in-patient mental health settings have been around for over 200 years. Indeed, as noted earlier, public asylums were set up primarily because of concerns about abuse and neglect in private madhouses (Parry-Jones, 1988). Since the 19th century, various groups have been set up to detect and remedy abuse and monitor quality; these have included parliamentarians, doctors, lay inspectors, professional administrators and multiprofessional teams. None has been particularly successful. In England there have been three different national inspectorates of healthcare since 2001 – the Commission for Health Improvement (2001–04), the Healthcare Commission (2004–09) and the Care Quality Commission (CQC) (2009 onwards). The CQC is a super-regulator with responsibility for both health and social care settings.

The evidence in favour of the effectiveness of these large (and expensive), centralised bureaucracies in improving quality is very weak (Walshe, 2003). At the time of two recent abuse cases in England (Winterbourne View and Mid-Staffordshire Foundation Trust), the CQC was in contact with the facilities concerned, but either did not detect the problems or failed to address them (or both). Why is this? What does it tell us about systems for monitoring standards and improving quality?

In the first place, it suggests that these problems are an intrinsic risk in settings in which human beings are placed in positions of power and authority over others who are weak and vulnerable. Violence, sexual exploitation, financial malpractice, neglect, oppression and so on can and do happen – see Farquharson's (2004) 'How good staff become bad'. Fortunately, such incidents are rare, but the danger is always present. The effective remedies to manage such risk are also clearly identified. Units need to have good leadership, and to be reasonably well resourced and subject to the checks and balances that are part of proper management and supervision. Above all, they should not be allowed to become physically or organisationally isolated (Martin, 1984). The second lesson is that the issues that led to poor practice and abuses of care are complex and difficult to address. There is certainly no correlation between the amount of resources devoted to the problem and the effectiveness of the systems set up to address it. Finally, it tells us that we should be careful to distinguish between two very different manifestations of problems with the quality of care – what we might call 'flagrant abuse' and 'low standards'. They are both concerned with 'failures' but differ in terms of their severity. They also differ with respect to a number of other characteristics that make it necessary to apply very different kinds of remedies to address them, in terms of both style and content.

In cases of flagrant abuse, which are rare, one does not need a great deal of technical expertise to determine that abuse has happened. It is clear that hitting patients, or sexually assaulting them, or stealing their money, is wrong. If it can be established that a particular member of staff has committed such acts, then she or he deserves to be punished – with either disciplinary or legal sanctions – and that is the end of it. By contrast, low standards of care are much more common, but it is more difficult to establish that they prevail in particular instances. It may require research investigations to define a consensus of expert opinion, then further studies of the reliability and validity of measuring instruments, how to implement them and the most effective methods of change. Successfully raising standards (improving the quality of care) then depends on collaboration between staff, service users and carers to develop new ideas and to apply them to their own, unique situation (Miller *et al*, 2009). This gives the sense of local ownership that is so vital to the success of quality improvement programmes.

Sometimes the process can be facilitated by having access to a respected figure, from within or outside the organisation, who can provide expert opinion and a degree of objectivity. Often it is sufficient simply to give staff the time to discuss the problem and come up with their own solutions, or to arrange for them to meet another staff team who have been grappling with similar problems.

The Royal College of Psychiatrists' Centre for Quality Improvement runs peer accreditation networks for in-patient mental health services, including rehabilitation services, that incorporate these principles (the 'Assessment of In-patient Mental Health Services' or 'AIMs' programmes). Clinicians and experts by experience agree standards of quality for their services, carry out inspections of each other's services and assess these against the standards using a combination of quantitative and qualitative evidence. Quality improvement then becomes a continuous journey where standards may be progressively raised – even radically reformulated – as people increase their expectations as to what might be possible. It is noteworthy that the CQC intends to incorporate the Royal College of Psychiatrists' service accreditations (http://www.rcpsych.ac.uk/workinpsychiatry/ qualityimprovement.aspx) into its processes for inspecting health services.

The Quality Indicator for Rehabilitative Care (QuIRC)

The AIMS programme for in-patient rehabilitation services incorporates two standardised measures, the Good Milieu Index described earlier and the Quality Indicator for Rehabilitative Care (QuIRC). The latter tool was developed during a 3-year collaboration funded by the European Commission involving ten countries at different stages of deinstitutionalisation (Bulgaria, Czech Republic, Germany, Greece, Italy, the Netherlands, Poland, Portugal, Spain and the UK). Its content was derived from triangulation of the results from three sources in order to identify the components of care that are most important for the recovery of people living longer term in mental health facilities. These included a review of the relevant care standards in each of the ten countries, a systematic literature review (Taylor et al, 2009) and an international Delphi exercise with mental health professionals, service users, carers and mental health advocates from each of the ten countries (Turton et al, 2010). The QuIRC was refined through piloting and reliability testing in over 200 facilities across Europe (Killaspy et al, 2011) and cross-validated against over 1750 service users' experiences of care (Killaspy et al, 2012). The final version is available as a web-based application (http:// www.quirc.eu), to be completed by the manager of a facility. It produces a printable report on their facility's performance on each of seven domains of care (living environment, therapeutic environment, treatments and interventions, promotion of self-management and autonomy, promotion of social integration, human rights and recovery-based practice) and shows the average performance for similar units in the same country. It also provides further information about how the unit could improve the quality of care it provides. It is available in ten languages and can be used for local, regional, national or international audit and research. As well as being incorporated into the AIMS-rehab programme in the UK, the QuIRC is being used for similar national quality improvement activities for longer-term mental healthcare facilities in Portugal, the Netherlands, Germany, Czech Republic and Bulgaria.

Quality improvement

Raising standards through quality improvement programmes depends critically on staff being prepared to share their ideas and experiences, including those that might be characterised as 'failures'. This culture has been established in the air transport industry, where there is a general recognition of the positive value attached to a detailed analysis of crashes or 'near misses' using an analytical framework (root cause analysis) that aims to reveal both human error and system failure. As has been noted by many commentators recently, this is not the culture in health services at present. Most staff are frightened of discussing incidents openly because they assume that when it comes to apportioning 'blame' (a very loaded word) the organisation will err on the side of attributing it to human error, rather than system failure. It can be argued that this is a direct result of activities by organisations like the CQC, which seem to approach all examples of poor standards of care as if they were incidents of 'flagrant abuse'. The use of external inspectors who do not have recognised expertise in the field, the focus on individual responsibility and punitive consequences, and the treatment of each incident as an isolated example to be quickly remedied have all contributed to a culture where staff are reluctant to engage in the kind of collaborative process necessary to produce meaningful and long-lasting quality improvement. Hence, health settings are deprived of being 'learning organisations' (Senge, 1990); ironically, therapeutic community approaches to mental healthcare share many similarities with 'learning organisations' (Davies, 1999). Quality is, truly, everyone's business and the responsibility for improving quality must lie within the services themselves.

The future: a whole-systems approach; quality and austerity; guarding against failure

The evidence now exists that a comprehensive local rehabilitation system, with good links to more specialist providers in care pathways (e.g. secure brain injury), is cheaper and more effective than cutting back local services and relying on a multiplicity of providers not linked to local services. This model of dispersed care also infringes a basic human right to private and family life, enshrined in article 8 of the European Convention on Human Rights, disrupted by placements away from community and carers. There is also evidence that better-quality services, measured by validated instruments and promoted through well-developed accreditation processes such as AIMS-Rehab, and which involve professionals and service users, do positively influence outcomes (Killaspy *et al*, 2013), a finding not, so far, replicated in physical medicine.

The temptation in times of austerity, particularly with new commissioning arrangements not well suited to understanding long-term complex psychiatric conditions, is to take short–term decisions and cut back on seemingly less acute and rigorous services such as community rehabilitation units or to cut back on therapeutic interventions such as occupational therapy and psychology. Earlier experience, such as the 'new long stay' crisis of the 1990s, when acute wards were blocked by patients needing rehabilitation that was not locally available, acts as a warning of the consequences. The problem with out-of-area treatments (OATs) in the late 1990s and the 2000s was an inadequate response to this, which often led to poor care and breakdown of community links, leading to longer lengths of stay (and increased costs). Recent developments such as national surveys of OAT usage and models of local service development and repatriation (Royal College of Psychiatrists, 2005, 2012) show that local rehabilitation systems are cost and clinically effective.

The answer in times of austerity or out is to take a long-term strategic view, accept that those with long-term complex conditions exist and recognise that they will require services either in a planned way or as distressed purchasers of secure placements when something goes wrong. It is necessary to invest in a quality rehabilitation system with the therapeutic resources to ensure people move through the services at the optimum rate and with community components that include rehabilitation teams and supported accommodation, to ensure blockages do not occur in expensive parts of the system (or out of area). The other message from the time of post-war austerity and the origins of the therapeutic community movement is to involve people as much as possible in their own recovery, individually and in groups, and for the rehabilitation system to be sufficiently resourced in management terms to engage with and develop community resources such as voluntary organisations and social enterprises.

In terms of the recommendations of the Francis report (2013), to avoid further failures of care we need to understand our history and learn from the mistakes identified in previous inquiries into failures of care because 'those who cannot remember the past are condemned repeat it' (Santayana, 1905). In rehabilitation we already have the tools and instruments such as the QuIRC and GMI and professional- and user-led accreditation networks to use as a cultural barometer. The main concerns for mental health rehabilitation services at present in the UK, and elsewhere, are that recurrent reconfigurations of services and the processes for commissioning services tends to impede the ability of hard-pressed managers to maintain a culture of openness, transparency and candour in the face of political and financial pressures. Substandard in-patient care, like the poor, will always be with us, but a socialised healthcare system in a modern Western democracy has the resources, as well as the material and intellectual ability, to guard against them if it has the will to do so and, as recommended by the Berwick report, 'to make sure pride and joy in work, not fear, infuse the NHS' (National Advisory Group on the Safety of Patients in England, 2013).

References

Clark D (1996) *The Story of a Mental Hospital: Fulbourn 1858–1983.* Process Press.

Clark D, Meyers K (1970) Themes in a therapeutic community. *British Journal of Psychiatry,* 117: 389–95.

Cowan C, Meaden A, Commander M, *et al* (2012) In-patient psychiatric rehabilitation services: survey of service users in three metropolitan boroughs. *The Psychiatrist,* 36: 85–9

Cresswell J, Beavon M, Davies S, *et al* (2012) *Standard Development and Accreditation Process for In-patient Rehabilitation Units.* CCQI, Royal College of Psychiatrists. At http://www.rcpsych.ac.uk/pdf/AIMS-Rehab%20Accreditation%20Process%20-%20July%202012.pdf (accessed December 2014).

Davies S (1999) Therapeutic community treatment of personality disorder: is organisational culture a psychosocial treatment? *Clinician in Management,* 8: 37–43.

Davies S (2004) Toxic institutions. In *From Toxic Institutions to Therapeutic Environments: Residential Settings in Mental Health Services* (eds P Campling, S Davies, G Farquarson): 20–31. Gaskell.

Department of Health (1999) *National Service Framework for Mental Health Modern Standards and Service Models.* Department of Health (https://www.gov.uk/government/uploads/system/uploads/attachment_data/file/198051/National_Service_Framework_for_Mental_Health.pdf).

Department of Health Commissioning Development (2011) PCT Programme Budget Benchmarking Tool, available from http://www.dh.gov.uk/prod_consum_dh/groups/dh_digitalassets/@dh/@en/documents/digitalasset/dh_132501.zip (accessed December 2014).

Farquharson G (2004) How good staff become bad. In *From Toxic Institutions to Therapeutic Environments: Residential Settings in Mental Health Services* (eds P Campling, S Davies, G Farquarson): 12–19. Gaskell.

Francis R (2013) *Report of the Mid-Staffordshire NHS Foundation Trust Public Inquiry: Executive Summary.* TSO (The Stationery Office).

Goffman E (1961) *Asylums: Essays on the Social Situation of Mental Patients and Other Inmates.* Doubleday/Anchor Books.

Harrison T, Clark D (1992) The Northfield experiments. *British Journal of Psychiatry,* 160: 698–708.

Howells K, Tonkin M, Milburn C, *et al* (2009) The EssenCES measure of social climate: a preliminary validation and normative data in UK high secure hospital settings. *Criminal Behaviour and Mental Health,* 19: 308–20.

Joint Commissioning Panel for Mental Health (2012) *Guidance for Commissioners of Rehabilitation Services for People with Complex Mental Health Needs.* Royal College of Psychiatrists.

Killaspy H, Meier R (2010) A fair deal for mental health rehabilitation services. *The Psychiatrist,* 34: 265–7.

Killaspy H, Harden C, Holloway F, *et al* (2005) What do mental health rehabilitation services do and what are they for? A national survey in England. *Journal of Mental Health,* 14: 157–66.

Killaspy H, White S, Wright C, *et al* (2011) The Development of the Quality Indicator for Rehabilitative Care (QuIRC): a measure of best practice for facilities for people with longer term mental health problems. *BMC Psychiatry*, **11**: 35.

Killaspy H, White S, Wright C, *et al* (2012) Association between service user experiences and staff rated quality of care in European facilities for people with longer term mental health problems. *PLoS One*, **7** (6): e38070.

Killaspy H, Marston L, Omar R, *et al* (2013) Service quality and clinical outcomes: an example from mental health rehabilitation services in England. *British Journal of Psychiatry*, **202**: 28–34.

Leff J, Trieman N (2000) Long stay patients discharged from psychiatric hospitals. Social and clinical outcomes after five years in the community. TAPS Project 46. *British Journal of Psychiatry*, **176**: 217–23.

Martin JP (1984) *Hospitals in Trouble*. Blackwell.

Miller V, Rosen A, Gianfrancesco P, *et al* (2009) Australian national standards for mental health services – a blueprint for improvement. *International Journal of Leadership in Public Services*, **5**: 25–42.

National Advisory Group on the Safety of Patients in England (2013) *The Berwick Report. A Promise to Learn – A Commitment to Act: Improving the Safety of Patients in England*. At https://www.gov.uk/government/publications/berwick-review-into-patient-safety (accessed December 2014).

NHS Confederation (2012) *Defining Mental Health Services: Promoting Effective Commissioning and Supporting QIPP*. At http://www.nhsconfed.org/Publications/reports/Pages/Defining-mental-health-services-QIPP.aspx (accessed December 2014).

NHS England (2013) Beds time series – 1987–88 to 2009–10; Beds time-series 2010–11 onwards. At http://www.england.nhs.uk/statistics/statistical-work-areas/bed-availability-and-occupancy/bed-data-overnight (accessed December 2014).

Parry-Jones W (1988) Asylum for the mentally ill in historical perspective. *Psychiatric Bulletin*, **12**: 407–10.

Poole R, Ryan T, Pearsall A (2002) The NHS, the private sector, and the virtual asylum. *BMJ*, **325**: 349–50.

Powell E, Minister of Health (1961) The water tower speech. At http://studymore.org.uk/xpowell.htm (accessed December 2014).

Priebe S, Badesconyi A, Fioritti A, *et al* (2005) Reinstitutionalisation in mental health care: comparison of data on service provision from six European countries. *BMJ*, **330**: 123–6.

Royal College of Psychiatrists (2005) *Out of Area Treatments for Working Age Adults with Complex and Severe Psychiatric Disorders: Review of Current Situation and Recommendations for Good Practice* (Working Group Report, Faculty of Rehabilitation and Social Psychiatry). Royal College of Psychiatrists. At http://www.rcpsych.ac.uk/pdf/FR_RS_02.pdf (accessed December 2014).

Royal College of Psychiatrists (2009) *Enabling Recovery for People with Complex Mental Health Needs. A Template for Rehabilitation Services* (Rehabilitation and Social Psychiatry Faculty Report FR/RS/01). Royal College of Psychiatrists.

Royal College of Psychiatrists (2012) *A Guide to Good Practice in the Use of Out-of-Area Placements* (Rehabilitation and Social Psychiatry Faculty Report FR/RS/07). Royal College of Psychiatrists.

Santayana G (1905) *The Life of Reason. Vol. 1*. At Project Gutenberg, http://www.gutenberg.org/files/15000/15000-h/vol1.html#CHAPTER_I_THE_BIRTH_OF_REASON (accessed December 2014).

Senge PM (1990) *The Fifth Discipline – The Art and Practice of Learning Organisations*. Random House.

Taylor T, Killaspy H, Wright C, *et al* (2009) A systematic review of the international published literature relating to quality of institutional care for people with longer term mental health problems. *BMC Psychiatry*, **9**: 55.

Thompson DG (1914) The presidential address on the progress of psychiatry during the past hundred years, together with the history of the Norfolk County Asylum during the same period, delivered at the seventy-third annual meeting of the Medico-Psychological Association, held at Norwich, on July 14th and 15th, 1914. *Journal of Mental Science*, **251**: 541–72.

Timko C, Moos RH (2004) Measuring the therapeutic environment. In *From Toxic Institutions to Therapeutic Environments: Residential Settings in Mental Health Services* (eds P Campling, S Davies, G Farquarson): 143–56. Gaskell.

Trieman N, Leff J (2002) Long-term outcome of long-stay psychiatric in-patients considered unsuitable to live in the community: TAPS Project 44. *British Journal of Psychiatry*, **181**: 428–32.

Tuke S (1813) *Description of The Retreat, An Institution near York for Insane Persons of the Society of Friends*. BiblioBazaar (2009).

Tuke S. (1814) *Samuel Tuke on Insanity, The Critical Review or Annals of Literature*. Series IV, Vol 6, p. 25. J. Souter, 1 Paternoster Row, London.

Turton P, Wright C, White S, *et al* (2010) Promoting recovery in long term mental health institutional care: an international Delphi study. *Psychiatric Services*, **61**: 293–9.

Walshe K (2003) *Regulating Healthcare – A Prescription for Improvement*. Open University Press.

CHAPTER 18

Community-based rehabilitation and recovery

Sridevi Kalidindi and Frank Holloway

Introduction

This chapter provides an account of the work of community mental health teams that aim to promote the rehabilitation and recovery of the people they are serving. Both rehabilitation and recovery are 'everyone's business' and the principles and practices discussed in the chapter are relevant to all community mental health services. The roles of specialised teams offering assertive outreach, early intervention in psychosis and, in particular, community rehabilitation are, however, described in some detail.

It is important at the outset to emphasise three issues that are often overlooked. First, services are not in themselves treatments – they are, rather, vehicles for delivering treatment and care. Second, a vital element of good treatment and care is the therapeutic relationship between those providing services (the individual practitioner, the treatment team and the wider care system) and the person receiving services (the patient, client or service user) and her or his support network. Third, high-quality work within rehabilitation and recovery almost invariably takes place in the context of effective team working. Effective teams are supportive of the practitioner, have a positive therapeutic culture, reflect on their work and make use of the skills and experience of all team members.

Principles

Rehabilitation services must strive to ensure they work collaboratively and in a recovery-focused, person-centred way. The key aims are to support service users in attaining their goals and moving towards self-management of their mental health condition, while ensuring that the challenges they face are adequately addressed. These challenges include risks such as social isolation, self-neglect, relapse into acute illness, challenging behaviours, comorbid substance misuse, inability to cope, exploitation in the community and co-occurring physical health problems (Kalidindi *et al*, 2012). To put the laudable aims of rehabilitation services into practice, effective engagement, assessment, formulation and care planning are essential.

Involvement of family, carers and others in the social network of the service user is likely to be important in bringing about sustained positive change. Families need information, advice and support from statutory services and, sometimes, specific interventions such as family work or therapy (see Chapter 10, 'Family interventions').

All teams that offer rehabilitation, particularly those working in the community, need to invest time and energy in working alongside other organisations within the health and social services and the independent and voluntary sector to facilitate the 'whole-system approach' that is required if users of their service are to succeed in achieving their goals and living and staying well. Part of the team's remit will be managing transitions to and from differing levels of supportive setting with an ultimate goal, when possible and in keeping with the service user's wishes, of a move into independent accommodation (with domiciliary support if necessary).

Key is the ability to ensure that the right person receives the right care at the right time. This routinely involves managing the processes of movement in and out of funded placements. Advice should be given to other teams that support people with severe mental health issues around options when living independently in the community appears no longer to be working. Rehabilitation teams should facilitate access to the right sort of supported placement by working with funding panels, reviewing people in out-of-area placements or treatments (OATs) in order that the placement provides the necessary treatment, and planning the return to local provision whenever achievable. It is necessary for specialist teams to have an overview of all the service users in high-support care in a locality and changes in their service needs over time. It is also important to develop, in conjunction with commissioners and others, appropriate local services.

Engagement

Engagement is a term that is both 'over-used and under-defined' (Burns & Firn, 2002) in the community-care literature. Burns & Firn describe the various activities that staff use to foster engagement. First and foremost is an attempt to work constructively with the person (and the family) by befriending, offering advocacy and practical support (addressing needs for accommodation, finances, employment and leisure activities) and adopting a collaborative, non-judgemental and strengths-focused approach. Meetings may be at home or in the community and the person is supported to make use of mainstream activities. A second strand to engagement is an 'informative' approach, which involves the use of a variety of techniques to ensure there is a good understanding of the person's welfare and needs. These include an assertive approach to maintaining contact, if necessary 'door-stepping' the person with unannounced visits, and having contact with the person's care network, including family, general practitioner and housing officer. The final strand to engagement is more coercive and includes the use of statutory powers under mental health legislation, such as compulsory treatment orders and appointeeship.

Assessment

Assessment issues are discussed in detail in Chapter 4, 'A comprehensive approach to assessment in rehabilitation settings'. A thorough, systematic assessment can help engagement. Flexibility is key, however, as many people will be unable to tolerate in-depth assessments in settings outside their usual living environment. Assessment tools such as the Camberwell Assessment of Need – Clinical Version (Slade *et al*, 1999) and the Social Functioning Questionnaire (Clifford & Morris, 1983) can be helpful. The Health of the Nation Outcome Scale is a summary outcome measure that focuses mainly on symptoms (Wing *et al*, 1996). In England its descendant, the Mental Health Clustering Tool (Department of Health, 2013a), is used to assign people to a 'care cluster' which in theory should give an indication of the type of illness, severity and care pathway with incumbent resource each individual will require. 'Care clustering' is in readiness for 'payment by results', or whatever term will eventually be used, to provide a tariff for episodes of care and interventions provided as part of this (Department of Health, 2013b). Assessment tools can be repeated at timely intervals to demonstrate improved outcomes in terms of needs being met and independent living skills being improved.

Key assessment domains include mental health (including comorbidities), physical health, family and personal relationships, daytime activities, housing, occupation and education (including functional skills), risk issues, substance misuse, medication (including side-effects) and insight, early-warning signs, relapse indicators and contingency plans. Carers' assessments can identify and address the enormous burden often placed on those closest to the patient, with the hope that they are able to stay involved in the lives of those they care for and support them in their recovery journey.

This approach is one that statutory organisations will regularly take, but those who work in the non-statutory sector who espouse a more recovery-based stance may argue that focusing on needs leads to a deficits view. A more radically person-centred assessment may be more effective at identifying personal goals, offer a more strengths-based view and be empowering. Non-statutory organisations are, of course, readily able to move people out of their services when levels of risk or disturbance to others become unacceptable.

The goal of assessment is a formulation. Formulating how and why people have reached the position they are now in should provide an understanding of the individual and offer the basis for thinking with the care team, carers and the individual about how to plan the necessary care.

Care planning

The traditional way of formulating care plans in statutory services is based around a list of headings that cover areas of a person's life that are felt to be important, with an aim of providing a holistic approach to each individual. In England, documentation will be in accordance with the Care Programme Approach (CPA). CPA is sometimes perceived by service users as more for the benefit of services than users.

At present, 'recovery and support plans' are being used, which are very similar to the Wellness Recovery Action Plan® (Copeland, 2002). Here the emphasis is very much on the care plan and goals being developed and owned by the service user. An outline of the recovery and Support plan used in the South London and Maudsley (SLaM) National Health Service Foundation Trust is shown in Box 18.1.

There is a distinct difference between the approach taken within a recovery and support plan and the CPA. The service user may experience a higher level of ownership and personal responsibility when using a recovery and support plan compared with the CPA form. Empowerment, personal responsibility and increased self-management can be better facilitated and encouraged, but staff training in its use is required.

Also essential to the effectiveness of a recovery and support plan as a joint care plan is a section that allows the professional working with the service user to discuss any issues he or she feels are missing from the plan. This discussion needs to be taken forward in as collaborative a way as possible, with the service user adding it to the plan if he or she wishes or the professional working with him or her recording it in the service user's electronic record on his or her behalf.

The recovery and support plan also provides an opportunity to 'contract' with others, including family and other important people in the service user's life (with the service user remaining as much as possible in charge of the process). This may help a carer to make positive contributions to the person's life in ways that everyone has agreed and feels comfortable with – including the carer's role in crises.

Another tool that can assist in care planning and indeed with engagement and mapping progress is the Recovery STAR (see http://www.mhpf.org.uk/programmes/mh-and-recovery/the-recovery-star). Although there are concerns over its utility as a recovery outcome measure (Killaspy *et al*, 2012), as opposed to an engagement and coaching tool, it can be helpful in facilitating discussions between the service user and staff about needs, which can then feed into collaborative care and support planning. It enables a more personal and self-rated perspective on quality of life or progress in reaching personal goals or recovery as defined by the individual.

Reframing treatment and care planning in an educational context, for example through recovery colleges as in the USA and in the UK in Nottingham and South West London, can support a paradigm shift

Box 18.1 Outline contents of a SLaM recovery and support plan

- Whether on Care Programme Approach (CPA)/has a personal budget

Freeform recovery and support plan: recovery and staying well

Write, audio/video record or draw your plan in your own style. Try to include as many/all of the questions within the freeform plan.

- What is important to me?
- What does staying well mean to me?
- What if anything, would I like to be different in my life?
- How will I stay in control and safe?
- What supports me to communicate more easily with others?
- What am I going to do each day to stay well and achieve my goals? What I do, time, why I do it?
- Types of support that have helped in the past
- Preferred medications and why
- Are there any medications and/or treatments that you prefer not to have
- Personal budget – how it will be spent
- Goals and aspirations:
  - Describe what a personal goal is and how you'll know when you've achieved it
  - You then need to describe how you plan to achieve your goal including any support you might receive
  - Mention who will provide the support if any
- Comments – disagreements about what's in your plan or other comments
- Agreements and signatures
- Information-sharing agreement
- Agreement to use personal budget solely for support and services agreed in this plan
- Agreement that user was involved in writing the recovery and support plan and that user understands what it is
- Date, signatures, date when it will be reviewed
- Copy given/offered to service user

for both users and providers of mental health services. This approach emphasises that the service users can be in control of the direction their lives, 'co-production' being key.

Trusting relationships are central to helping service users reach their targets and develop the ability to self-manage their condition. There is a role for a coaching approach to foster the development of interests and strengths (Bora, 2012). The building of such relationships requires continuity of care over longer periods of time, a taking of the 'long view' and also a sense of hope, even in the face of very slow improvements and multiple attempts to achieve certain goals.

Personal goal-setting implies a strengths-based approach. The implication of change being possible may in itself engender hope. Engaging patients, families and carers, working together towards their goals and finding meaning in their lives other than just managing the severe mental illness that they have, enables them to move towards recovery.

Working with the care network

In order to be effective in guiding service users to greater independence, meaningful occupation and social inclusion, it is necessary for a community mental health team to have excellent knowledge of and strong connections across a broad range of other mental health services and agencies. The 'whole-system approach' this book emphasises as necessary for successful rehabilitation includes primary care, other secondary mental health and social care services, the staff at supported accommodation (nursing/residential care, supported tenancies with support on site or floating outreach) leading on to independent tenancies and services that support social inclusion, such as vocational rehabilitation (sheltered and supported employment, voluntary work, welfare benefits advice), education, advocacy services, peer support and cultural and leisure services (Joint Commissioning Panel for Mental Health, 2012). Collaborative working can facilitate incremental improvements in service users' functional ability and their ability to self-manage their condition.

Community rehabilitation (and recovery) teams should form an important element of the local care system, often working particularly closely with the local in-patient rehabilitation services. Rehabilitation in-patient units will receive referrals from local acute in-patient units, intensive-care units and low- and medium-secure services. When the system is working well, patients can move readily between the in-patient and community rehabilitation services.

Key skills for members of a community rehabilitation team are to build relationships across the care network, to avoid splitting, to support the service user and family to manage transitions and to identify gaps in services. The team will need to work with commissioners to address these gaps.

The personalisation agenda in England, which seeks to encourage the allocation of social care and more recently health budgets to individuals based on their wants and needs, presents significant challenges to all community mental health services (see Chapter 3, 'Rehabilitation as a values-led practice'). It may have major implications for how services are run, given that there is an expectation that service users will be making more personal choices as to which service they would prefer to employ to provide the support, interventions and outcomes they would like to see. The outcomes sought by commissioners of services and by service users are likely to overlap, but not completely, and services will need to be mindful of ensuring they satisfy all buyers.

Risk management in community mental health services

A thorough and fit-for-purpose risk assessment, relating not only to the mental illness the individual has, but also to the personal and social context of the service user, is at the core of enabling a good formulation of and subsequent management of those risks. (These issues are discussed in more detail in Chapter 26, 'Risk management in rehabilitation practice'.) The Mental Capacity Act 2005 can be used where people do not have capacity to make an informed decision about an aspect of their care or the risks that their actions or inactions may incur. The risk to someone suffering diabetes mellitus of eating sugary foods or refusing anti-diabetic medication is an example of such decisions. Where there is concern about vulnerability because of lack of capacity, the route of involving family or an independent mental capacity advocate in a 'best interests' meeting should be followed. The meeting leads to an agreed plan of action. It is important to ensure that, when appropriate, 'deprivation of liberty' safeguards are in place and reviewed at least annually.

Positive risk-taking, when undertaken well, can promote personal learning and growth for the individual and the care team. There is potentially a tension when taking more of a recovery approach in risk assessment and management. For example, a formal approach to risk for someone attending a recovery college may be replaced only by explicit expectations of behaviour in the form of a 'student charter', without formal risk assessment of each student attending (Perkins *et al*, 2012).

Risks such as self-neglect, fire-setting, vulnerability to exploitation and challenging behaviours are not uncommon among users of rehabilitation services, as is a forensic history. Understanding the context of the risk behaviour, for example whether it occurred at a time of deteriorating mental health or when engaging in substance misuse, or is due to criminality itself, enables the service user and team to work together to take considered positive risks.

Challenges for community teams

Mental health teams working in the community face particular challenges depending on their client group and specific remit. There are, however, a number of challenges common to all teams working with people who have longer-term and complex needs relating to a psychotic illness. One is 'comorbidity' – more than one psychiatric problem coexisting with the psychotic illness. Important and very common comorbidities are anxiety disorders (including panic disorder, post-traumatic stress disorder and obsessive–compulsive disorder) and depression (Buckley *et al*, 2009). These comorbidities are under-recognised and often require specific pharmacological or psychological treatment. Anxiety symptoms may be particularly socially disabling but can respond to quite simple behavioural interventions.

Community teams are certainly well aware of the importance of comorbid substance misuse – estimated as occurring in 47% of people with a diagnosis of schizophrenia. Substance misuse is associated with a range of adverse consequences, which include worsening of positive symptoms, increased tendency to relapse, increased risks of violence and suicide, greater medical comorbidities and a higher risk of contact with the criminal justice system (Buckley *et al*, 2009). It is important to note that risky substances include cigarettes, alcohol and over-the-counter analgesics, all of which contribute to the excess mortality rates seen in people with psychotic illnesses. Practical options for working with comorbid substance misuse are presented in Chapter 12, 'Working with coexisting substance misuse'. The key messages are that the team needs to be aware of substance misuse issues, be prepared to work with the patient on the substance misuse and access whatever additional resources are available.

There are other important, if less common, comorbidities relating to acquired brain injury (see Chapter 24, 'Rehabilitation and acquired brain injury') and autistic spectrum disorder (see Chapter 25, 'Autism spectrum disorder'). Staff working in non-specialist teams will need to have an understanding of the issues that these problems present to patients and carers and may need to draw in additional expertise in developing an effective care plan.

A second set of challenges that teams working with people suffering from psychosis face flow from the illness itself, which is not only manifested in the 'positive' symptoms of psychosis that tend to interest psychiatrists and the lay understanding of mental illness. Severe psychosis is also associated with 'negative' symptoms and cognitive impairment – nicely described as 'disabling cognitive and motivational impairments' (van Os & Kapur, 2009). Addressing these impairments is a core skill of rehabilitation practice.

Community teams also frequently struggle to engage people with services and the consequences of non-adherence with medication. A patient's failure to engage with mental health services and to adhere to treatment are not in themselves manifestations of an illness but may reflect a breakdown in communication or a lack of common ground between the patient and the clinicians. Though this may be influenced by the degree to which the patient has insight into the condition, being able to work constructively when there is a difference of opinion about or perspective on the causes and consequences of the patient's experiences and symptoms is a key clinical skill. We do know that engagement can be improved by the techniques routinely employed by assertive outreach teams (see below).

Engaging with services for physical healthcare and adhering to treatments for comorbid physical health conditions is another area where people with severe psychosis often need extensive support. The management of physical health conditions when a patient lacks capacity to consent to investigations and treatment is an area that requires the specific knowledge and specialist skills of the team. Chapter 15, 'Physical healthcare', covers these issues in depth.

A final challenge for community teams of any description is working effectively with families, which goes beyond the delivery of psycho-educational packages (see Chapter 10, 'Family interventions'). Traditionally, mental health services have had enormous difficulty in engaging families and implementing evidence-based family interventions that can assist patients in their recovery.

Rehabilitation and the community mental health team

In England there is a current trend to separate generic community mental health teams (CMHTs) into an assessment and short-term treatment team and a longer-term team, sometimes called a 'recovery team'. The traditional CMHT served a catchment area and worked with a designated in-patient unit, assessing and treating all comers. There is some evidence that a well-run CMHT that is focused on the functional outcomes of patients referred to the service can have results for people with severe mental illness at least as good as and possibly better than the assessment and brief treatment/longer-term team model (Thornicroft *et al*, 1998). However, the direction of travel for community mental health services since the publication of the National Service Framework for Mental Health (Department of Health, 1999) has been resolutely towards increasing differentiation of services within a 'functional' model. This included, in addition to the generic CMHT, crisis resolution/home treatment teams, assertive outreach teams (AOT) and early intervention in psychosis (EIP) teams (Department of Health, 2001).

Teams with interest and expertise in working with people experiencing psychotic illness, whether they be a traditional 'catch-all' team or a designated long-term team, can be very effective. This is particularly true if the CMHT knows the area and works effectively with other local services (e.g. primary care, housing and domiciliary care providers, educational institutions and, for vulnerable people, community safety arrangements). Local teams will need to take on the 'step-down' care of people with highly complex conditions, some of whom may have committed serious offences. To do this effectively, the team must have an understanding of the legal frameworks that apply to offender patients.

There is one important limitation to what generic services can do. Experience suggests that managing the placement of someone who requires expensive residential or hospital care requires rather specific expertise best located within a specialist community rehabilitation team (see below).

The assertive outreach team

Assertive community treatment (ACT) was developed by Leonard Stein and Mary-Ann Test in the USA (Stein & Test, 1980). It is a form of intensive community support that seeks to enable people at high risk of readmission to stay out of hospital. Stein & Test based their service model on a set of requirements they believed were necessary for successful tenure in the community, which included: material resources (food, shelter, clothing, basic medical care); basic functional skills (e.g. budgeting, shopping and cooking); motivation to enable people to cope with stress; education and support of members of the community who interact with vulnerable patients; a system of assertive support; and what they described as 'freedom from dependent relationships'. ACT staff were expected to work with patients *in vivo* – in their environment of need – rather than in some artificial setting such as a day hospital or team base. Over time, the ACT model was refined to the extent that there now is a widely used schedule for assessing a team's fidelity to the model – the DACTS (Teague *et al*, 1998). Key components of DACTS are low staff–patient ratios, a team approach to care, effective management of crisis and hospital admission, and staff members who address substance misuse and vocational rehabilitation working within the team.

The assertive outreach team (AOT), as it is known in England, was a core element of the 'functionalised' services set up as a result of the National Health Service Plan in England (Department of Health, 2001). Many AOTs were developed out of 'rebadged' functioning community rehabilitation teams (Killaspy *et al*, 2009*a*). The remit of the AOT service was to work with people who are socially chaotic and hard to engage and who have experienced repeated in-patient admissions. AOT proved to be a model of care that was popular with clinicians, patients and carers.

However, research undertaken in the UK has consistently shown that ACT/AOT does not deliver improved clinical or social outcomes compared with 'standard' treatment provided by a CMHT, although engagement with services and satisfaction with care are better for people receiving ACT/AOT (Killaspy *et al*, 2006, 2009*b*; Burns, 2009). A study of ACT in the Netherlands, which like the UK has a well developed system of community mental health services, had very similar findings (Sytema *et al*, 2007). Such evidence data, along with the harsh economic climate, has resulted in significant disinvestment in AOT in recent years.

The AOT/ACT story has not yet reached a conclusion. It seems clear that with adequate resources, motivation and leadership a generic CMHT can work well with people with long-term mental illness (Thornicroft *et al*, 1998), adopting many of the techniques and principles that make ACT so attractive to clinicians, patients and carers. However, the reality in many settings is that CMHTs are overburdened and often have to focus their energies on assessment of new referrals and managing crises. One intriguing approach, which was first developed in the Netherlands but is gaining increasing attention across Europe, is the FACT model (Veldhuizen, 2007). A 'functional' ACT is a hybrid community mental health team focused on people with a severe mental illness which can provide assertive outreach and extended-hours care to a subgroup of patients who, at a particular time, require the intensive 'whole team' approach offered by ACT. Most patients receive a more standard level of case management – care is titrated to current need (in contemporary parlance, 'zoned'). The FACT model has not been subject to anything like the volume of research that ACT has received, although there is encouraging evidence available about the outcome for patients moving from an ACT service to FACT (Firn *et al*, 2013).

The early intervention in psychosis team

Dedicated services to provide 'early intervention in psychosis' (EIP) are based on pioneering work in Melbourne, Australia (McGorry & Jackson, 1999). EIP services were developed across England following the National Health Service Plan (Department of Health, 2001), although they were not uniformly resourced to treat everyone within a catchment area newly presenting with a psychotic illness. The EIP concept was developed in the knowledge that there is often a very long delay between onset of illness and actual receipt of treatment. It has long been known that long delays in receiving treatment are associated with poorer outcomes. However, the causal relationship is far from clear since the factors associated with delays in receiving treatment may in themselves be predictive of poor outcomes.

There are four components to a comprehensive EIP service:

- identification of people at high risk of developing psychosis, either because they have non-specific symptoms suggestive of an incipient psychotic illness or because of high genetic loading
- a systematic attempt to ensure that people developing a psychotic illness are identified and referred for assessment and treatment, which might be achieved through public education, specific education of general practitioners and other agencies (notably schools), and provision of accessible services that can rapidly undertake an assessment
- addressing age-specific and phase-specific issues (the needs of someone newly presenting with a psychosis at 13 years of age, which can happen, are very different from those of people who first develop a psychosis in their 30s, by which time they may well have developed a significant amount of life experience and social capital, and differ again with the person presenting to services after decades of untreated psychosis)
- providing a comprehensive range of treatments (including psychological treatments and family interventions) and, if necessary, offering an assertive-outreach approach.

There is enormous face validity to the development of dedicated EIP services. The EIP model, with its focus on maintaining the social world of a person experiencing a psychotic illness, is entirely compatible with the principles of psychiatric rehabilitation. Advocates of EIP have produced clinical practice guidelines that encourage early identification, community education, phase-specific care, cautious pharmacological treatment, access to psychosocial interventions and engagement of patients and carers (International Early Psychosis Association Writing Group, 2005). One important issue for EIP services is working through with patients and carers the implications of a diagnosis of psychosis, attempting to address the perils of either outright denial of the illness on the one hand or catastrophic despair and disruption of social networks on the other. Skilled workers can forge and maintain close links with family, who are, as already emphasised, an important and often neglected resource (see Chapter 10, 'Family interventions').

The EIP movement has undoubtedly improved the recognition and treatment of psychosis in children and young people. Intervention in 'at risk' individuals who have not become overtly psychotic remains highly controversial. A meta-analytic review concluded that there is modest evidence that psychological treatments may delay or prevent transition to psychosis (Stafford *et al*, 2013). The suggestion that dedicated EIP services improve outcome has, though, rather lukewarm support (Marshall & Lockwood, 2011). What is clear is that gains over standard care from EIP are lost when support from the service is withdrawn (Gafoor *et al*, 2010). EIP services, even if of good quality, do not abolish the long-term disabilities that some people with psychosis experience (Castle, 2012) and as a consequence some people will require very high levels of support in the early stages of their illness (Craig *et al*, 2004).

The specialist community rehabilitation team

Community rehabilitation teams (CRTs) were originally developed to support patients leaving long-stay hospitals and in-patient rehabilitation services. Contemporary CRTs now receive referrals from early-intervention and assertive-outreach services, generic CMHTs and a wide range of in-patient services. Although some CRTs support people who are living independently, albeit with continuing problems with daily living skills, the commonest model is for the CRT to work with patients who have been placed in residential and nursing homes and 'Supporting People' placements (Kalidindi *et al*, 2012) (see Chapter 19, 'Housing', for a description of the Supporting People initiative).

Important functions of the CRT are: to give expert advice on placement options to other teams; to provide direct care coordination; to work with clients who are moving from hospital to supported accommodation and from higher to lower support; and to work collaboratively with local providers of accommodation, education and vocational rehabilitation (Joint Commissioning Panel for Mental Health, 2012). In some areas, senior members of the CRT are involved in funding panels, gate-keeping referrals and working formally with commissioners to ensure appropriate move-on of patients to greater levels of independence.

To achieve these aims there are a number of tasks that CRT members undertake. They work directly with clients to enable them to gain confidence in everyday living skills and self-manage their condition, intervene to improve their social network and support them in engaging in meaningful occupation. Maintaining therapeutic optimism and helping people develop and meet achievable goals are key tasks. The CRT will need to provide or arrange access to the range of therapeutic interventions documented elsewhere in this book, including access to appropriate physical healthcare (see Chapter 15, 'Physical healthcare'). The CRT will offer practical support to maintain a placement or tenancy – which will frequently involve detailed discussion with the housing provider and problem-solving when difficulties are encountered.

In helping people move through the rehabilitation care pathway, teams can develop bespoke packages of community care that address specific clinical or social needs, funded through personal budgets (now termed self-directed support) (Newbronner *et al*, 2011).

Managing out-of-area placements

In England, a large number of patients are placed out of area (and in independent hospitals that happen to be local). Out-of-area placements (commonly known as OATs – the 't' is for 'treatment') will be into residential and hospital provision. OATs are more expensive than local provision. It is estimated that in 2009/10 £690 million was spent on them in England (National Mental Health Development Unit, 2011), which is over 20% of spending on longer-term adult mental healthcare (Edwards *et al*, 2012). In the past, it was often a case of 'out of sight, out of mind' – although some local health and social care economies have long been aware of the value, in terms of both expenditure and quality of care, of closely managing OAT placements. Good-practice guidance is now available on the use of OATs (National Mental Health Development Unit, 2011; Edwards *et al*, 2012). Health and social care economies are investing in either dedicated OAT teams or (probably more effectively) resourcing the local CRT to develop rehabilitation care pathways for people already placed in OATs and develop clear pathways for people who are being considered for an out-of-area placement. Strong care coordination by the placing service is vital and much welcomed by the higher-quality OAT providers, which are motivated to support people moving through the care system.

Conclusion

Community-based rehabilitation and recovery can be undertaken in teams with different service models. The key factors that enable success include a collaborative, strengths-based, hopeful and person-centred approach by services that is inclusive of the person's social network. People can be enabled to move towards recovery by working with them on their goals and helping them find meaning in their lives separate from their severe mental illness (Davidson, 2003). Goals need to be realistic and achievable and progress should be reviewed regularly. We have noted the potential value of reframing treatment in an educational context, for example through the recovery college model.

We have also noted the importance of trusting relationships in helping service users reach their targets and develop the ability to self-manage their condition. Building relationships requires continuity of care over longer periods of time, a taking of the 'long view' and also a sense of hope, even in the face of very slow improvements and multiple attempts to achieve certain goals. Each attempt should be seen as a learning process and not as a failure, which can be built upon to ensure the next try at attaining a particular goal is more likely to be successful. Peer workers, with their lived experience and their own recovery status, may be particularly effective at sustaining hope in this scenario.

Service users, helped by those around them, may have worked incredibly hard over a long time to move forwards with their lives. It is often at such moments that a move to a more independent setting or to a different team may be mooted. Moving to less intensive levels of support will allow scarce resources to be devoted to others in greater need within a local area but it can be challenging. Careful management of transitions is imperative if deterioration in functional level and mental health are to be avoided. Planning with good, psychologically informed thinking around minimising anxiety and working in a joined-up way across the interfaces involved is important.

By working as part of a wider system (Kalidindi *et al*, 2012), rehabilitation in the community can quite literally, as one service user stated after moving to a special sheltered flat of his own after decades of living in residential care homes, 'give people their lives back'.

References

Bora R (2012) *Empowering People: Coaching for Mental Health Recovery*. Rethink Mental Illness.

Buckley PF, Miller BJ, Lehrer D, *et al* (2009) Psychiatric comorbidities and schizophrenia. *Schizophrenia Bulletin*, **35**: 383–402.

Burns T (2009) End of the road for treatment-as-usual studies? *British Journal of Psychiatry*, **195**: 5–6.

Burns T, Firn M (2002) *Assertive Outreach in Mental Health*. Oxford University Press.

Castle DJ (2012) The truth, and nothing but the truth, about early intervention in psychosis. *Australian and New Zealand Journal of Psychiatry,* **46**: 10–13.

Clifford P, Morris I (1983) *The Social Functioning Questionnaire.* Research and Development for Psychiatry.

Copeland ME (2002) Overview of WRAP: wellness recovery action plan. *Mental Health Recovery Newsletter,* **3**: 1–9.

Craig TK, Garety P, Power P, et al (2004) The Lambeth Early Onset (LEO) Team: randomised controlled trial of the effectiveness of specialised care for early psychosis. *BMJ,* **329**: 1067.

Davidson L (2003) *Living Outside Mental Illness: Qualitative Studies of Recovery in Schizophrenia.* New York University Press.

Department of Health (1999) *National Service Framework for Mental Health.* Department of Health.

Department of Health (2001) *Mental Health Policy Implementation Guide.* Department of Health.

Department of Health (2013a) *Mental Health Clustering Booklet v. 3* (Gateway Reference 18768). Department of Health.

Department of Health (2013b) *Mental Health Payment by Results Guidance for 2013–14* (Gateway Reference 18768). Department of Health.

Edwards T, Wolfson P, Killaspy H (2012) *A Guide to Good Practice in the Use of Out-of-Area Placements* (Faculty Report FR/RS/06). Royal College of Psychiatrists.

Firn M, Hindhaugh K, Hubbeling D, et al (2013) A dismantling study of assertive outreach services: comparing activity and outcomes following replacement with the FACT model. *Social Psychiatry and Psychiatric Epidemiology,* **48**: 997–1003.

Gafoor R, Nitsch D, McCrone P, et al (2010) Effect of early intervention on 5-year outcome in non-affective psychosis. *British Journal of Psychiatry,* **196**: 372–6.

International Early Psychosis Association Writing Group (2005) International clinical practice guidelines for early psychosis. *British Journal of Psychiatry,* **187** (suppl 48): s120–4.

Joint Commissioning Panel for Mental Health (2012) *Guidance for Commissioners of Rehabilitation Services for People with Complex Mental Health Needs.* JCP-MH.

Kalidindi S, Killaspy H, Edwards T (2102) *Community Psychosis: The Role of Community Mental Health Rehabilitation Teams* (FR/RS/07). Royal College of Psychiatrists.

Killaspy H, Bebbington P, Blizard R, et al (2006) The REACT study: randomised evaluation of assertive community treatment in north London. *BMJ,* **332**: 815.

Killaspy H, Mountain D, Holloway F (2009a) Mental health rehabilitation services in the UK in 2007. *Psychiatric Bulletin,* **33**: 215–18.

Killaspy H, Kingett S, Bebbington P, et al (2009b) Randomised evaluation of assertive community treatment: 3-year outcomes. *British Journal of Psychiatry,* **195**: 81–2.

Killaspy H, White S, Taylor TL, et al (2012) Psychometric properties of the Mental Health Recovery Star. *British Journal of Psychiatry,* **201**: 65–70.

Marshall M, Lockwood A (2011) Assertive community treatment for people with severe mental disorders. *Cochrane Database of Systematic Reviews [electronic resource],* **4**: CD001089.

McGorry P, Jackson HJ (1999) *The Recognition and Management of Early Psychosis. A Preventative Approach.* Cambridge University Press.

National Mental Health Development Unit (2011) *In Sight and In Mind: A Toolkit to Reduce the Use of Out of Area Mental Health Services.* Royal College of Psychiatrists. At http://www.rcpsych.ac.uk/pdf/insightandinmind.pdf (accessed December 2014).

Newbronner L, Chamberlain R, Bosanquet K, et al (2011) *Keeping Personal Budgets Personal: Learning from the Experiences of Older People, People with Mental Health Problems and Their Carers* (SCIE Report 40). At http://www.scie.org.uk/publications/reports/report40 (accessed 12 May 2013).

Perkins R, Repper J, Rinaldi M, et al (2012) *Implementing Recovery Through Organisational Change (IMRoC), 1. Recovery Colleges.* Centre for Mental Health and Mental Health Network, NHS Confederation.

Slade M, Thornicroft G, Loftus L, *et al* (1999) *CAN: Camberwell Assessment of Need – A Comprehensive Needs Assessment Tool for People with Severe Mental Illness.* Gaskell.

Stafford MR, Jackson H, Mayo-Wilson E, *et al* (2013) Early interventions to prevent psychosis: systematic review and meta-analysis. *BMJ*, **346**: 1185.

Stein LI, Test MA (1980) Alternative to mental hospital treatment. I. Conceptual model, treatment program, and clinical evaluation. *Archives of General Psychiatry*, **37**: 392–7.

Sytema S, Wunderink L, Bloemers W, *et al* (2007) Assertive community treatment in the Netherlands: a randomized controlled trial. *Acta Psychiatrica Scandinavica*, **13**: 105–12.

Teague GB, Bond GR, Drake RE (1998) Program fidelity in assertive community treatment: deployment and use of a measure. *American Journal of Orthopsychiatry*, **68**: 216–32.

Thornicroft G, Wykes T, Holloway F, *et al* (1998) From efficacy to effectiveness in community mental health services: the PRiSM Psychosis Study (10). *British Journal of Psychiatry*, **173**: 423–6.

van Os J, Kapur S (2009) Schizophrenia. *Lancet*, **374**: 635–45.

Veldhuizen J (2007) FACT: a Dutch version of ACT. *Community Mental Health Journal*, **43**: 421–33.

Wing J, Curtis E, Beever AS (1996) *Health of the Nation Outcome Scales (HoNOS).* Research Unit, Royal College of Psychiatrists.

CHAPTER 19

Housing: a place to live

Helen Killaspy, Stefan Priebe and Geoff Shepherd

Introduction

This chapter describes the history, development and evidence for supported accommodation for people with mental health problems. Clearly, people with mental health problems who do not reside in supported accommodation also need somewhere to live and support to remain as well as possible and maintain their home successfully: in the UK most live alone, although many do live with family. People living in supported accommodation will require the interventions described in Part 2 of this book ('Treatment approaches'), delivered by the community-based services described in Chapter 18, 'Community-based rehabilitation and recovery'; these are not reiterated here.

Specialist supported accommodation for people with mental health problems includes nursing and residential care homes, group homes, hostels, blocks of individual or shared tenancies with staff on site, and independent tenancies with 'floating' or outreach support from staff. In 2006 it was estimated that around 12 500 people with mental health problems in England were in a nursing or residential care home (National Statistics, 2006), although a recent 'freedom of information' enquiry to the organisations commissioning these services – local authorities and National Health Service (NHS) primary care trusts – puts the figure much higher, at around 30 000 (Killaspy & Meier, 2010). This discrepancy could be due to changes in the registration processes for these kinds of facilities, which have led to an increase in the number of homes formally registered, rather than an increase in the actual number of people residing in them, although there has also been greater use of nursing and residential care for people with longer-term mental health problems in the UK in recent years owing to disinvestment in local rehabilitation services (on the 'virtual asylum', see Chapter 17, 'Rehabilitation in hospital settings'). In 2006, around 160 000 people in England were receiving floating outreach services, of whom around 15% (24 000) were classified as receiving a specialist mental health floating outreach service (Department of Communities and Local Government, 2006).

The people who require specialist mental health supported-accommodation services will have complex needs and functional impairments that affect their ability to manage activities of daily living, either consistently or during periods of relapse. Most have severe, enduring mental health problems such as schizophrenia. Many have active symptoms of illness despite medication and experience impairments in cognition affecting their organisational skills and everyday functioning (Holloway, 2005). The support they need to live successfully in the community includes assistance to manage their medication, personal care, laundry, bills, shopping, cooking and cleaning. Although they live in the community, this in itself does not equate with social inclusion; most are unemployed, socially isolated and do not participate in civil and political processes (Boardman *et al*, 2010). Many therefore also require encouragement and support to access community resources and to remain in touch with family and friends.

The annual cost to the public purse of supported accommodation in England runs into the hundreds of millions of pounds. In 2010, the estimated average cost of providing floating outreach to one tenant was around £150 per week and a place in residential care was around £500 per week, giving an estimated total annual cost of around £1 billion. Although, historically, nursing care has been considered an NHS financial responsibility and other forms of supported accommodation were considered the responsibility of local authorities, the 'mixed economy' of provision, and greater integration of mental health and social care services in general, has led to a blurring of this distinction. In addition, many patients require care packages that include health and social care inputs. Mental health services will provide care coordination and additional input to the residents and staff of supported accommodation through the Care Programme Approach (Department of Health, 2008*a*). It is therefore not meaningful to separate 'health' and 'social care' investment in mental health supported accommodation.

A brief history of the development of supported accommodation

The UK

The NHS Hospital Plan of 1962 laid out the process of deinstitutionalisation in England and Wales and the development of community-based mental healthcare (Ministry of Health, 1962). Shepherd & Macpherson (2011) have observed that the number of long-stay beds, excluding patients in forensic settings, reduced from over 150000 in 1955 to less than 3000 in 2010. This process was accompanied by investment in specialist accommodation in the community providing varying levels of support, from 24-hour staffed 'hospital hostels', residential care and nursing homes, to hostels with less intensive on-site support and group homes with visiting staff. Subsequent policy changes moved the responsibility for provision of mental health supported accommodation from regional health authorities to local authorities, which have, in turn, subcontracted responsibility for provision to the independent sector (both 'for profit' and 'not for profit'). NHS mental health services continue to support residents in this new range of housing and there has been an increasing emphasis on partnership working between statutory, voluntary and independent sectors.

Other European countries

Other European countries have established various forms of supported accommodation as part of the process of deinstitutionalisation. For some patients, all that changed was the designation of part of the former asylum as 'supported accommodation', resulting in them staying in exactly the same place but receiving poorer quality care than before the hospital closure. However, in some places there was a clear programme of investment in supported living in the local community, often influenced by the local context. For example, in Berlin, flat-sharing was very popular among young people and similar arrangements were often made for four or five patients to move to a flat together. In Trieste, a city considered a pioneer in the process of deinstitutionalisation, buildings of the former asylum were converted into group homes for those with the highest level of needs, while a range of apartments in the city provided accommodation for those who were able to manage with less support, with staff being either on site or visiting. Other patients moved in with family members. Buildings in the former asylum campus were also converted for mainstream use (e.g. to university departments, administration blocks, nurseries and cafés), thereby bringing the community into the grounds of the former asylum as well as moving patients into the city.

In many European countries the number of places in supported accommodation has been rising since 1990. It has been argued that this increase might reflect the 'reinstitutionalisation' of people with more severe mental health problems. Bearing in mind that data are incomplete and not wholly reliable, five possible reasons for this phenomenon have been suggested: increasing morbidity; less family support; greater societal concern about the risks posed by people with mental health problems; the economic interests of provider organisations; and a shift of care costs from the health sector to the social care sector (Priebe *et al*, 2008; Mundt *et al*, 2012). Others have called the process 'trans-institutionalisation', where patients who were or would have been long-term hospitalised in the past are now cared for in other forms of institution, including private hospitals, nursing and residential care homes and various types of supported housing (Priebe & Fioritti, 2004; Priebe *et al*, 2008).

Funding for supported accommodation

In England, alongside changes in the nature of residential services and the responsibilities of different agencies, there have also been important changes to funding arrangements for supported accommodation. Early community developments were mainly funded through NHS monies that had previously been spent on the old institutions. These could be transferred as 'dowry' payments which accompanied patients as they left hospital and continued until they died, supplemented by their welfare benefit entitlements. This mechanism was not available for the next generation of people with long-term and severe mental health problems who had not spent long periods of time in hospital: accommodation providers became increasingly dependent on funding through the welfare benefit system combined with national grants.

The 'Supporting People' initiative was launched in 2003 to provide additional funding to support people in 'ordinary housing' and to try to increase their independence. It represented a bold attempt by government to bring together various funding streams to house vulnerable groups (older people, those with mental health problems, the homeless, women at risk of domestic violence) under a single grant, administered by local authorities and provided through voluntary sector organisations and housing associations. However, for people with serious mental health problems, it has been something of a mixed blessing.

As originally conceived, 'Supporting People' aimed to prevent individuals experiencing crises and requiring more costly service interventions, and to enable them to live as independently as possible through the provision of housing-related support. At the outset it seemed an attractive new budget that could be used for multiple purposes. New schemes were rapidly established and old schemes were relabelled to meet the 'Supporting People' criteria. This caused some problems as the criteria of 'social care' sat uneasily with NHS staff, who saw themselves as primarily providing health interventions that might or might not make the person more independent. Inevitably, different local authorities also drew different boundaries between health and social care provision, but generally the initiative was popular and the demands on the 'Supporting People' budget quickly grew.

In fact, they grew rather too quickly and by 2006 schemes were beginning to be cut back and people who were formerly considered eligible were no longer considered so. This caused distress for both residents and staff, but worse was to come. In 2009, the ring-fencing of the 'Supporting People' budget within local authorities was removed. People with long-term and severe mental health problems were therefore in a position of having to compete not only with other vulnerable groups for housing support, but also with all the other services that local authorities were required to provide.

The story of 'Supporting People' funding is an instructive one. It contains the familiar ingredients of policy changes which are made with the best of intentions, but turn out to have unintended, adverse consequences. It also underlines the practical difficulties of achieving effective partnership working between statutory agencies with different ideologies and responsibilities, which are then required to make invidious decisions regarding the prioritisation of different kinds of need in a climate of diminishing resources.

Across Europe, the way in which supported accommodation for people with mental health problems is organised is driven by economic considerations. Where mental health supported-accommodation costs are attributed to the social services budget rather than the health sector budget (whether paid for through insurance or state-funded systems), people who were originally placed in urban areas tend be rehoused in rural or suburban areas, where accommodation costs are much lower. In the UK, the current wave of welfare reforms seems likely to result in many people with mental health problems being unable to afford inner-city rents and being, effectively, forced out of their homes. The negative impact of this in terms of distress to individuals, disruption of their support networks (both professional and personal) and the extra burden of care on health and social care systems in the areas to which they move is likely to be far-reaching.

In England, individual placements in other forms of supported accommodation (hospital, nursing and residential care) are funded through a separate process. Specialist placement funding panels, which should include senior clinicians with appropriate expertise (often rehabilitation psychiatrists) and representatives of the NHS and local authorities that provide the funding (service commissioners, managers and finance directors), meet to review and agree whether a specific placement is appropriate for an individual. The lead clinician (usually the care coordinator) provides details of the individual's needs and the ability of the proposed placement to meet them. Agreement about whether the placement should be funded by the NHS or local authority budget (or a combination of both) is made. The most expensive placements are usually required for individuals with the highest needs and these are assessed against so-called 'continuing care' criteria. Most of these will be NHS-funded hospital or nursing home placements (Department of Health, 2012). Some areas pool their health and social care resources, while others operate separate systems and panels. Further complexity is introduced when an individual has a combination of physical and mental health problems and a referral to a separate physical disability funding panel has to be made and a cost-share agreed.

Disinvestment in local rehabilitation and supported-accommodation services in recent years in the UK has meant that local stocks of supported housing do not always meet local need. This has led to the use of 'out of area' placements (nursing/residential care outside the service user's area of origin), which have been criticised for their lack of rehabilitative ethos and the disruption they can cause to an individual's recovery through social dislocation (Killaspy & Meier, 2010). Although some use of specialist out-of-area facilities is necessary for people with very complex problems (where small numbers require regional rather than local provision), a survey of those placed out of area by one local authority and its associated mental health service found few differences in needs, social functioning and challenging behaviours compared with those using local rehabilitation services and supported accommodation (Killaspy *et al*, 2009). The fact that out-of-area placements cost, on average, around two-thirds more than similar local facilities (Killaspy & Meier, 2010) has provided a lever for this issue to be addressed through recently published guidance to commissioners of services that explicitly encourages local investment in local supported-accommodation services (National Mental Health Development Unit, 2011; Joint Commissioning Panel for Mental Health, 2012).

The evidence for the effectiveness of supported accommodation

Despite massive investment in supported accommodation, there has been very little high-quality research investigating the effectiveness of different models to guide service planners and providers (Fakhoury *et al*, 2002). The only rigorous systematic literature review that has considered evidence for mental health supported accommodation found that no trials of adequate quality had been carried out (Chilvers *et al*, 2002). This is understandable given the ethical and logistical difficulties of research in this area. Randomisation to different types of supported accommodation may be resisted by clinicians who feel that service users require a staged process, moving from higher to lower supported settings as their skills and confidence increase, and by service users who may have clear preferences for particular services.

Evidence from the studies that have attempted to investigate the effectiveness of mental health supported accommodation suggests benefits for residents of supported accommodation compared with long-term hospitalisation. Research on deinstitutionalisation has repeatedly shown that when long-stay hospital patients are resettled into supported community placements, the majority experience improvement in functioning, reduction in challenging behaviours and greater satisfaction with care. In the 1990s, the Team for the Assessment of Psychiatric Services (TAPS) undertook a large-scale follow-up of 700 long-stay patients discharged to the community following the closure of the two large mental hospitals in north London. The majority were not only able to sustain community tenure but gained skills and confidence that enabled them to move to less-supported settings over the following 5 years (Leff & Trieman, 2000). Of those considered to have the most complex and challenging behaviours who were placed in highly supported and specialist settings to begin with, 40% were able to move on to less supported settings (Trieman & Leff, 2002). Similarly, a review of the effectiveness of the 'hospital hostel' concluded that there were benefits for around 40% with regard to social functioning and successful move-on (Macpherson & Jerrom, 1999). Observational studies in other countries have also found positive outcomes for patients moved from long-stay hospitals into different types of supported community housing. For example, the Berlin Deinstitutionalisation Study found that patients' quality of life improved after moving to the community (Priebe et al, 2002).

A recent study of 141 people under the care of one trust's mental health rehabilitation service found that, of the 124 still alive 5 years later, 40% had successfully moved on from hospital to supported community accommodation (or from a more supported to a less supported placement in the community), without requiring readmission to hospital and without any breakdown in their community placement. Of these, 13 (10% overall) successfully progressed to independent (unsupported) accommodation. However, over a quarter remained in the same placement throughout the 5 years (or one with a similar level of support) and 38% moved to a more supported placement or were admitted to hospital. Those who were noted to have any episode of non-adherence with medication during the 5 years were eight times more likely not to progress to a less supported setting or to be readmitted to hospital (Killaspy & Zis, 2013).

As well as the proportion of individuals who move on successfully to sustain community tenure in a less supported setting, it is important to assess other clinical outcomes. These include the degree to which the supported-accommodation service promotes service users' autonomy towards achieving successful move-on, service users' satisfaction with the support they receive, improvements in service users' quality of life, and the degree to which they have the opportunity to engage in activities that they enjoy and find rewarding (such as leisure, education, work and social activities).

A review of floating outreach commissioned by the Department of Communities and Local Government (2006: p. 39) commented:

> Success cannot be measured in terms of the number of clients who no longer require support. Factors such as sustained tenancies, rates of hospital readmission, attendance at day centres, voluntary work, training courses and employment should be taken into account ... there is a need to undertake more comprehensive and longer term studies to evaluate the impact of floating support services.

Although very little research has been undertaken reporting on these outcomes, one qualitative study found that staff acknowledged the importance of supporting the social inclusion of their service users (Hogberg et al, 2006).

The only survey of mental health supported accommodation to be carried out to date in England found few differences in characteristics of service users in different types of setting and heterogeneity in the support offered (Priebe et al, 2009). The survey sampled 12 nationally representative regions, identified a total of 481 projects and 250 were randomly sampled. Of these, 153 responded to a postal survey; 57 were nursing/residential care homes (with a mean of 16 residents), 61 were individual or shared flats with on-site staff support (with a mean of 13 service users) and 30 provided floating outreach to (a mean of 34) service users in their own independent flats, usually rented from the local authority or a housing association. Staff provided anonymised data on 414 service users. The majority were male, 80% had a diagnosis of a psychotic disorder and 48% also had a history of substance misuse. There were no discernible differences between service types in the characteristics of the service users. Around 40% of those in supported housing or receiving floating outreach were participating in some form of community activity (compared with 25% of those in residential care) but similar numbers of hours were spent by service users across all settings in education or work (a mean of 13 hours per week) and only 3% were in open employment. Between four and six service users (18–25%) moved on from each service annually. Although residential care settings had a higher proportion of trained mental health staff than the other services, almost all service users in all types of setting were prescribed medication and all services provided support with personal care and activities of daily living. The costs of these services appeared to be driven by the local tradition of provision rather than clinical need: the development of local supported accommodation seemed to be largely determined by history, the sociodemographic context of the area and the support available from primary care and secondary mental health services (Shepherd & Macpherson, 2011).

Over the past 20 years or so there has been increased investment in supported flats rather than group settings, since many services users prefer their own self-contained living space to shared facilities (Massey & Wu, 1993; Tanzman, 1993; Killaspy et al, 2009). Studies have identified discrepancies between service users' and staff views on the level of support required, with service users tending to prefer more independent accommodation while mental health staff and family members tend to prefer the service users to be in staffed environments (Minsky et al, 1995; Friedrich et al, 1999; Piat et al, 2008). An important criticism of staffed settings is the maintenance of institutional regimes and impaired facilitation of service users' autonomy through over-support and a poor rehabilitative culture (Ryan et al, 2004). Conversely, some service users and family members have reported that more independent settings such as supported single tenancies are socially isolating (Friedrich et al, 1999; Walker & Seasons, 2002).

Most areas have systems of supported accommodation where service users move to more independent settings as their skills improve. This allows for graduated 'testing', but many users dislike repeated moves. It often takes a number of years for service users to move successfully through each step of the care pathway owing to the severity and complexity of their mental health needs. They may need to make repeated attempts to transition successfully from a higher to a lower level of support. An alternative is to provide flexible support to service users living in their own, permanent tenancy. In the USA, the 'train and place' approach (which provides a constant level of staffing on site to a number of flats, with the expectation that service user will move on as they gain independent living skills) has been compared in a quasi-experimental study to the 'place and train' approach (which provides floating outreach support of flexible intensity to service users living in an independent, time-unlimited tenancy). The place and train approach was found to facilitate greater community integration and gave more service user satisfaction (Corrigan & McCracken, 2005).

A programme of research, funded by the National Institute for Health Research in England, that commenced in 2012 will attempt to address some of the evidence gaps in this field. This 5-year programme (Quality and Effectiveness of Supported Tenancies for people with mental health problems – QuEST) includes investigation of the provision, quality and clinical- and cost-effectiveness of different forms of mental health supported accommodation and a feasibility trial comparing supported housing and floating outreach services (see http://www.ucl.ac.uk/quest).

Quality of supported-accommodation services

Recent government policy defines service quality as incorporating the effectiveness and safety of care alongside a positive experience for the people using the service (Department of Health, 2008b). With regard to supported accommodation, quality of care can be assessed in terms of the degree to which support and treatment are provided that are acceptable to the service user and that facilitate improvements in symptoms, functioning and quality of life. Quality includes structures (e.g. the built environment and the intensity and type of staffing), processes (e.g. the degree to which treatment and support are supervised and tailored to each service user's needs) and the culture of the service (e.g. the expectation that service users will gain skills for more independent living and move on).

Nursing and residential care homes have to meet certain standards to achieve registration with the Care Quality Commission (CQC). However, there is no formal registration process for other supported-accommodation services (supported housing and floating outreach) and, unlike in-patient mental health services, no nationally recognised process for peer assessment and review of standards of care. One aspect of the QuEST research programme is the adaptation of an existing standardised quality assessment tool used in mental health rehabilitation services to make it suitable for assessing the quality of supported accommodation. Such a tool could then be used for national benchmarking of the quality of these services and contribute to a more robust process for driving up the quality of care. It is not unreasonable to consider that peer quality networks and accreditation systems, similar to the Royal College of Psychiatrists' AIMS programme for in-patient wards (described in Chapter 17, 'Rehabilitation in hospital settings'), could be developed for use across specialist mental health supported-accommodation services in the future.

The role of statutory mental health services in working with supported-accommodation services

Supported-accommodation services do not operate in isolation. They work with statutory community mental health services (often a community mental health team, community mental health rehabilitation team or another team that specialises in working with people with longer-term and severe mental health problems) to ensure that service users are able to make a success of their placement. This input from statutory mental health services is vital from the point of referral and throughout the person's stay. These services are involved in agreeing that there is a possible 'match' between the service user's needs and the support available at the supported accommodation prior to referral. They facilitate informal visits for service users to the accommodation and support them through the referral and any assessment process. This may take a number of visits and adequate time must be allowed for the sharing of clinical and risk information and to address any anxieties on the part of the service user, carers and the supported-accommodation service before the service user is accepted for a place. There will then often be a period of graduated leave to allow the person to become familiar with the new environment and for staff to identify any issues that they may require further help with before the person's move is finalised.

Once the service user moves in, the community mental health team will continue to visit and support the service user and staff. The aim should be to help tailor individualised care plans to enable the service user to gain skills and confidence for more independent living (e.g. managing medication more independently, self-catering, budgeting, accessing community resources, contact with family and friends, engaging in leisure activities, education and work). This may require very detailed, graduated care planning. Focusing on strengths rather than areas of difficulty is important in building up a person's confidence. This work requires skilled mental health staff and staff working in supported accommodation to work together to encourage service users to take responsibility for their own decisions and to manage their mental health and other aspects of their life to their best of their ability.

The mental health team will also provide more intensive support during periods of crisis and attempt wherever possible to avoid placement breakdown or hospital admission. Helping the service user and staff of the accommodation to identify early signs of relapse is particularly important.

Liaison with other services may also be needed (e.g. the local crisis resolution team). Expertise from statutory mental health services will also be required for service users who are subject to a statutory framework. In England and Wales relevant legislation includes the Mental Capacity Act, which has specific provisions for deprivation of liberty, and the Mental Health Act, which provides powers of guardianship and supervised community treatment. Assessment and application of legal processes such as these and those relating to the safeguarding of vulnerable adults is another responsibility for the statutory mental health service.

Conclusions

A significant proportion of people with severe mental health problems reside in supported accommodation of varying types. The types of facility and the systems for funding and providing them have evolved over recent decades alongside the process of deinstitutionalisation and vary from one country to another. In England, the system of supported accommodation is now quite complex (and imperfect) and specialist expertise is required at all levels to ensure it continues to provide the right kind of support to enable individuals to achieve their optimum level of independence and engagement in their local community. The specific skills of rehabilitation practitioners are needed to ensure that commissioners invest in the right kinds of specialist mental health supported accommodation to meet the needs of the local population, and to provide clinical expertise to those living in supported accommodation and those providing these services.

References

Boardman J, Currie A, Killaspy H, *et al* (eds) (2010) *Social Inclusion and Mental Health.* Royal College of Psychiatrists.

Chilvers R, Macdonald G, Hayes A (2002) Supported housing for people with severe mental disorders. *Cochrane Database of Systematic Reviews*, 4: CD000453.

Corrigan P, McCracken S (2005) Place first, then train: an alternative to the medical model of psychiatric rehabilitation. *Social Work*, 50: 31–9.

Department of Communities and Local Government (2006) *Research into the Effectiveness of Floating Support Services for the Supporting People Programme. Final Report.* Department of Communities and Local Government.

Department of Health (2008a) *Refocusing the Care Programme Approach: Policy and Practice Guidance.* Department of Health.

Department of Health (2008b) *High Quality Care for All: NHS Next Stage Review Final Report.* Department of Health.

Department of Health (2012) *National Framework of NHS Continuing Healthcare and NHS-Funded Nursing Care.* Department of Health.

Fakhoury WKH, Murray A, Shepherd G, *et al* (2002) Research in supported housing. *Social Psychiatry and Psychiatric Epidemiology*, 37: 301–15.

Friedrich R, Hollingsworth B, Hradeck E, *et al* (1999) Family and client perspectives on alternative residential settings for persons with severe mental illness. *Psychiatric Services*, 50: 509–14.

Hogberg T, Magnusson HT, Lutzen K (2006) Living by themselves? Psychiatric nurses' views on supported housing for persons with severe and persistent mental illness. *Journal of Psychiatric and Mental Health Nursing*, **13**: 735–41.

Holloway F (2005) *The Forgotten Need for Rehabilitation in Contemporary Mental Health Services* (Position Statement from the Executive Committee of the Faculty of Rehabilitation and Social Psychiatry). Royal College of Psychiatrists. At http://www.rcpsych.ac.uk/college/faculty/rehab/frankholloway_oct05.pdf (accessed December 2014).

Joint Commissioning Panel for Mental Health (2012) *Guidance for Commissioners of Rehabilitation Services for People with Complex Mental Health Needs.* Royal College of Psychiatrists.

Killaspy H, Meier R (2010) A fair deal for mental health rehabilitation services. *The Psychiatrist*, **34**: 265–7.

Killaspy H, Zis P (2013) Predictors of outcomes of mental health rehabilitation services: a 5-year retrospective cohort study in inner London, UK. *Social Psychiatry and Psychiatric Epidemiology*, **48**: 1005–12.

Killaspy H, Rambarran D, Harden C, *et al* (2009) A comparison of service users placed out of their local area and local rehabilitation service users. *Journal of Mental Health*, **18**: 111–20.

Leff J, Trieman N (2000) Long stay patients discharged from psychiatric hospitals. Social and clinical outcomes after five years in the community. TAPS Project 46. *British Journal of Psychiatry*, **176**: 217–23.

Macpherson R, Jerrom W (1999) Review of twenty-four-hour nursed care. *Advances in Psychiatric Treatment*, **5**: 146–53.

Massey OT, Wu L (1993) Important characteristics of independent housing for people with severe mental illness: perspectives of case managers and consumers. *Psychosocial Rehabilitation Journal*, **17**: 81–92.

Ministry of Health (1962) *The Hospital Plan for England and Wales* (Cmnd, 1604). HMSO.

Minsky S, Riesser GG, Duffy M (1995) The eye of the beholder: housing preferences of inpatients and treatment teams. *Psychiatric Services*, **46**: 173–6.

Mundt AP, Franciskovic T, Gurovich I, *et al* (2012) Changes in the provision of institutionalized mental health care in post-communist countries. *PLoS One*, **7**: e38490 (Epub).

National Mental Health Development Unit (2011) *In Sight and in Mind: A Toolkit to Reduce the Use of Out of Area Mental Health Services.* Royal College of Psychiatrists. At http://www.rcpsych.ac.uk/PDF/insightandinmind.pdf (accessed December 2014).

National Statistics (2006) *Community Care Statistics 2006. Supported Residents (Adults), England.* Information Centre, Government Statistical Service.

Piat M, Lesage A, Boyer R, *et al* (2008) Housing for persons with serious mental illness: consumer and service provider preferences. *Psychiatric Services*, **59**: 1011–17.

Priebe S, Fioritti A (2004) Dopo la deistituzionalizzazione: stiamo imboccando il cammino contrario? [The era of reinstitutionalization: is it really coming?] *Psichiatria di Comunita*, **3**: 137–44.

Priebe S, Hoffmann K, Iserman M, *et al* (2002) Do long-term hospitalised patients benefit from discharge into the community? *Social Psychiatry and Psychiatric Epidemiology*, **37**: 387–92.

Priebe S, Frottier P, Gaddini A, *et al* (2008) Mental health care institutions in nine European countries, 2002 to 2006. *Psychiatric Services*, **59**: 570–3.

Priebe S, Saidi M, Want A, *et al* (2009) Housing services for people with mental disorders in England: patient characteristics, care provision and costs. *Social Psychiatry and Psychiatric Epidemiology*, **44**: 805–14.

Ryan T, Pearsall A, Hatfield B, *et al* (2004) Long term care for serious mental illness outside the NHS: a study of out-of-area placements. *Journal of Mental Health*, **13**: 425–9.

Shepherd GW, Macpherson R (2011) Residential care. In *Oxford Textbook of Community Mental Health* (eds G Thornicroft, G Szmukler, KT Mueser, RE Drake): 178–87. Oxford University Press.

Tanzman B (1993) An overview of surveys of mental health consumers' preferences for housing and support. *Hospital and Community Psychiatry,* **44**: 450–5.

Trieman N, Leff J (2002) Long-term outcome of long-stay psychiatric inpatients considered unsuitable to live in the community: TAPS Project 44. *British Journal of Psychiatry,* **181**: 428–32.

Walker R, Seasons M (2002) Supported housing for people with serious mental illness: resident perspectives on housing. *Canadian Journal of Community Mental Health,* **21**: 137–51.

CHAPTER 20

Work and employment

Jed Boardman

Introduction

Historically, work and employment have played an important role in the rehabilitation of people with severe mental health problems. Work, employment and engagement in other rewarding activities are central factors in the recovery of people with mental health problems and their inclusion in broader society (Boardman *et al*, 2010). This chapter examines the importance of work and employment for people with mental health problems. It focuses on people with severe mental health problems and the supported-employment model, for which there is more evidence than for other models that it does help to increase the opportunities for this group to obtain open employment.

Work, leisure, employment and occupation

The traditional definitions of work emphasise that it is an activity that involves the exercise of skills and judgement and that it takes place within set limits prescribed by others (Bennett, 1970). Work is therefore essentially something you 'do' for other people. By contrast, in most leisure activities you can 'please yourself'.

'Employment' is work you get paid for. Most childcare, housework, looking after elderly or sick relatives is clearly 'work', in the sense that the tasks and outcomes are defined by others, but they do not, at present, usually attract formal payments. This distinction between 'work' and 'employment' is very important in the context of mental health problems because the overwhelming majority of people with these problems want to 'work', that is, to be engaged in some kind of meaningful activity which uses their skills and meets the expectations of others. However, not all wish to be 'employed', with all the additional stresses and responsibilities that entails. Occupation may be considered as a general term that refers to engagement in activities, tasks and roles for the purpose of meeting the requirements of living.

The terms *open* or *competitive* employment are often used in the context of people with mental health problems or disabilities. These jobs are *competitive* in that they pay at least the minimum wage and the same wages that others receive for performing the same work. They are *open* jobs as they are based in settings alongside others without disabilities and are not reserved for people with disabilities (Drake *et al*, 2012).

Work and people with mental health problems

Work plays a central role in all people's lives and is generally considered to be beneficial to health and well-being (Waddell & Burton, 2006). The main arguments for the value of work are shown in Box 20.1. In most

---

Box 20.1 Why is work important?

Work as a social and health benefit

- Provides a monetary reward
- Provides non-financial gains – 'latent benefits' (Warr, 1987):
  - social identity and status
  - social contacts and support
  - means of structuring and occupying time
  - activity and involvement
  - a sense of personal achievement
- Enhances quality of life (Hatfield *et al*, 1992; Hill *et al*, 1996)
- Promotes social inclusion, linking the individual to society (Boardman *et al*, 2010)
- Unemployment is linked with:
  - premature death (Brenner, 1979; Bartley, 1994)
  - development of mental health problems (Warr, 1987; Warner, 2004)
  - increased use of mental health services (Wilson & Walker, 1993; Warner, 2004)
  - increased risk of suicide (Platt & Kreitman, 1984)

Work as a rights issue

- Article 23 of the United Nations Declaration of Human Rights states: 'everyone has a right to work, to free choice of employment, to just and favourable conditions of work and to protection against unemployment'
- Valuing people with disabilities includes promoting respect, self-determination and empowerment
- Prejudice and discrimination are major obstacles to people with mental health problems gaining work (Manning & White, 1995)

Work as an economic issue

- A large proportion of public money is spent on welfare benefits for the unemployed and almost 25% of invalidity payments are paid to people with mental health problems
- Further costs to society come in the form of loss of productivity due to absenteeism and presenteeism (Sainsbury Centre for Mental Health, 2007)

---

industrialised economies, people with long-term mental health problems are disadvantaged in the labour market; in general, they are less likely to be in employment than those without such problems (Marwaha & Johnson, 2004; Marwaha *et al*, 2007); this is especially so for people with long-term and severe mental disorders.

Box 20.2 Barriers to employment

The impact of mental health problems on the individual

The features of the conditions, especially periods of overwhelming symptoms and rapidly fluctuating conditions, may prevent work for periods of time. The impact of the condition may lead to loss of motivation and confidence. Side-effects of medication may prohibit work (Marwaha *et al*, 2007; Perkins *et al*, 2009)

Disincentives produced by the welfare system – the 'benefits trap'

The complexities of the benefits system and the loss of some benefits after return to work may deter people from trying open employment. People may fear that they will be without access to benefits if the job does not work out. They may be better off on benefits rather than in low-paid employment (Perkins *et al*, 2009)

Attitudes of employers and public

The disadvantages faced by people with a history of mental illness in the open employment market include stigma, a reluctance to employ them, public perception of risk, and a lack of understanding of mental health conditions (Manning & White, 1995; Shaw Trust, 2010; Little *et al*, 2011; Brohan *et al*, 2012)

Attitudes of health professionals

Mental health professionals and others tend to underestimate the capacities and skills of their clients and possibly to overestimate the risk to employers (Marwaha *et al*, 2009)

Fears and low expectations of self among people with mental health problems

People may fear that work will lead to a worsening of their mental health. Poor experiences at work, the effects of prejudice and discrimination and feedback from health professionals may contribute to lack of self-belief and self-stigma. There is often a fear of failure should there be a return to work (Corrigan & Watson, 2002; Corrigan *et al*, 2009)

Dominance of an approach by mental health services

There is an approach that emphasises episodes and 'cure' as opposed to one that focuses on the disabilities of people with long-term mental illness. A social model of disability and a recovery-oriented approach may be more beneficial (Boardman, 2003)

Lack of appropriate support and services

Evidence-based supported employment schemes are generally poorly implemented. There is limited evidence for benefits of government back-to-work schemes and welfare reform. There is a lack of an integrated approach (Bevan *et al*, 2013; Boardman & Rinaldi, 2013)

While there is evidence to suggest that some clinical features are associated with unemployment, particularly the negative symptoms of schizophrenia and associated cognitive problems, the most consistently noted individual predictors of success in employment are motivation, self-efficacy and employment history (Marwaha & Johnson, 2004; Marwaha *et al*, 2007; Catty *et al*, 2008). Indeed, the desire to have a job is one of the best predictors of future employment (Marwaha & Johnson, 2004).

People with mental health conditions, like all people who experience an acute episode of illness, will have times when they are unable to work. Those with long-term conditions will typically experience fluctuations in their health and may need support and adjustments to allow them to work consistently; they may also need time off during periods of relapse. However, long-term conditions and continuing fluctuating symptoms are not in themselves a barrier to employment. People with mental health problems face more significant barriers to gaining open employment than most other disabled people, the most important of which are external social factors (see Box 20.2).

Approaches to vocational rehabilitation

The use of 'constructive occupation' has formed a part of the care for people who are mentally ill since the development of the mental hospitals (Tuke, 1813; Connolly, 1847). In the 20th century, many of the vocational rehabilitation schemes were associated with the large mental hospitals, for example industrial rehabilitation units that offered courses of training in industrial skills and work habits. Later, sheltered-employment factories and workshops were subsidised to allow for a lower productivity, and offered permanent or interim employment. The success of these schemes was limited: they did not lead to many people returning to open employment and they were not adaptable to changing industrial conditions.

With the demise of the large asylums in many countries and the shift to community-based services in the later years of the 20th century, new approaches to vocational rehabilitation developed, such as club houses and transitional employment programmes, which use graduated skills training and temporary work placements to help individuals become 'work ready' (Beard *et al*, 1982). Over recent decades, a greater optimism has emerged as to the achievable outcomes for people with schizophrenia and the possibilities of them achieving open employment. Alternatives to sheltered work and transitional employment schemes emerged in the 1980s and are usually referred to as supported employment (Drake *et al*, 2012). These involve placing people in a 'real' employment setting and providing direct support to them, and their employer, while in the workplace. There are a number of different models of supported employment (Bond *et al*, 1997), but the most effective and most widely researched is individual placement and support (IPS) (Drake *et al*, 2012).

Individual placement and support

Individual placement and support differs from other types of vocational rehabilitation, which have traditionally been 'train and place', based on a stepwise approach to finding open structured vocational activity for service users. The latter typically focus time and resources on countering people's deficits, providing skills training and supporting people to learn and develop new skills in segregated or sheltered environments. In contrast, the primary goal of the IPS approach is to find a job on the open labour market and then provide continued support – a 'place and train' approach.

The main principles of IPS are shown in Box 20.3. Essentially, it offers an individual approach to employment, focusing on the preferences of service users and their strengths and work experiences. They have primary authority in deciding on their vocational goals and the methods to achieve these. There are no eligibility criteria for entry into an IPS scheme except that the person wants to find open employment. People are not excluded, for example, on the basis of their job readiness, the severity of their disorder or their substance misuse or forensic history. There is no lengthy pre-employment assessment and in the early stages of working with a service user the focus is on building up a picture of choices, strengths, skills and past work. This leads quickly to searching for a suitable job (not rapid job placement), which may involve the employment worker, with or without the client, liaising with suitable employers and job agencies. While employment workers may not be employed directly by the mental health services, they should be integrated into mental health service clinical teams. This means including them within the clinical team and work base, which aids communication and the provision of a consistent approach to the client. This also allows for the continuing input of the clinical team, for example to provide medicines management or continuing therapy, or early intervention and crisis management if necessary. Integration of

---

Box 20.3 The individual placement and support (IPS) approach – key principles

- Competitive employment is the goal
- Eligibility is based on individual choice – there are no exclusions
- Rapid job search is used (with minimal pre-vocational training)
- Supported employment is integrated with the work of the clinical team
- Attention to client preferences is important. Job finding and support are tailored to the individual's needs
- Job finding is proactive, with an emphasis on relationships with employers
- Support is available for an unlimited period
- Financial planning is provided. Benefits counselling is provided to help people maximise their welfare benefits

---

mental healthcare and employment support ultimately benefits the person whose goal it is to gain employment; however, bringing these different specialisms together to develop a common language and purpose is not always straightforward. Lessons from the IPS implementation literature have shown that effective integration takes clinical and managerial leadership, expertise in IPS to provide training and support, and time to bring about the cultural changes required to integrate the IPS and clinical expertise successfully.

A major problem faced by people going into work is the threat to their loss of welfare benefits. It is thus important that there is provision of benefits counselling to give information and advice about the effects of working on social security provision. The support given to the client is not time limited. In reality, the support is more intensive during the early stages of employment, with the employment worker providing support to the client and liaison with the employers and clinical team. The type and length of the support are dependent on the person's individual needs and circumstances.

Evidence for IPS

Systematic reviews of supported employment trials all conclude that IPS is effective in achieving open employment for people with severe mental disorders (e.g. Crowther *et al*, 2001; Twamley *et al*, 2003; Bond, 2004; Bond *et al*, 2008*a*) and recent overviews of the randomised trials of IPS conclude that the evidence for its effectiveness is strong and consistent (Bond *et al*, 2012; Drake *et al*, 2012). IPS has been internationally evaluated in a diverse group of randomised controlled trials. The results of 16 have been reported and all show a positive effect of IPS over control services in attaining open employment. There is a variation in the rates of success of IPS, with two trials achieving weak results (Lehman *et al*, 2002; Heslin *et al*, 2011). Overall, IPS delivers rates of open employment of just over 60%, compared with rates of around 25% in the control services across a range of territories including the USA, Canada, Australia, Europe and Hong Kong (Bond *et al*, 2012; Drake *et al*, 2012). IPS has also been shown to be effective in delivering positive employment outcomes for people with first-episode psychosis (Killackey *et al*, 2008; Nuechterlein *et al*, 2008).

In addition:

- The IPS trials have low drop-out rates.
- IPS improves several employment outcomes – getting people into work quicker, working more hours per week and achieving longer job tenure (Drake *et al*, 2012). Many remain in steady employment or make successful transitions between jobs (Becker *et al*, 2007; Bond & Kukla, 2011).
- IPS schemes are well regarded by service users (Clevenger, 2008; Dunn *et al*, 2008).

313

- Placing people successfully in employment produces good personal outcomes, including better self-esteem, relationships, social functioning and personal management of their illness (Bond *et al*, 2001; Becker *et al*, 2007; Drake *et al*, 2012; McHugo *et al*, 2012).
- The schemes can be cost saving. The European multicentre trial of IPS (EQOLISE trial – Burns *et al*, 2007) showed significantly lower admission rates during follow-up in the IPS group and, consequently, for health and social services costs; compared with standard vocational services, IPS was cost-effective as a means of getting people with severe mental disorders into open employment (Knapp *et al*, 2013).

An important determinant of the success of IPS is adherence to its key components or principles (often referred to as 'fidelity to the model') (Becker *et al*, 2001; McGrew & Griss, 2005). The two trials that have demonstrated the weakest effects of IPS (Lehman *et al*, 2002; Heslin *et al*, 2011) may be due to low fidelity. The Lehman *et al* (2002) study used entry criteria that did not require participants to have a goal of competitive employment. Lack of support and follow-up of clients by employment staff and lack of integration of employment workers into the clinical team probably explains the low success rate of the IPS service in the SWAN study (Latimer, 2010; Heslin *et al*, 2011).

The skills of employment workers and the quality of their relationship with service users are crucial in achieving success (Catty *et al*, 2008; Taylor & Bond, 2014). The desirable attributes of the employment workers include transmitting hope, liaising with employers, showing initiative, empathy and passion, persistence, hardiness, a team orientation and professionalism (Gowdy *et al*, 2003; Whitley *et al*, 2010).

IPS schemes can be effective in routine practice (Cook *et al*, 2008; Rinaldi *et al*, 2011). The introduction of an IPS scheme in mental health services in south-east London showed a significant rise in rates of competitive employment among people using those services in an area that had high rates of unemployment (Perkins & Rinaldi, 2002; Rinaldi *et al*, 2011). Rinaldi *et al* (2004) showed that the integration of an IPS worker into an early-intervention service for young people with first-episode psychosis could be done with good fidelity and increased the proportion of clients engaged in work or educational activity.

Implementation of IPS

IPS schemes offer much for vocational rehabilitation: they are evidence based; the approach assumes that people with severe mental health conditions are able to work in normal competitive employment settings; they directly tackle the lack of integration of mental healthcare and employment services and the disconnection of different specialists; and they have shifted the focus of the mental health system away from treatment onto employment, by demonstrating much better employment outcomes.

Despite strong and consistent evidence from randomised controlled trials and from routine practice across several countries (something unusual in psychosocial interventions and uncommon in vocational rehabilitation), IPS has proved difficult to implement internationally (King *et al*, 2006; van Erp *et al*, 2007; Becker *et al*, 2008; Boyce *et al*, 2008; Hasson *et al*, 2011). This seems to be influenced by the effects of welfare benefits systems (the 'benefits trap') and labour market conditions, the use of IPS schemes that do not adhere to the IPS model (low-fidelity schemes) and a lack of organisational commitment (see Boardman & Rinaldi, 2013).

Improving implementation

The effect of organisational culture on the development of new and innovative services has been noted by Whitely *et al* (2009). Their study of the implementation of illness management and recovery programmes across 12 community settings highlighted the importance of training, supervision, leadership and a culture of innovation in determining their success. Training on its own was ineffective and it was where these factors were present together and acted synergistically that success was achieved. This suggests a need to direct attention to changing the organisation and its values. Other reviews of implementation have reached similar conclusions and have pointed to the importance of having 'champions' or 'purveyors' to support and encourage the implementation of innovative programmes within organisations (e.g. Fixsen *et al*, 2005).

In the USA, the National Evidence-Based Practices Project (Bond *et al*, 2008*b*) and the Mental Health Treatment Study (Frey *et al*, 2011) both demonstrated that it is possible to implement local IPS schemes with high fidelity through the use of local support to champion good practice, feedback of the findings of fidelity reviews and encouragement of integration of employment workers in clinical teams. The learning collaborative in the Johnson & Johnson–Dartford County Mental Health Programme created state trainers to help networks of hospitals or clinical teams to share good practice, and to set benchmarks and targets to attain and measure progress to monitor success (Becker *et al*, 2008, 2011).

In the UK, the Department of Health has produced commissioning guidance for the development of vocational services (Department of Health & Department of Work and Pensions, 2006). The Centre for Mental Health has developed a version of the Dartford programme – the *Centres of Excellence Programme* – and piloted a regional trainer (Centre for Mental Health, 2012). These approaches attempt to facilitate cultural change within the organisation, for example by encouraging an acceptance of employment as an integral parts of a person's recovery. They also use IPS fidelity reviews to determine how well the principles of IPS are applied in practice and feedback of these results to promote improvement in working practices.

What would a good vocational service look like?

The main elements of a good vocational service are shown in Box 20.4. These are consistent with the principles of IPS and the current evidence base for vocational schemes and recovery-oriented services (Warner, 2010). The service should focus on getting people into competitive jobs and supporting them while in work. There is an emphasis on the development of an integrated approach between clinical services (including occupational health), employment services (including job centres and welfare benefits) and employers (Perkins *et al*, 2009). This integration is required at individual, local and national levels.

The use of peer support is an important addition to facilitating recovery for people with mental health problems (see Chapter 21, 'Peer support in mental health services'). There is increasing evidence for the effectiveness of peer support workers employed within mental health services (Repper & Carter, 2011; Trachtenberg *et al*, 2013). One pertinent role is to support people into work by, for example, encouraging job applications, organising buddying or mentoring systems, providing a model for someone who has gained employment, and sharing recovery stories.

Box 20.4 Elements of a good vocational service

- The focus is on open employment, job attainment and retention, and early intervention
- Services are open to all and are based on choice; people are not selected for support on the basis of 'employability' or 'work readiness'
- Comprehensive, coherent support is provided, with integration of employment support and clinical treatment and social support; this integration is at all levels (individual, local, national)
- Early job search is based on client preferences and interests; treatment and employment are supported in parallel
- Relationships with employers are established to help with proactive job finding; employers are approached with the needs of individuals in mind
- Individualised support is provided, tailored to the person's needs and preferences, with promotion of self-management
- Personalised support at the time of need is provided to both individuals and their manager/employer, with early intervention, sustaining jobs, building careers
- Support to negotiate necessary adjustments is provided, under fluctuating conditions
- Employers are helped to develop mentally healthy workplaces and to attend to health and well-being of all employees
- Peer support and lived experience are engaged to give access to the expertise of people with mental health conditions; lived experience is actively valued and central to the design and delivery of services
- High-quality support is provided for welfare benefits and financial planning

Early intervention can be crucial. This may mean incorporating IPS services in early-onset psychosis teams or it can mean working with people as soon as possible after they become unemployed or stop working. Liaison with employers is an important part not only of getting people into work but also of supporting them while there. Clinicians can advise about the appropriate adjustments to support a person in work and liaise with occupational health clinicians if the company has them. The employer has a responsibility to develop a healthy workplace in which employees can thrive.

The role of mental health clinicians

Mental health clinicians need not be experts in employment support, but they need to be aware of the importance of employment in a person's recovery journey and their role in supporting a person into or back to work. Clinicians should adopt an approach that provides treatment and work support in parallel and does not wait for clinical recovery before raising the issue of work.

Some suggestions for clinicians are given in Box 20.5. A useful structure for promoting the benefits of employment is provided by Perkins *et al* (2009: p. 46 – adapted from the '3 Rs' developed by the Bridge Building Services that form part of Glasgow Employability Partnership) in the form of the 4 Rs:

*   *Raise* the issue of employment with people who have a mental health condition and convey a positive view about the person's skills and ability to work

---

Box 20.5 Championing employment – suggestions for clinicians

*   Follow the 4 Rs: *Raise, Respond, Recommend, Refer*
*   Promote the benefits of employment
*   Challenge inaccurate assumptions
*   Focus on people's strengths – not what they cannot do
*   Help people to manage their condition in the work context
*   Adjust medication to fit with the work context
*   Refer for specialist support – employment and benefits
*   Help draw up agreements with employers about how to support the person in the workplace
*   Encourage the use of wellness recovery action plans in the workplace
*   Liaise with the occupational health department
*   Encourage patients to keep in touch with their employer during sickness absence
*   Discuss with patients how to manage disclosure of their mental health conditions at work
*   Provide appropriate reports for employers, occupational health and benefit agencies
*   Provide advice on 'reasonable adjustments'

- *Respond* positively to people's questions about work
- *Recommend* that the right sort of work is good for mental health, point out the deleterious consequences of unemployment and encourage people to think through what they may be able to do
- *Refer* the person to people or agencies that may be able to help them in their journey to employment.

Mental health clinicians are often asked to provide clinical reports for patients by their employer's occupational health department, either before employment or when the person goes off work for sickness reasons. It is important to provide these in a timely manner, as delay may result in the person not being appointed or losing the job. Suggestions for compiling these reports are given in Box 20.6.

Box 20.6 Occupational health reports from mental health professionals to occupational health staff: suggestions for good practice

1. Background to report
- Relationship of author to patient
- Means by which relationship first established (e.g. general practitioner referral)
- Duration and frequency of contact (individual and team)
- Whether report is based on consultation and/or clinical records

2. Body of report
- Provide the information requested and add the following if relevant:
  - outline of clinical condition (not normally though a detailed psychiatric report)
  - treatment plan, including details of any medication
  - estimate of clinical prognosis
  - perceived barriers to return to work or progress of other employment issues
  - suggested means of overcoming barriers
  - flag any significant risk of harm to the patient
- Do not repeat unsubstantiated allegations by the patient as fact
- Do not suggest causal links between work and health without firm evidence
- Do not make employment recommendations unless qualified to do so
- Do not comment on financial matters (e.g. sick pay or medical retirement benefits)
- Ensure that opinion is justified by rational argument and is not reported as fact
- Remember that clinical risk aversion often results in job loss
- Remember that keeping a job is much easier than finding a new one
- Remember that unemployment is a potent cause of mental ill-health

3. Procedural issues
- Ensure that the consent provided is appropriate and contemporaneous
- Offer to show, or give, a copy of the report, to the patient before it is sent

Taken from Royal College of Psychiatrists' website, pages on 'Supporting good communication between health professionals, employee and employer' (http://www.rcpsych.ac.uk/usefulresources/workandmentalhealth.aspx)

Box 20.7 Examples of 'reasonable adjustments' in the workplace

Working hours or patterns

- Take a flexible approach to start and finish times and shift patterns
- Allow use of paid or unpaid leave for medical appointments
- Phase the return to work after sickness absence (e.g. offering temporary part-time hours)
- Give an equal amount of break time, but in shorter, more frequent chunks
- Allow someone to arrange annual leave so that it is spaced regularly throughout the year
- Allow the possibility to work from home at times
- Where a person found that the stress of a formal interview exacerbated his or her mental health condition, allow him or her instead to work (unpaid) to assess suitability for the job
- Allow a person who has difficulty travelling on crowded trains to start early and finish early to avoid the rush hour
- Avoid contact with the public if this aggravates the mental health condition
- Change shift patterns to allow a longer period of night shifts if changing the schedule of medication in the transfer from day to night shifts is problematic
- Arrange for someone who became very drowsy after monthly medication to take a day off and make up the hours elsewhere
- Enable people to arrange their hours to permit them to attend therapy sessions
- Permit people to take 10 minutes out of the office when they become particularly anxious
- Create the possibility of part-time working and job-share arrangements for someone who is unable to work full time

Physical environment

- Minimise noise (e.g. by providing a private office, room dividers, partitions, or by reducing the pitch or volume of telephone ringtones)
- Provide a quiet space for breaks away from the main work space
- Offer a reserved parking space
- Allow for increased personal space
- Move the workstation (e.g. to avoid having a client's back to the door)
- For someone who found the distractions of an open-plan office detracted from work performance, arrange for them to have the desk in a quieter area

Support with workload

- Increase the frequency of supervision
- Support someone to prioritise the work
- Allow the individual to focus on a specific piece of work
- Consider job sharing
- Ensure that a manager, for example, who found the pressure of large meetings difficult can arrange for there to be at least 15 minutes between meetings
- Provide written instructions for someone who is very anxious about forgetting to do things that were expected
- Allow someone who becomes particularly paranoid at times to call a friend or support worker for support and reassurance
- Allow temporary reallocation of some tasks

Support from others

- Provide a job coach
- Appoint a 'buddy' or 'mentor' – someone on a similar grade and outside the usual management structure – to show the new employee the ropes and help in settling in to the workplace
- Provide mediation if there are difficulties between colleagues

Adapted from Perkins *et al* (2009) and Department of Health (2012)

Employers often wish to know what 'reasonable adjustments' can be made to support the employee. The Equality Act 2010 outlines an employer's duty to make reasonable adjustments for people with disabilities in order that they may have the same access as a non-disabled person to everything that involves gaining or retaining employment. From the definition in the Act, a people are defined as disabled if they have a mental or physical condition that has a substantial long-term (more than 12 months) effect on their normal day-to-day activities. A reasonable adjustment is defined as a 'change or adjustment to a person's needs that will enable them to do their job'. For many people with mental health problems these adjustments are concerned with helping them negotiate the social and interactional aspects of work and may involve changes in working hours or patterns, support with their workload and support from others. Some examples of useful adjustments are listed in Box 20.7. These need to be tailored to fit the individual and many may need no adjustments at all.

Conclusions

Work has always been a central feature of rehabilitation practice, and today open employment can be a realistic goal for vocational rehabilitation. Nevertheless, the majority of people with long-term mental health problems are not in open employment despite a considerable body of evidence that supported-employment schemes improve their chances of gaining work. People with mental health problems want to live meaningful and satisfactory lives and have the opportunity to engage in valued activities. Employment has an important role in people's recovery journeys and offers a means for their improved participation in their local communities.

Mental health professionals and services can play a role in helping people gain and retain employment, by promoting the health benefits of work, championing supported-employment schemes and liaising with employers, job centres and work schemes, welfare advisors, occupational health departments and general practitioners. Work and employment are not merely add-ons to a person's health and well-being: they are core outcome indicators for the quality of mental health services.

References

Bartley M (1994) Unemployment and ill health: understanding the relationships. *Journal of Epidemiology and Community Health*, **48**: 333–7.

Beard JH, Propst RN, Malamud TJ (1982) The Fountain House model of rehabilitation. *Psychiatric Rehabilitation Journal*, **5**: 47–53.

Becker DR, Smith J, Tanzman B, *et al* (2001) Fidelity of supported employment programs and employment outcomes. *Psychiatric Services*, **52**: 834–6.

Becker D, Whitley R, Bailey EL, *et al* (2007) Long-term employment trajectories among participants with severe mental illness in supported employment. *Psychiatric Services*, **58**: 922–8.

Becker DR, Lynde D, Swanson SJ (2008) Strategies for state-wide implementation of supported employment: the Johnson & Johnson-Dartmouth community mental health program. *Psychiatric Rehabilitation Journal*, **31**: 296–9.

Becker DR, Drake RE, Bond GR, *et al* (2011) A mental health learning collaborative on supported employment. *Psychiatric Services*, **62**: 704–6.

Bennett D (1970) The value of work in psychiatric rehabilitation. *Social Psychiatry*, **5**: 224–30.

Bevan S, Gulliford J, Steadman K, *et al* (2013) *Working with Schizophrenia: Pathways to Employment, Recovery and Inclusion*. The Work Foundation.

Boardman J (2003) Work, employment and psychiatric disability. *Advances in Psychiatric Treatment*, **9**: 599–603.

Boardman J, Rinaldi M (2013) Difficulties in implementing supported employment for people with severe mental health problems. *British Journal of Psychiatry*, **203**: 247–9.

Boardman J, Currie A, Killaspy H, *et al* (2010) *Social Inclusion and Mental Health*. Royal College of Psychiatrists.

Bond GR (2004) Supported employment: evidence for an evidence-based practice. *Psychiatric Rehabilitation Journal*, **27**: 345–59.

Bond GR, Kukla M (2011) Is job tenure brief in individual placement and support (IPS) employment programs? *Psychiatric Services*, **62**: 950–3.

Bond GR, Drake RE, Mueser KT, *et al* (1997) An update on supported employment for people with severe mental illness. *Psychiatric Services*, **48**: 335–46.

Bond GR, Resnick SG, Drake RE, *et al* (2001) Does competitive employment improve non-vocational outcomes for people with severe mental illness? *Journal of Consulting and Clinical Psychology*, **69**: 489–501.

Bond GR, Drake RE, Becker DR (2008a) An update on randomized controlled trials of evidence-based supported employment. *Psychiatric Rehabilitation Journal*, **31**: 280–90.

Bond GR, McHugo GJ, Becker DR, *et al* (2008b) Fidelity of supported employment: lessons learned from the National Evidence-Based Practices Project. *Psychiatric Rehabilitation Journal*, **31**: 300–5.

Bond GR, Drake RE, Becker DR (2012) Generalizability of the individual placement and support (IPS) model of supported employment outside the US. *World Psychiatry*, **11**: 32–9.

Boyce M, Secker J, Floyd M, *et al* (2008) Factors influencing the delivery of evidence-based supported employment in England. *Psychiatric Rehabilitation Journal*, **31**: 360–6.

Brenner MH (1979) Mortality and the national economy. *A review*, and the experience of England and Wales. *Lancet*, **ii**: 685–99.

Brohan E, Henderson C, Wheat K, *et al* (2012). Systematic review of beliefs, behaviours and influencing factors associated with disclosure of a mental health problem in the workplace. *BMC Psychiatry*, **12**: 11.

Burns T, Catty J, Becker T, *et al* (2007) The effectiveness of supported employment for people with severe mental illness: a randomised controlled trial in six European countries. *Lancet*, **370**: 1146–52.

Catty J, Lissouba P, White S, *et al* (2008) Predictors of employment for people with severe mental illness: results of an international six-centre randomised controlled trial. *British Journal of Psychiatry*, **192**: 224–31.

Centre for Mental Health (2012) *Implementing What Works. The Impact of the Individual Placement and Support Regional Trainer*. Centre for Mental Health.

Clevenger N (2008) In favor of science. *Psychiatric Rehabilitation Journal*, **31**: 277–9.

Cook JA, Blyler CR, Leff HS, *et al* (2008) The Employment Intervention Demonstration Program: major findings and policy implications. *Psychiatric Rehabilitation Journal*, **31**: 291–5.

Connolly J (1847) *The Construction and Government of Lunatic Asylums and Hospitals for the Insane*. Dawsons of Pall Mall (1968).

Corrigan P, Watson AC (2002) Understanding the impact of stigma on people with mental illness. *World Psychiatry*, **1**: 16–20.

Corrigan P, Larson JE, Rusch N (2009) Self-stigma and the 'why try' effect: impact on life goals and evidence-based practices. *World Psychiatry*, **8**: 75–81.

Crowther RE, Marshall M, Bond GR, *et al* (2001) Helping people with severe mental illness to obtain work: systematic review. *BMJ*, **322**: 204–8.

Department of Health (2012) *Advice for Employers on Workplace Adjustments for Mental Health Conditions*. Department of Health.

Department of Health & Department for Work and Pensions (2006) *Vocational Services for People with Severe Mental Health Problems: Commissioning Guidance*. Department of Health.

Drake RE, Bond GR, Becker DR (2012) *Individual Placement and Support. An Evidence-Based Approach to Supported Employment*. Oxford University Press.

Dunn EC, Wewiorski NJ, Rogers ES (2008) The meaning and importance of employment to people in recovery from serious mental illness: results of a qualitative study. *Psychiatric Rehabilitation Journal*, **32**: 59–62.

Fixsen DL, Naoom SF, Blase KA, *et al* (2005) *Implementation Research: A Synthesis of the Literature* (FMHI Publication 231). University of South Florida, Louis de la Parte Florida Mental Health Institute, National Implementation Research Network.

Frey WD, Drake RE, Bond GR, *et al* (2011) *Mental Health Treatment Study: Final Report*. Westat. At http://www.socialsecurity.gov/disabilityresearch/mentalhealth.htm (accessed December 2014).

Gowdy EA, Carlson LS, Rapp CA (2003) Practices differentiating high-performing from low performing supported employment programs. *Psychiatric Rehabilitation Journal*, **26**: 232–9.

Hasson H, Andersson M, Bejerholm U (2011) Barriers in implementation of evidence-based practice: supported employment in Swedish context. *Journal of Health Organization and Management*, **25**: 332–45.

Hatfield B, Huxley P, Mohamad H (1992) Accommodation and employment. A survey into the circumstances and expressed needs of users of mental health services in a northern town. *British Journal of Social Work*, **22**: 60–73.

Heslin M, Howard L, Leese M, *et al* (2011) Randomized controlled trial of supported employment in England: 2 year follow-up of the Supported Work and Needs (SWAN) study. *World Psychiatry*, **10**: 132–7.

Hill RG, Hardy P, Shepherd G (1996) *Perspectives on Manic Depression. A Survey of the Manic Depression Fellowship*. Sainsbury Centre for Mental Health.

Killackey E, Jackson HJ, McGorry PD (2008) Vocational intervention in first-episode psychosis: individual placement and support v. treatment as usual. *British Journal of Psychiatry*, **193**: 114–20.

King R, Waghorn G, Lloyd C, *et al* (2006) Enhancing employment services for people with severe mental illness: the challenge of the Australian service environment. *Australian and New Zealand Journal of Psychiatry*, **40**: 471–7.

Knapp M, Patel A, Curran C, *et al* (2013) Supported employment: cost-effectiveness across six European sites. *World Psychiatry*, **12**: 60–8.

Latimer E (2010) An effective intervention delivered at sub-therapeutic dose becomes an ineffective intervention. *British Journal of Psychiatry*, **196**: 341–2.

Lehman AF, Goldberg RW, Dixon LB, *et al* (2002) Improving employment outcomes for persons with severe mental illness. *Archives of General Psychiatry*, **59**: 165–72.

Little K, Henderson C, Brohan E, *et al* (2011) Employers' attitudes to people with mental health problems in the workplace in Britain: changes between 2006 and 2009. *Epidemiology and Psychiatric Sciences*, **20**: 73–81.

Manning C, White PD (1995) Attitudes of employers to the mentally ill. *Psychiatric Bulletin*, **19**: 541–3.

Marwaha S, Johnson S (2004) Schizophrenia and employment. *Social Psychiatry and Psychiatric Epidemiology*, **39**: 337–49.

Marwaha S, Johnson S, Bebbington P, *et al* (2007) Rates and correlates of employment in people with schizophrenia in the UK, France and Germany. *British Journal of Psychiatry*, **191**: 30–7.

Marwaha S, Balachandra S, Johnson S (2009) Clinicians' attitudes to the employment of people with psychosis. *Social Psychiatry and Psychiatric Epidemiology*, **44**: 349–60.

McGrew JH, Griss ME (2005) Concurrent and predictive validity of two scales to assess the fidelity of implementation of supported employment. *Psychiatric Rehabilitation Journal*, **29**: 41–7.

McHugo GJ, Drake RE, Xie H, *et al* (2012) A 10 year study of steady employment and non-vocational outcomes among people with serious mental illness and co-occurring substance use disorder. *Schizophrenia Research*, **138**: 233–9.

Nuechterlein KH, Subotnik KL, Turner LR, *et al* (2008) Individual placement and support for individuals with recent-onset schizophrenia: integrating supported education and supported employment. *Psychiatric Rehabilitation Journal*, **31**: 340–9.

Perkins R, Rinaldi M (2002) Unemployment rates among patients with long-term mental health problems. A decade of rising unemployment. *Psychiatric Bulletin*, **26**: 295–8.

Perkins R, Farmer P, Litchfield P (2009) *Realising Ambitions: Better Employment Support for People with a Mental Health Condition*. Department for Work and Pensions.

Platt S, Kreitman N (1984) Trends in parasuicide among unemployed men in Edinburgh 1968–82. *BMJ*, **289**: 1029–32.

Repper J, Carter T (2011) A review of the literature on peer support in mental health services. *Journal of Mental Health*, **20**: 392–411.

Rinaldi M, McNeil K, Firn M, *et al* (2004) What are the benefits of evidence-based supported employment for patients with first-episode psychosis? *Psychiatric Bulletin*, **28**: 281–4.

Rinaldi M, Montibeller T, Perkins R (2011) Increasing the employment rate for people with longer-term mental health problems. *The Psychiatrist*, **35**: 339–43.

Sainsbury Centre for Mental Health (2007) *Mental Health at Work: Developing the Business Case* (Policy Paper 8). Sainsbury Centre for Mental Health.

Shaw Trust (2010) *Mental Health: Still the Last Workplace Taboo?* Shaw Trust.

Taylor AC, Bond GR (2014) Employment specialist competencies as predictors of employment outcomes. *Community Mental Health Journal*, **50**: 31–40.

Trachtenberg M, Parsonage M, Shepherd G, *et al* (2013) *Peer Support in Mental Health Care: Is It Good Value for Money?* Centre for Mental Health.

Tuke S (1813) *Description of The Retreat, An Institution Near York for Insane Persons of the Society of Friends*. Dawsons of Pall Mall (1964).

Twamley EW, Jeste DV, Lehman AF (2003) Vocational rehabilitation in schizophrenia and other psychotic disorders: a literature review and meta-analysis of randomised controlled trials. *Journal of Nervous and Mental Disease*, **191**: 515–23.

van Erp NHJ, Giesen FBM, van Weeghel J, *et al* (2007) A multisite study of implementing supported employment in the Netherlands. *Psychiatric Services*, **58**: 1421–6.

Waddell G, Burton AK (2006) *Is Work Good for Your Health and Well-being?* TSO (The Stationery Office).

Warner R (2004) *Recovery from Schizophrenia: Psychiatry and Political Economy* (3rd edn). Brunner-Routledge.

Warner R (2010) Does the scientific evidence support the recovery model? *The Psychiatrist*, 34: 3–5.

Warr P (1987) *Work, Unemployment and Mental Health*. Oxford University Press.

Whitley RE, Gingerich S, Lutz WJ, *et al* (2009) Implementing the illness management and recovery program in community mental health settings: facilitators and barriers. *Psychiatric Services*, **60**: 202–9.

Whitely RE, Kostick K, Bush P (2010) The desirable attributes of supported employment specialists: an empirically-grounded framework. *Administration and Policy in Mental Health and Mental Health Service Research*, **37**: 509–19.

Wilson S, Walker G (1993) Unemployment and health. A review. *Public Health*, **107**: 153–62.

CHAPTER 21

Peer support in mental health services

Julie Repper and Emma Watson

Introduction

It is likely that people have valued the support of others who share their experiences and challenges since time began. Whether it occurs in informal friendships, self-help groups or statutory services, mutual support is a key tenet in stories of recovery from all kinds of experiences, traumas and loss. Many such accounts come from people who have mental health conditions (see e.g. Deegan, 1997) and as the value of peer support has been recognised by mental health services, peer support roles have been developing across both the Western world and in lower-income countries. Guidance on peer support workers has been developed along with accredited training in England (Repper, 2013*a*, 2013*b*, 2013*c*) and in Scotland (Scottish Recovery Network, 2011). In the USA, 27 states have collaborated to create a scoping and guidance document for peer support (Daniels *et al*, 2010). In Canada, standards and guidelines for peer support have been developed by the Mental Health Commission (Sunderland *et al*, 2013). Peer workers have been employed in various roles and settings in Australia (Franke *et al*, 2010), New Zealand (Scott *et al*, 2011), parts of Europe (Castelein *et al*, 2008) – and although less is published about the ongoing work in the low- and middle-income countries, peer workers are increasingly employed there to augment professional support.

This chapter first seeks to define peer support, focusing largely upon peer support in statutory services, and then reviews the evidence that supports it. It goes on to illustrates peer support in practice, with personal reflections from a peer support worker with 3 years' experience of employment in in-patient and community mental health services.

Defining peer support

Peer support occurs when people who have common concerns draw on their own experiences to offer emotional and practical support to help each other move forwards. Peer support may be defined simply as offering and receiving help, based on shared understanding, respect and mutual empowerment between people in similar situations (Mead *et al*, 2001). The 'shared understanding' may relate to the specific challenge or symptoms, or it may be due to a common response to a trauma or change (Sunderland *et al*, 2013). The help that is offered and received is often most useful if both parties have other things in common, such as cultural background, religion, age, gender or a shared history of oppression or exclusion (Faulkner & Kalathil, 2012).

Peer support encompasses a personal understanding of the frustrations experienced with the mental health system and serves to confirm recovery as making sense of what has happened and moving on, rather than identifying and eradicating symptoms and dysfunction (Bradstreet, 2006; Adams & Leitner, 2008). One of the core features of peer support is the hope that can be inspired when meeting someone who has moved on following a crisis similar to one's own, or (re)built a meaningful life with ongoing mental health challenges. It is through this trusting relationship, which offers companionship, empathy and empowerment, that feelings of isolation and rejection can be replaced with hope, a sense of agency and belief in personal control (Repper & Carter, 2010).

Types of peer support

Three broad types of peer support have been identified (Davidson *et al*, 1999; Bradstreet, 2006): 'informal' (naturally occurring) support; peers participating in consumer, or peer-run, programmes alongside formal mental health services; and people with lived experience employed in formal positions within statutory services. However, Repper (2013*a*) suggests that the distinctions between these types of peer support are not clear, as peer support varies along a number of dimensions whatever the setting. First, peer support can be provided on a group or individual basis. For example, a peer-run support group may be available only on a group basis whether it occurs on an in-patient ward or in a self-help setting, whereas buddy systems, recovery aides and peer workers – in a statutory or peer-run service – might provide individualised support. Second, the degree of choice over worker varies. Some peer support schemes offer a choice over which worker provides the support, but no service offers open choice over which housing worker, day centre staff member or co-counsellor provides support as there is a usually a very limited staff team. Third, the standards, expectations and rules governing peer-to-peer relationships vary in whatever setting peer support is offered. Fourth, the extent to which the parties involved are in the same place in their recovery varies. In statutory services, it is generally expected that peer workers are further on in their recovery journey, but recovery is not a linear process, so at different points in time one person may be further on, but then experience a setback, so reversing roles.

Table 21.1 The core principles of peer support

Principle	Features
1. Mutual	The experience of peers who give and gain support is never identical. However, peer workers in mental health settings share some of the experiences of the people they work with. They have an understanding of common mental health challenges, the meaning of being defined as a 'mental patient' in our society and the confusion, fear and hopelessness that can ensue
2. Reciprocal	Traditional relationships between mental health professionals and the people they support are founded on the assumption of an expert (professional) and a non-expert (patient/client). Peer relationships involve no claims to such special expertise, but a sharing and exploration of different world views and the generation of solutions together
3. Non-directive	Because of their claims to special knowledge, mental health professionals often prescribe the 'best' course of action for those whom they serve. Peer support is not about introducing another set of experts to offer prescriptions based on their experience, such as 'You should try this because it worked for me'. Instead, workers help people to recognise their own resources and seek their own solutions. 'Peer support is about being an expert in not being an expert and that takes a lot of expertise' (Recovery Innovations training materials, from http://www.recoveryinnovations.org)
4. Recovery focused	Peer support workers engage in recovery-focused relationships by: • inspiring *hope* – they are in a position to say 'I know you can do it' and to help generate personal belief, energy and commitment with the person they are supporting • supporting people to take back *control* of their personal challenges and define their own destiny • facilitating access to *opportunities* that people value, enabling them to participate in roles, relationships and activities in the communities of their choice
5. Strengths based	Peer support involves a relationship where the person providing support is not afraid of being with people in their distress. But it is also about seeing within that distress the seeds of possibility and creating a fertile ground for those seeds to grow. It explores what people have gained from their experiences, seeks out their qualities and assets, identifies hidden achievements and celebrates what may seem like the smallest steps forward
6. Inclusive	Being a 'peer' is not just about having experienced mental health challenges; it is also about understanding the meaning of such experiences within the communities of which the person is a part. This can be critical among those who feel marginalised and misunderstood by traditional services. Someone who knows the language, values and nuances of those communities obviously has a better understanding of the resources and the possibilities. This equips her or him to be more effective in helping others become a valued member of their community

7. Progressive	Peer support is not a static friendship, but progressive mutual support in a shared journey of discovery. The peer is not just a 'buddy', but a travelling companion, with both travellers learning new skills, developing new resources and reframing challenges as opportunities for finding new solutions
8. Safe	Supportive peer relationships involve the negotiation of what emotional safety means to both parties. This can be achieved by discovering what makes each other feel unsafe, sharing rules of confidentiality, demonstrating compassion, authenticity and a non-judgemental attitude and acknowledging that neither has all the answers

Adapted from Repper (2013*b*).

Roles of peer workers

Peer support workers have been employed in many different roles within mental health services: as additional staff in existing teams (e.g. new posts may be created in community mental health teams to support other staff); in new roles (e.g. peer workers are employed in Nottinghamshire Healthcare Trust in the UK to facilitate earlier discharge from acute in-patient wards); or as a substitute for existing team members (in Central and North West London Trust healthcare assistant posts have been converted into peer worker posts on acute in-patient wards). Peer workers have also been employed in substance misuse, eating disorder, older people's and criminal justice teams (see Repper, 2013*a*). In addition, peer workers are employed within recovery colleges as trainers, in research teams, in business development posts and in human resources departments.

The core defining feature of the peer worker role, whatever the setting, is the explicit use of their own experiences in providing support, training or development for others who are facing similar challenges. Repper (2013b) has drawn on the experience of many different organisations employing peer workers to provide a summary of other defining features of peer support workers (see Table 21.1). This concurs with similar lists developed in guidelines for peer support elsewhere (e.g. Daniels *et al*, 2010; Scottish Recovery Network, 2012; Canadian Mental Health Commission, 2013).

What difference does peer support make?

It is difficult to draw hard and fast conclusions about the impact of peer support because the evidence base is varied in terms of the definition of peer support, weak in terms of the quality of research undertaken and inconsistent in terms of outcomes measured. Repper & Carter (2011) have reviewed the literature and reported on seven randomised controlled trials. They found that trials comparing the employment of peer support workers with care as usual or other case management conditions report either improved outcomes or no change and concluded that people in recovery are able to offer support that maintains admission rates at a comparable level to professionally trained staff. A more recent Cochrane review was able to identify 11 randomised controlled trials (Pitt *et al*, 2013) and similarly concluded that outcomes across a range of domains were no different from when services had been provided by professionals – but could cost considerably less. The question of cost has been considered in more depth by Trachtenberg *et al* (2013), who identified six studies in the research literature that provided some evidence of a relationship between peer support and in-patient bed use. They aggregated and reanalysed these data and concluded that the financial benefits of employing peer support workers do indeed exceed the costs, in some cases by a considerable margin.

It is worth looking beyond trials to the broader body of literature to explain these findings and explore further the effects of peer support on those who receive it. Repper & Carter (2010) reviewed the findings of trials, observational studies, naturalistic comparison studies and long-term follow-up research to reveal a more promising picture of the impact of peer support.

Admission rates

Wider evidence on admission rates suggests that peer support tends to reduce admission rates. Chinman *et al* (2001) compared a peer support out-patient programme with traditional care and found a 50% reduction in rehospitalisation compared with the general out-patient population. Forchuk *et al* (2005) evaluated a model of discharge involving peer support and reported significantly reduced readmission rates and increased discharge rates. In a longitudinal comparison group study, Min *et al* (2007) reported that consumers involved in a peer support programme demonstrated longer community tenure and had significantly less rehospitalisation over a 3-year period. Finally, in an evaluation of an Australian mental health peer support service providing hospital-avoidance and early-discharge support to consumers of adult mental health services, Lawn *et al* (2008) reported that in the first 3 months of operation more than 300 bed-days were saved when peers were employed as supporters for people at this stage of their recovery.

Self-efficacy

An improved sense of self-efficacy has been reported in several studies of peer support (Dummont & Jones, 2002; Corrigan, 2006; Resnick & Rosenheck, 2008). In a qualitative follow-up study, Ochocka *et al* (2006) reported that participation in peer support as both a provider and a recipient resulted in an increased sense of independence and empowerment. Participants reported gaining control of their symptoms and problems by researching their illness independently and consequently becoming more involved in their treatment, thereby moving away from the traditional role of 'mental patient'.

Social isolation

Social isolation is one of the most significant challenges faced by individuals with mental health problems. Yanos *et al* (2001) found that individuals involved in consumer-run services had improved social functioning compared with individuals involved in traditional mental health services. Nelson *et al* (2006) reported that at 3-year follow-up, consumers continuously involved in peer support programmes scored significantly higher than comparison groups on a measure of 'community integration'.

Sense of acceptance

An important aspect of peer support is the sense of acceptance and real empathy that the peer gains through a sharing relationship (Davidson *et al*, 1999). In a qualitative study exploring the peer support relationships within mental health, Coatsworth-Puspoky *et al* (2006) found that consumers believed that the experiential knowledge provided by peer workers created a 'comradery' and a 'bond', which made them feel that their challenges were better understood. Similarly, Paulson *et al* (1999) demonstrated through qualitative data that there were significant differences in the focus of consumer and non-consumer providers of assertive community treatment (ACT). Specifically, the consumer providers emphasised 'being' with the client, whereas the non-consumer providers emphasised the importance of 'doing' tasks.

Stigma

Ochocka *et al* (2006) found that participants involved in peer support were less likely to identify stigma as an obstacle to getting work and were more likely to have employment. When patients are in frequent contact with peer support workers, their stability in employment, education and training has been shown to increase (Ochocka *et al*, 2006). Mowbray *et al* (1998) reported that peer workers recognised that through engaging in peer support they were altering attitudes to mental illness and as such were breaking down the stigma and fostering hope in the peers they were working with.

Hope

One of the essential benefits gained from peer support is the sense of hope – a belief in a better future – created through meeting people who are recovering, people who have found ways through their difficulties and challenges (Davidson *et al*, 2006). The inspiration provided by successful role models is hard to overstate. So many people who have been supported by peers describe their surprise when meeting others who have had similar experiences (Ratzlaff *et al*, 2006).

Benefits for the peer workers

In addition to the benefits for those receiving the service, there is evidence of benefits for the peer workers themselves. They feel more empowered in their own recovery journey, have greater confidence and self-esteem, feel more valued and less stigmatised, and have a more positive sense of identity (Mowbray *et al*, 1998; Salzer & Shear, 2002; Repper & Carter, 2011).

Recovery-focused approach within organisations

Finally, the introduction of peer workers is a powerful way of driving a more recovery-focused approach within organisations (Repper, 2013c). Just as peer workers provide hope and inspiration for service users, so they can challenge negative attitudes of staff and provide an inspiration for all members of the team. Their example demonstrates to everyone that people with mental health problems can make a valued contribution to their own and others' recovery if they are given the opportunity. They also have a valuable role in bringing their own experience-based perspective to bear on routine practices, procedures, paperwork, policies and language.

Peer support from the inside: reflections from a peer support worker

In the following account, Emma Watson reflects on her role: what makes it different, how it affects those receiving support and the essential aspects of training, management and supervision of peer workers.

Over the past 3 years I have worked in both in-patient and community settings and I am drawing on this experience to consider how peer support makes a difference, how peers can be supported to make a difference, and what can be learnt from peers for the rest of the organisation. As I am writing about my experiences of peer support, I have made reference to the practice of other staff based on my working relationships. It is not my intention to criticise current practice or to idealise peer support workers, merely to reflect upon how this approach differs from other approaches. These reflections are based on the majority of my peer support relationships. However, it has to be stressed that the power of peer support does not extend to all people or situations. There are certainly some who are indifferent to the thought of working with a peer support worker, some who actively choose professionals over peer support and some situations where lived experience may not have a place. The following sections are a general consideration of my own understanding of peer support, which does seem to contain something powerful and unique.

The magic ingredients – a light bulb and a reframe

There is often a magic moment which occurs the first time somebody meets a peer support worker. Although the worker is a relative stranger to the person she or he meets, it seems as if some barrier dissolves when both parties recognise the other as having lived experience. The instant connection between peer support worker and peer over time can develop into a powerful bond built upon a shared knowledge of darker times. It is difficult to pin down what is so different about a peer support relationship, although from the inside the difference is clear. From my experience I have come to understand that there are two extremely powerful components of peer support relationships: the 'light bulb' and the 'reframe'.

The 'light bulb' is the moment when the person hears that you too have been through the mental health mill but have come out the other side. A degree of formality is lifted by the fact that you have disclosed something so personal. The act of sharing shows that you have put your trust in the person, you have viewed them as somebody worth sharing with – an equal. A relationship where both parties have lived experience is likely to feel less stigmatising. When I meet somebody who has lived experience, a knot of tension loosens within me. The best way for me to explain the reason for this is with my own experience.

On my visits to the clinic where I received support, I would talk to the same person every week. Every week I would try to find ways to describe to her how I was feeling. I would try to put into words the motivations that were driving me to do or feel certain things. Every week she would respond with a sound, logical reason why I was wrong:

Me: I feel like everyone's watching me.
Her: In actual fact they're probably too wrapped up in their own lives.
Me: I haven't opened the post because I'm scared I'm in trouble.
Her: You're not in trouble; you shouldn't leave post unopened.

And it wasn't just her that this happened with: my family, my friends, my general practitioner – all of them would feel the need to remind me that what I was saying didn't make sense. And the scary thing was I *knew* it didn't make sense, but that didn't stop me from feeling it.

A peer support worker's presence doesn't remind people all the time of how wrong they are, and there is no reason to feel ashamed of what you're feeling because they have felt it too. So it's natural, if you have felt ashamed and foolish for so long, to feel a light bulb turn on when you meet a peer support worker. Suddenly you are with someone who can hear your words and know your meaning.

The 'reframe' comes after the light bulb, as the peer support relationship develops (see Table 21.2). Peer support workers who have survived their own mental health problems and who continue to manage their well-being can provide a real reason for someone to have hope. Part of their role is to

Table 21.2 Peer support: the reframe

So a ...	becomes a ...
A shameful experience	A strength
A personal failure	A normal part of emotional growth
Recovery as impossible and illusive	Recovery as in one's control
Wellness as not worth it	Wellness as desirable
Other people fixing me	My responsibility
A hopeless situation	The potential for growth
A wasted life	An inspiring feat of survival

model positivity, focus on strengths and use language in a way that reflects this. In this way, peer support relationships have the potential to reframe a person's whole life in terms of possibility instead of deficit.

Practicalities of peer support

Training

Any person who has lived experience may be considered a peer to another. Quite often people do share their experiences of recovery, or illness, when talking to others. This may be peer support. Peer support workers are a step on from such informal support. In a statutory service, it is important that they share their lived experience in a 'safe' way. Lived experience is not enough to qualify a person for the role of peer support worker; it simply provides the essential base on which other, equally essential skills may rest.

It is important that a peer can *frame* recovery in such a way as is helpful for the listener. A training course or other learning experience that facilitates this is crucial. The Institute of Mental Health (IMH) runs the first nationally accredited peer support training course in England and this has set the precedent for what such a course must entail. A key element of the approach is the use of co-production, co-facilitation and co-learning. All the training is delivered by two trainers, who between them have lived experience of distress and clinical expertise, grounded in an academic understanding of recovery and peer support. Consistently co-producing training courses creates an inclusive learning environment where everybody can learn from one another. During course sessions a 'recovery environment' is created by encouraging ongoing discussions about how stigma and discrimination can create environments where hope and recovery are impossible. By focusing on individual strengths, the trainers acknowledge that everyone is able to contribute something to the shared learning process.

The role of the training is fundamentally to help students harness the parts of their story that enable them to empathise and work towards the recovery of others. Core components include:

- an introduction to recovery
- identifying personal strengths
- active listening
- early warning signs and triggers
- problem-solving
- story-sharing
- setbacks and challenges
- giving and receiving feedback
- working with a range of experiences
- ethics, values and principles.

Supervision and wellness plans

It is one of the common assumptions of other mental health professionals that peer support workers, when employed alongside other staff, will require more intensive, regular supervision than other employees. While this may be the case for some (and indeed some staff of all disciplines). it is not true as a general rule. What may be more accurate is the idea that peer support workers require a different approach to supervision than is currently offered in conventional services. Integral to this are 'wellness plans'.

Similarly, it is commonly assumed that peer support workers require greater levels of support than other staff, as they are more vulnerable to mental health challenges, and therefore more likely to take time off sick. I am not convinced that this is the case; I have not known any member of the team of peer support workers with whom I work to take any significant time away from work as a result of their mental health. As a team we are as reliable as any other and sickness statistics demonstrate lower levels of sickness absence than other staff groups (Repper, 2013c). This may be due to several factors. First, the open and accepting culture fostered within a peer support worker team means that we have the freedom to discuss exactly what we are feeling without having to witness the shocked or uncomfortable faces of those around us. Having 'outed' ourselves in becoming peer support workers we have fewer shameful secrets to keep from other team members regarding our mental health. Second, as individuals we do not expect others to look after our mental health if we are not prepared to first. We are all required to have reflected on our own patterns of mental health and become aware of our triggers and early warning signs. We refer to this as wellness planning.

All peer support workers have their own wellness plan, which includes not only their triggers and early warning signs but also what they themselves will do to address these. For example, if I notice that my sleep pattern is beginning to slip (an early warning sign for me), I will first make an effort to prioritise sleep, perhaps by avoiding caffeine or eating late, perhaps even a visit to the general practitioner for some sleeping tablets. It is only after I have done everything in my power to help myself that I will ask for support from my employers. The support I ask for will relate to my wellness plan and will be a specific 'reasonable adjustment'. In this case the reasonable adjustment I request is a change in my working hours from 9–5 to 10–6 for a short time to allow for morning lethargy. Reasonable adjustments differ for all the peer support workers within the team. They can be as simple as adjusting the office temperature to avoid one peer support worker from feeling too hot (a trigger for her) or a change of working days to allow for recovery from stressful events.

This approach to maintaining well-being is very different from reaching a crisis and begging for non-specific help. It is empowering for the peer support worker and is a skill in itself which we hope to pass on to those we work with. The times when we may not be the first to notice our own early warning signs are also considered within team wellness plans so that those around us may know how to communicate their concerns to us and how best to support us if we are struggling.

Management

There are many who believe that the managers of peer support workers should themselves have had some personal experience of mental ill-health. In this way managers might be able to provide peer-to-peer supervision, to create an environment of acceptance and openness between themselves and the peer support worker and to empathise with themes of well-being and disclosure. However, just as is true for the peer support worker, lived experience alone does not determine the competence of the manager. Our peer support team has been managed by several different people since it was established, all with very different approaches. What they had in common was an awareness of and commitment to the values of recovery – this may be the one essential component of a peer support team manager. The values base allows for a flexible, compassionate management approach. For the power of peer support to be harnessed well, a manager must echo the relationships that peer support workers build with clients. By being non-directive, strengths-based and flexible, peer support workers can begin to trust in their own instincts with an awareness of organisational support.

Conclusion: peer support from the inside

The approaches that I have described above are those that I have experienced as part of a peer support worker team. However, it is likely that if other teams were trained using the same values base, given flexible, tailored supervision and were required to reflect regularly on their own well-being and support needs, it would improve their working environment, job satisfaction and morale, and even reduce sickness absence.

I believe that peer support relationships provide a unique opportunity for people to share experiences with the certain knowledge that they will be met with true understanding and positive regard. The power of peer support makes it an essential component of mental health teams. However, the implementation of this must be considered. Lived experience is necessary but not sufficient: it must be well placed and accompanied by a recovery philosophy. This philosophy can be developed through training, management and supervision structures. New structures and pathways to support peer workers as they are employed and as they continue to progress may require some creative thinking but it is now time that these support structures were adapted for all staff teams. It is not just peer support workers who need reasonable adjustments: the workforce as a whole should be modelling the values of recovery and personal well-being that we continue to advocate to those we serve.

References

Adams AL, Leitner LM (2008) Breaking out of the mainstream: the evolution of peer support alternatives to the mental health system. *Ethical Human Psychology and Psychiatry*, **10**: 146–62.

Bradstreet S (2006) Harnessing the 'lived experience'. Formalising peer support approaches to promote recovery. *Mental Health Review*, **11**: 2–6.

Canadian Mental Health Commission (2013) *Guidelines for the Practice and Training of Peer Support*. Mental Health Commission of Canada.

Castelein S, Bruggeman RJ, van Busschbach JT, *et al* (2008) The effectiveness of peer support groups in psychosis: a randomized controlled trial. *Acta Psychiatrica Scandinavica*, **118**: 64–72.

Chinman MJ, Weingarten R, Stayner D, *et al* (2001) Chronicity reconsidered: improving person-environment fit through a consumer-run service. *Community Mental Health Journal*, **37**: 215–29.

Coatsworth-Puspoky R, Forchuk C, Ward Griffin C (2006) Peer support relationships: an unexplored interpersonal process in mental health. *Journal of Psychiatric and Mental Health Nursing*, **13**: 490–7.

Corrigan PW (2006) Impact of consumer-operated services on empowerment and recovery of people with psychiatric disabilities. *Psychiatric Services*, **57**: 1493–6.

Daniels A, Grant E, Filson N, *et al* (2010) *Pillars of Peer Support: Transforming Mental Health Systems of Care Through Peer Support Services*. At http://www.pillarsofpeersupport.org (accessed December 2014).

Davidson L, Chinman M, Kloos B, *et al* (1999) Peer support among individuals with severe mental illness: a review of the evidence. *Clinical Psychology Science and Practice*, **6**: 165–87.

Davidson L, Chinman M, Sells D, *et al* (2006) Peer support among adults with serious mental illness: a report from the field. *Schizophrenia Bulletin*, **32**: 443–5.

Deegan PE (1997) Recovery and empowerment for people with psychiatric disabilities. In *Social Work In Mental Health: Issues and Trends* (ed U Aviram): 11–24. Haworth Press.

Dummont JM, Jones K (2002) Findings from a consumer/survivor defined alternative to psychiatric hospitalization. *Outlook*, spring: 4–6.

Faulkner A, Kalathil K (2012) *The Freedom To Be, The Chance To Dream: Preserving User-Led Peer Support in Mental Health*. Together.

Forchuk C, Martin ML, Chan YCL, *et al* (2005) Therapeutic relationships: from psychiatric hospital to community. *Journal of Psychiatric and Mental Health Nursing*, **12**: 556–64.

Franke C, Paton B, Gassner L (2010) Implementing mental health peer support: a South Australian experience. *Australian Journal of Primary Health*, **16**: 179–86.

Lawn S, Smith A, Hunter K (2008) Mental health peer support for hospital avoidance and early discharge: an Australian example of consumer driven and operated service. *Journal of Mental Health*, **17**: 498–508.

Mead S, Hilton D, Curtis L (2001) Peer support: a theoretical perspective. *Psychiatric Rehabilitation Journal*, **25**: 134–41.

Min S, Whitecraft J, Rothband AB, *et al* (2007) Peer support for persons with co-occurring disorders and community tenure: a survival analysis. *Psychiatric Rehabilitation Journal*, **30**: 207–13.

Mowbray C, Moxley D, Colllins M (1998) Consumers as mental health providers: first person accounts of benefits and limitations. *Journal of Behavioural Health Services and Research*, **25**: 397–411.

Nelson G, Ochocka J, Janzen R, *et al* (2006) A longitudinal study of mental health consumer/survivor initiatives: Part 1 – Literature review and overview of the study. *Journal of Community Psychology*, **34**: 247–60.

Ochocka J, Nelson G, Janzen R, *et al* (2006) A longitudinal study of mental health consumer/survivor initiatives: Part 3 – A qualitative study of impacts of participation on new members. *Journal of Community Psychology*, **34**: 273–83.

Paulson R, Herinckx H, Demmler J, *et al* (1999) Comparing practice patterns of consumer and non-consumer mental service providers. *Community Mental Health Journal*, **35**: 251–69.

Pitt V, Lowe D, Hill S, *et al* (2013) Consumer providers of care for adult clients of statutory mental health services. *Cochrane Database of Systematic Reviews*, **3**: CD004807.

Ratzlaff S, McDiarmid D, Marty D, *et al* (2006) The Kansas consumer as provider program: measuring the effects of a supported education initiative. *Psychiatric Rehabilitation Journal*, **29**: 174–82.

Repper J (2013a) *Peer Support Workers: Theory and Practice* (Briefing Paper 5). ImROC Publications.

Repper J (2013b) *Peer Support Workers: A Practical Guide to Implementation* (Briefing Paper 7). ImROC Publications.

Repper J (2013c) *Introducing Peer Support in Mental Health Services. Final Report for 'Closing the Gap through Changing Relationships' Programme*. Health Foundation.

Repper J, Carter T (2010) *Using Personal Experience to Support Others with Similar Difficulties: A Review of the Literature on Peer Support in Mental Health Services*. Together, University of Nottingham, NSUN.

Repper J, Carter T (2011) A review of the literature on peer support in mental health services. *Journal of Mental Health*, **20**: 392–411.

Resnick SG, Rosenheck RA (2008) Integrating peer-provided services: a quasi-experimental study of recovery orientation, confidence, and empowerment. *Psychiatric Services*, **59**: 1307–17.

Salzer M, Shear S (2002) Identifying consumer-provider benefits in evaluations of consumer-delivered services. *Psychiatric Rehabilitation Journal*, **25**: 281–8.

Scott A, Doughty C, Kahi H (2011) *Peer Support Practice in Aotearoa, New Zealand*. University of Canterbury.

Scottish Recovery Network (2011) *Experts by Experience: Guidelines to Support the Development of Peer Worker Roles in the Mental Health Sector*. At http://www.recoverydevon. co.uk/download/Guidelines_on_developing_peer_support_-_Scotland.pdf (accessed December 2014).

Scottish Recovery Network (2012) *Values Network for Peerworking*. SRN.

Sunderland K, Mishkin W, Peer Leadership Group, Mental Health Commission of Canada (2013) *Guidelines for the Practice and Training of Peer Support*. Mental Health Commission of Canada. At http://www.mentalhealthcommission.ca (accessed December 2014).

Trachtenberg M, Parsonage M, Shepherd G, *et al* (2013) *Peer Support in Mental Health Care: Is It Good Value for Money?* Centre for Mental Health.

Yanos TP, Primavera LH, Knight EL (2001) Consumer-run service participation, recovery of social functioning, and the mediating role of psychological factors. *Psychiatric Services*, **52**: 493–500.

CHAPTER 22

Leadership, management and service development in rehabilitation practice

Tom Edwards and Frank Holloway

Introduction

This chapter is about leadership, management and service development in rehabilitation services. These issues were not discussed in the first edition of *Enabling Recovery*. In the intervening years, it has become clear that senior rehabilitation practitioners require specific skills in order to manage, lead and ensure the development of effective services. Psychiatric rehabilitation is in many ways a complex business. By definition, its clients have complex problems that require sophisticated multidisciplinary and multi-agency approaches to treatment and care. In the UK, rehabilitation and long-term care services operate in a marketplace that continues to evolve rapidly and without the benefit of a high-level strategy from government.

Although the distinction between management and leadership is frequently drawn, in reality they are inextricably linked. Leading, managing and developing services require a range of skills and personal qualities. It is a unique individual who has all these necessary skills and qualities, which is one of the reasons why we have management teams to run services and project teams that develop new services. There are, however, some basics: being able to get on with people; a passion about the need to improve services; an understanding of how the money underpinning the current service or a planned development works; and willingness to learn.

Leadership versus management?

Kotter (1990: p. 6) made an influential distinction between leadership and management. His essential thesis was that business organisations in the late 20th century were too concerned about management processes, at the expense of strategic vision and leadership. His conception is easiest to understand in terms of a specific project. This will begin with the creation of an agenda: the *leadership* task here is to establish direction, the *management* task to develop a detailed plan and budget. The next task is to develop a 'human resource network' for achieving the agenda (i.e. a project team): *leadership* involves aligning people to new directions, *management* providing organisation and staffing for the team. Executing the task involves motivating and inspiring (*leadership*) but also, just as importantly, bringing order to the work of the team and problem-solving (*management*). When the task is completed, the *leader* will have implemented and managed change, while the *manager* will have brought about a predictable and ordered outcome, for example a service that actually works.

The contemporary National Health Service (NHS) in England is much taken with the idea of leadership (NHS Institute for Innovation and Improvement & Academy of Medical Royal Colleges, 2010), particularly the 'transformational' aspects of leadership as described by Kotter, which relate to 'vision' and 'change'. In 2011 the Association of Medical Royal Colleges founded a Faculty of Medical Leadership and Management, which has as its vision 'to see excellence in medical leadership, driving continuous improvement in health and healthcare in the UK' (https://www.fmlm.ac.uk). Within mental health services, the Royal College of Psychiatrists has acknowledged the need for practitioners to develop and enhance their leadership skills (Brown & Brittlebank, 2013). Nurses, social workers, occupational therapists and psychologists aspiring to become 'approved clinicians', who can take charge of the care of a patient detained under the Mental Health Act, have to show competencies in leadership and multidisciplinary teamwork, which include being able to 'effectively lead a multidisciplinary team' (Mental Health Act 1983 Approved Clinician Directions 2008, Schedule 2).

'Transformational' leadership is associated with terms like 'vision', 'strategic direction', 'inspiring followership' and 'influencing skills' (Marshall, 2007). Management (which in the jargon is also sometimes called 'transactional' leadership) involves more mundane activities such as setting a budget and keeping to it; developing and implementing policies and procedures; recruiting staff and instituting disciplinary procedures; and providing information that is required for quality assurance.

Effective rehabilitation services will be managed well but are also dependent in the long term on a vision of what the service should be achieving. This vision needs to take account of emerging best practice, epidemiological realities, the prevailing economic context and current health and social care policy.

Leadership and management in rehabilitation psychiatry

Leadership competencies for rehabilitation services

The Medical Leadership Competency Framework (NHS Institute for Innovation and Improvement & Academy of Medical Royal Colleges, 2010) identifies five domains relevant to the planning, delivery and transformation of services: *personal qualities* (e.g. self-management and self-awareness); *working with others* (e.g. teamwork, encouraging others); *managing services* (managing resources, people, performance); *improving services*; and *setting direction*.

Senior rehabilitation practitioners need leadership skills in order to influence others in developing rehabilitation services. Service development that requires investment of capital or revenue needs to be based on a sound business case (put at its most crude, will the proposed capital and revenue investment provide an adequate return for the organisation?), knowledge of the emerging evidence for rehabilitation services and a keen awareness of local organisational priorities and national policy. Quality improvement does not necessarily require investment – and it is vital for a service to demonstrate a commitment to improvement.

There are particular dilemmas for rehabilitation psychiatrists, who are likely to practise in relative isolation compared with their colleagues. In these circumstances, it is essential that the clinician has a clear awareness of the goals that need to be achieved in order to maintain an adequate level of local provision and support service development when gaps become apparent. Involvement in a wider network of colleagues locally, nationally and internationally is invaluable. Rehabilitation psychiatrists also need to be able to recognise the limits of their own skills with the most complex of clinical cases and be able to know (for both themselves and the team) when to refer for a further opinion. The awareness of the limitations of the clinician's own competencies is in itself an important leadership skill.

Management within rehabilitation services

In *Management for Doctors*, the General Medical Council (2006) defines management as 'getting things done well through and with people, creating an environment in which people can perform as individuals and yet co-operate towards achieving group goals, and removing obstacles to such performance'. Effective care for people with severe and enduring mental illness requires working in partnership with many agencies.

Operational and strategic management

Operational management relates to the day-to-day tasks of the service, while strategic management is concerned with issues of service provision and development, which become ever more acute in this increasingly competitive area of mental healthcare. Strategic management is often conflated with leadership. However, effective operational managers also have to show qualities of leadership and some strategic managers may not be that good at aspects of leadership.

In the longer term, effective operational management can occur only within a well-defined strategy for a rehabilitation service. Strategy sets out a clear remit for the service and ensures that there are systems in place that can support efficient and effective operational and clinical practices.

This relationship may appear straightforward. However, the influences of political factors (both internal and external to the organisation), changes in policy and funding, and, increasingly, the introduction of competition into long-term care mean that strategy itself has to be constantly evolving. One key management skill is 'horizon scanning' – keeping on the lookout for emerging threats and opportunities.

Operational management considerations are particularly pertinent in rehabilitation psychiatry, given the complex nature of the patients under such a service and the numerous interfaces necessary to deliver comprehensive care. There is a need for rehabilitation services to embrace a whole-system approach, incorporating rehabilitation in-patient provision, community rehabilitation team support, a range of non-statutory supported accommodation in the community and an effective reviewing process for the monitoring of patients in out-of-area placements. Leaders of statutory rehabilitation services need to engage effectively with local third-sector organisations, which may involve joining management committees or boards of charities.

Teamworking

Leaders and managers of mental health services inevitably work within multidisciplinary teams (Jenkinson et al, 2013). Teamworking implies that individuals come together in a common enterprise. In the clinical setting, the task involves meeting the needs of patients and carers (Holloway & Chorlton, 2007). Clinical leadership encourages the team to find solutions to the particular problems that a patient presents. Maintaining the morale of the team, providing a positive role model and inspiring hope among team members are vital to the good running of a clinical team.

There are also important tasks that team managers or leaders must undertake. These include: recruiting and managing staff (which may well involve engaging in disciplinary processes); managing budgets; ensuring service quality and providing assurance information to the wider organisation; dealing with complaints and serious untoward incidents; and escalating concerns upwards within the organisation. Clinical leaders and managers need to be able to work effectively within their organisation since they are the representatives of the service to the wider organisation. This requires good communication skills and the ability to influence others.

Successful multidisciplinary working requires the senior practitioner to be competent, available, responsive to the concerns of colleagues, and able to listen to others and work effectively within the broader organisation. Senior practitioners who are rude, inconsistent, unwilling to take responsibility, fail to acknowledge and learn from mistakes, and are ignored or disliked by senior management are likely to fail in their role.

Significant service change and development will require project management, which involves a group of people coming together in a team to achieve a specific time-limited goal. Effective project management requires planning, leadership, teamwork and specific skills that relate to the project at hand.

Managing the 'rehabilitation pathway'

The 'care pathway' is a dominant theme in the contemporary organisation and funding of healthcare. Ideally, a care pathway will describe in detail the steps that are to be undertaken to achieve a particular healthcare goal (e.g. treat a fractured neck of femur) and benchmark the care that a particular patient receives against the template, with the aim of reducing variance and improving outcome (Evans-Lacko *et al*, 2010). Care pathways are being introduced with great confidence and vigour into mental health services in the UK (NHS Confederation, 2011*a*), as is the pathway-related funding mechanism 'payment by results' (Department of Health Payment by Results Team, 2012). That there is in fact very little evidence supporting the utility of care pathways in mental health (Centre for Reviews and Dissemination, 2011) has had no impact on policy.

The central tenet of the care pathway is that there is a predictable process that can be followed and benchmarked, with the pathway incorporating best practice as set out in evidence-based guidelines. Patients under the care of a rehabilitation service will tend to have exhausted traditional evidence-based guidelines, such as the schizophrenia guideline produced by the National Collaborating Centre for Mental Health (2010). These anyway have very little to say about the person suffering from chronic, severe disability. These patients have differing rates of recovery, which in some cases will mean that several years of intervention and support are required before patients can move on. At times, people go the wrong way down the pathway – requiring, for a period at least, a higher level of care. The varying and unpredictable 'throughput' for patients in rehabilitation services fits badly with a managerial culture that is focused on short-term interventions.

Rehabilitation practitioners are aware of the many factors that influence the rate of 'recovery', which in managerial practice means a step-down to a more independent setting (for an in-patient, in a rehabilitation unit or under the care of a community rehabilitation team). These include patient-related factors: treatment resistance to psychotropic medication, the patient's level of engagement with mental health services, the presence of ongoing substance misuse and slow progress in regaining daily living skills. Risk management may affect the amount of community leave a patient has from a rehabilitation in-patient facility or the intensity of support required to manage an individual patient's risks while residing in the community. The service itself may prove a barrier to move-on if essential aspects of assessment and treatment are not available (accessing psychological assessment and treatment is a perennial problem). Availability of appropriate move-on accommodation and an appropriate package of support will also impact on the possibility of people moving through the care system.

Specialist rehabilitation services have to adopt a long-term and strategic perspective on an individual patient's care. They are inevitably a 'low-volume, high cost' service that will be highly vulnerable to 'management by exception', a technique that looks at outliers in performance measures. It is therefore essential that individual services describe their rationale and have clear goals in terms of quality of care and throughput, against which their performance can be measured. In the current jargon this will be a rehabilitation care pathway.

Services also need to give serious consideration to their governance arrangements, which might include sign-up to external accreditation, for example AIMS-Rehab (College Centre for Quality Improvement, 2011). AIMS-Rehab, which is discussed in some detail in Chapter 17, 'Rehabilitation in hospital settings', provides information about the structure and process of care within an in-patient rehabilitation service. In the longer term, there is likely to be a requirement for services to develop governance arrangements that allow for comparison of outcomes between services.

The rehabilitation care pathway needs to take account of many interfaces, for example between 'acute' and 'rehabilitation' services; between 'adult' and 'forensic' services; between 'hospital' and 'community'; and between NHS-funded care and care funded by local authorities, or through other mechanisms.

Managing referrals

Rehabilitation services will either lie within a larger organisation (in England currently a mental health trust) or be a niche provider operating in the independent sector. In either case, they need to pay attention to maintaining positive relationships with other mental health teams and non-statutory services such as supported housing. It is important that referrals are responded to efficiently. This can be difficult when a referred patient has an extensive history and may have previously been under the care of mental health services in another part of the country or abroad.

The prompt acceptance of a patient 'stuck' on an acute ward into a rehabilitation in-patient unit will facilitate the patient's needs being met in an appropriate environment and ease pressures on acute in-patient services, which, from a managerial perspective, is an important function of specialist rehabilitation services. However, patients accepted for a service will commonly be placed on a waiting-list. Any waiting-list needs to have a clear timescale.

When a rehabilitation unit does not accept a referral, the patient, carers and the referring team may experience frustration and irritation. In these circumstances, the rehabilitation assessment should be offering a second opinion on possible alternative medication, suggestions about referral to a defined specialist opinion (for example when the presenting problem is autism spectrum disorder or acquired brain damage) or the consideration of an alternative rehabilitation service that is more appropriate to the patient's needs.

Influencing investment in rehabilitation services

Rehabilitation services are by their nature expensive, treating relatively small numbers of people over relatively long periods. As a consequence, they are under constant threat from the need to make immediate financial savings (Holloway, 2005). In reality, appropriate investment in the provision of local rehabilitation services will save money and improve individual outcomes (Killaspy *et al*, 2009). The ability to influence decisions within provider organisations and the commissioning process will become increasingly important in sustaining investment in rehabilitation services and promoting necessary service developments.

Out-of-area placements

Rehabilitation practitioners will be aware of the potential human, social and economic costs when patients are put in an out-of-area placement, often at considerable distance from their area of origin. Reliance on such placements has in the past all too frequently led to NHS trusts, local authorities and commissioners making decisions about the need for rehabilitation and continuing-care services based on an incomplete understanding of local needs (and costs of care). In 2010, local mental health economies in England spent £690 million on out-of-area services – purchased by the local authority, trusts or health commissioners. That was more than 10% of the total mental health spending that year (£6.3 billion). The publication *In Sight and In Mind* (National Mental Health Development Unit, 2011) provided authoritative guidance for health, social care and housing commissioners in developing and commissioning services which are as close to the patient's home as possible. *In Sight and In Mind* set out 'seven steps' to reducing local reliance on out-of-service placements (see Box 22.1). These 'seven steps' are important in their own right but also give an insight into the contemporary language used by commissioners and managers of mental health services. Those working within services who seek to influence or lead change need to be able understand and speak this specialist language.

There have long been examples of local rehabilitation services taking the initiative in 'repatriating' patients in out-of-area placements – with resultant financial savings, improved quality of care and increased investment in local services (Killaspy *et al*, 2009). However, it is only recently that the issue has become a matter of policy. In England, the Quality, Innovation, Productivity and Prevention (QIPP) agenda for mental health set as a major target a

---

Box 22.1 Seven steps to reduce out-of-service placement

1 *Stock take* – map current provider services (where they are, the cost levels, how effective people find them); analyse the options to expand the range and choice of local services
2 *Needs assessment* – what are the needs of people in the commissioner's area? How do current services meet, or not meet, need?
3 *Establish a planning structure* – to address the issues and outcomes to be achieved in a systematic, managed way, involving local leaders (clinical and political), front-line clinicians and practitioners, managers, people using the services, their families and carers
4 *Agree and communicate a whole-system strategy* – agree goals and timescales in a coherent development plan
5 *Implementation* – beginning with identifying options to develop:
   • clinical and commissioning systems (assessment, review, etc.), leadership and care pathways
   • data and information systems
   • service choice for people using the services and their clinicians or other practitioners (i.e. through market development, including procurement frameworks)
   • integrated service specifications and outcome measures across care pathways to build resilience and a whole system focused on providing best outcomes for people (i.e. recovery and maximum independence from services)
6 *Set up and monitor key processes* – e.g. quality assurance, case management and feedback, contracting systems, involvement of people who use the services and their carers
7 *Review and refine* – establish annual reviews of strategy, processes and services

From National Mental Health Development Unit (2011)

---

reduction in the use of out-of-area placements, by better management and review of placements and judicious local service development (NHS Confederation, 2011*b*). (QIPP is an attempt to combine saving money with improving service quality in an era of severe financial restraint.) However, it was agreed that within QIPP for some specialist conditions it will be necessary to deliver services to larger populations than a local health economy (NHS Confederation, 2011*b*).

The problem with England

The challenge of influencing investment differs between jurisdictions. It is particularly complex in England. The Health and Social Act 2012 introduced major changes to the structure of the NHS which affect the funding and management of mental health services (Holloway, 2012). Since April 2013, NHS England (a recent rebranding of the NHS Commissioning Board that was set up under the Act) has presided over four regions, which oversee 27 local area teams (branded, for example 'NHS South London'). These in turn relate to 211 clinical commissioning groups (CCGs). The CCGs are the commissioners of mainstream services, including the bulk of mental health services. Some 'highly specialist services' are commissioned nationally; importantly, these include a number of mental health services, such as secure/forensic mental health services (Clinical Advisory Group for Prescribed Services, 2012). At the time of writing, low-secure care lies within the national commissioning element, since it is considered to be a forensic mental health service.

There are immediate and obvious issues of scale within this commissioning landscape. The average population served by a CCG is in the region of 250 000, which in an area of low morbidity may not be able to support the commissioning of a dedicated rehabilitation in-patient unit and specialist expertise to undertake the functions of a community rehabilitation team. More refined gradations in an individual's rehabilitation pathway may well include low-secure care and step-down rehabilitation in-patient services, which cannot be commissioned locally. Providers therefore have to develop relationships with a range of commissioners at all levels of commissioning or induce local commissioners to work within larger consortia that make epidemiological sense. This is well understood by the independent sector, where services are generally 'spot purchased' on an individual basis by commissioners.

Working with commissioners and senior management

In arguing their case, leaders of rehabilitation services have an important resource: *Guidance for Commissioners of Rehabilitation Services for People with Complex Mental Health Needs* (Joint Commissioning Panel for Mental Health, 2012). It combines evidence-based content with consensual expert opinion and offers ten key messages, which are relevant both to commissioners of services and to management within a provider organisation (see Box 22.2). *Guidance for Commissioners of Rehabilitation Services for People with Complex Mental Health Needs* made use of earlier work that put the case for rehabilitation and complex care services (Holloway, 2005) and provided a template for these services (Wolfson *et al*, 2009). Three publications set out vital components of a local rehabilitation service: in-patient facilities (Edwards *et al*, 2010), community rehabilitation teams (Kalidindi *et al*, 2012) and an out-of-area placements service (Edwards *et al*, 2012). Effective rehabilitation services also lie within a wider network of provision that addresses the needs people have for work and meaningful occupation and a place to live (Wolfson *et al*, 2009). All these components are described in detail in Part 3 of the present volume.

Senior managers within NHS trusts may well not have a good understanding of rehabilitation psychiatry: the tendency to look on rehabilitation services as an easy target for financial savings has already been noted. Leaders and managers of rehabilitation services, seeking

---

Box 22.2 Guidelines for commissioners on rehabilitation services: ten key messages

1 Mental health rehabilitation services specialise in working with people whose long-term and complex needs cannot be met by general adult mental health services
2 Rehabilitation services are not the same as recovery services
3 There is an ongoing need for specialist rehabilitation services
4 People using rehabilitation services are a 'low volume, high needs' group
5 People with complex mental health problems often require a large proportion of mental health resources
6 There is good evidence that rehabilitation services are effective
7 Investment in a local rehabilitation care pathway is cost-effective
8 Commissioning a 'good' rehabilitation service includes components of care provided by the NHS, and the independent and voluntary sector
9 Mental health rehabilitation services require multidisciplinary staffing
10 The quality and effectiveness of rehabilitation service provision can be assessed with simple indicators and standardised outcome tools

From Joint Commissioning Panel for Mental Health (2012)

---

to defend valued existing services that are under threat or to argue for investment in new services, need to be able to convey the messages summarised in Box 22.2, in ways that are understandable, compelling and relevant to local circumstances. Leaders also have to be clear when disinvestment is appropriate: their aim should not be to maintain the status quo but to produce the best possible outcomes for the population they are serving, within the resources that are available.

Mapping local need and demand

Guidance for Commissioners on Rehabilitation Services for People with Complex Mental Health Needs and the documents listed above offer general recommendations about what services are required. These must be tailored to specific local needs, which will vary according to many factors, including the size of the local health economy, demand for rehabilitation and complex care services (which relate to demographic factors) and subtle contextual issues (e.g. the history of local services, inter-agency relationships and the capacity of the third sector).

Developing a business case

In complex organisations, some tasks and decisions are delegated to local managers (e.g. booking agency staff to cover a vacant shift, hiring to a vacant post, arranging a repair to the team photocopier or fax). Other decisions will require higher authorisation (e.g. establishing a new post, buying or renting a new photocopier). At times of financial stringency, the level of decision-making for any spending becomes higher. Agreement to a service change or other activity that involves significant commitment of resources is likely to require approval through a formal process. Good corporate practice suggests that the process should be through the presentation and agreement of a 'business case'.

The 'business case' might be on a rather small scale. An example would be establishing a new psychology post that will ensure a rehabilitation service meets guidelines from the National Institute for Health and Care Excellence in relation to cognitive–behavioural therapy and family interventions for schizophrenia. It might be on an intermediate scale, for example the establishment of a dedicated community rehabilitation team to manage people placed in local residential care and out-of-area placements. Business cases can also be on a large scale, such as the development of a new local high-dependency rehabilitation unit, which would have substantial capital costs and, for the organisation, large continuing revenue costs.

The 'business case' needs to put forward a convincing argument as to why the proposal represents the best possible use of the organisation's resources. (This involves the economic concept of opportunity cost – what else could we do with the money we spend on a particular activity, or would there be a better way of spending the money?) The process tends to be evolutionary, moving from an outline business case, through to a fully worked up proposal and, if successful, on to a funded project, which would need firm management.

In the context of rehabilitation, the organisation will be a service provider, although funding for any particular activity will ultimately come from commissioners. The independent sector (which, in England, receives a large proportion of the spending on rehabilitation and continuing care) will make business decisions in accordance with the market, which includes 'spot purchases' of a bed on an established unit and direct commissioning of a designated service. Similar principles apply, rather less transparently, to NHS providers. Inevitably, for a new service to be developed, senior management will have to commit resources to refining the business case and negotiating with commissioners, but practitioners can play a key role in making the initial business case. Edwards *et al* (2010) describe how to do this in relation to in-patient rehabilitation facilities.

In an era of financial restraint, service change may require disinvestment in one service and reinvestment in another. This can involve transfer of activity from an NHS or independent hospital provider to third-sector providers (usually in the local area), to offer various types of supported accommodation, as part of the comprehensive rehabilitation pathway.

Conclusions

This chapter has provided a brief overview of the leadership and management skills that are required by senior rehabilitation practitioners and an introduction to some of the resources available to support practitioners in influencing the shape and scope of rehabilitation services. The ultimate aim must not be the survival of any particular service but rather the welfare of the patients and the community it is seeking to serve.

References

Brown N, Brittlebank A (2013) How to develop and assess the leadership skills of psychiatrists. *Advances in Psychiatric Treatment*, **19**: 30–7.

Centre for Reviews and Dissemination (2011) *Evidence Briefing on Integrated Care Pathways in Mental Health Services*. Centre for Review and Dissemination, University of York.

Clinical Advisory Group for Prescribed Services (2012) *Final Recommendations* (Gateway Reference 17981). At https://www.gov.uk/government/uploads/system/uploads/attachment_data/file/141590/Clinical-Advisory-Group-for-Prescribed-Services.pdf (accessed 7 April 2013).

College Centre for Quality Improvement (2011) *AIMS – Rehab*. Royal College of Psychiatrists. At http://www.rcpsych.ac.uk/quality/qualityandaccreditation/psychiatricwards/aims/whygetaccredited/aims-rehab.aspx (accessed 3 April 2012).

Department of Health Payment by Results Team (2012) *Mental Health Clustering Booklet* (V2.03, 2012/13, Gateway Reference 17250). Department of Health.

Edwards T, Meier R, Killaspy H (2010) *Making the Case for a Rehabilitation Facility: Helping Psychiatrists to Work Together with Commissioners and Senior Service Managers* (Faculty Report FR/RS/05). Royal College of Psychiatrists. At http://www.rcpsych.ac.uk/pdf/Making%20the%20case_forweb2.pdf (accessed 7 April 2013).

Edwards T, Wolfson P, Killaspy H (2012) *A Guide to Good Practice in the Use of Out-of-Area Placements* (Faculty Report FR/RS/06). Royal College of Psychiatrists. At http://www.rcpsych.ac.uk/pdf/FR%20RS%2006_for%20web.pdf (accessed 7 April 2013).

Evans-Lacko S, Jarrett M, McCrone P, et al (2010) Facilitators and barriers to implementing clinical care pathways. *BMC Health Services Research*, **10**: 182.

General Medical Council (2006) *Management for Doctors*. GMC. At http://www.gmc-uk.org/Management_for_doctors_2006.pdf_27493833.pdf (accessed 7 April 2013).

Holloway F (2005) *The Forgotten Need for Rehabilitation in Contemporary Mental Health Services* (Faculty Report FR/RS/04). Royal College of Psychiatrists. At http://www.rcpsych.ac.uk/pdf/FR_RS_04.pdf (accessed 7 April 2013).

Holloway F (2012) The Health and Social Care Act 2012: what will it mean for mental health services in England? *The Psychiatrist*, **36**: 401–3.

Holloway F, Chorlton C (2007) Multidisciplinary teams. In *Management for Psychiatrists, 3rd Edition* (eds D Bhugra, S Bell, A Burns): 99–115. RCPsych Publications.

Jenkinson J, Oakley C, Mason F (2013) Teamwork: the art of being a leader and a team player. *Advances in Psychiatric Treatment*, **19**: 221–8.

Joint Commissioning Panel for Mental Health (2012) *Guidance for Commissioners of Rehabilitation Services for People with Complex Mental Health Needs*. At http://www.rcpsych.ac.uk/pdf/rehab%20guide.pdf (accessed 6 April 2013).

Kalidindi S, Killaspy H, Edwards T (2012) *Community Psychosis Services: The Role of Community Mental Health Rehabilitation Teams* (Faculty Report FR/RS/07). At http://www.rcpsych.ac.uk/pdf/FR%20RS%2007_for%20web_rev.pdf (accessed 7 April 2013).

Killaspy H, Rambarran D, Harden C, et al (2009) A comparison of service users placed out of their area and local rehabilitation services. *Journal of Mental Health*, **18**: 111–20.

Kotter JP (1990) *Force for Change. How Leadership Differs from Management*. Free Press.

Marshall S (2007) Leadership. In *Management for Psychiatrists* (eds D Bhugra D, S Bell, A Burns): 189–204. Royal College of Psychiatrists.

National Collaborating Centre for Mental Health (2010) *Schizophrenia. The NICE Guideline on Core Interventions in the Treatment and Management of Schizophrenia in Adults in Primary and Secondary Care*. British Psychological Society.

National Mental Health Development Unit (2011) *In Sight and In Mind: A Toolkit to Reduce the Use of Out of Area Mental Health Services*. NMHDU. At http://www.rcpsych.ac.uk/pdf/insightandinmind.pdf (accessed 6 April 2013).

NHS Confederation (2011a) *Efficiency in Mental Health Services. Supporting Improvements in the Acute Care Pathway* (Briefing, Issue 214). NHS Confederation.

NHS Confederation (2011b) *QIPP and Mental Health. Reducing the Use of Out of Area Services* (Briefing, Issue 220). NHS Confederation.

NHS Institute for Innovation and Improvement & Academy of Medical Royal Colleges (2010) *Medical Leadership Competency Framework: Enhancing Engagement in Medical Leadership* (3rd edn). NHS Institute for Innovation and Improvement.

Wolfson P, Holloway F, Killaspy H (2009) *Enabling Recovery for People with Complex Mental Health Needs: A Template for Rehabilitation Services* (Faculty Report FR/RS/01). Royal College of Psychiatrists. At http://www.rcpsych.ac.uk/pdf/fr_rs_1_forwebsite.pdf (accessed 7 April 2013).

Part 4

Special topics in psychiatric rehabilitation

CHAPTER 23

Special topics in psychiatric rehabilitation: overview

Frank Holloway, Sridevi Kalidindi, Helen Killaspy and Glenn Roberts

Up to this point this book has provided a review of the concepts surrounding rehabilitation and recovery in mental health services (in Part 1, 'Setting the scene'), described a range of therapeutic approaches that are important in rehabilitation practice (in Part 2, 'Treatment approaches') and set out the core components of an effective and comprehensive rehabilitation service (in Part 3, 'Key elements of a rehabilitation service').

All the contributors to Parts 1, 2 and 3 work in the UK, the majority as practitioners working in the National Health Service (NHS) or in academic positions. It is likely that any further edition of this or a future book with similar aspirations would include significantly more contributions from people working in independent and voluntary sector organisations and people with lived experience of severe mental illness.

Rightly, the focus of the book has been on people living with a diagnosis of major mental disorder – schizophrenia, schizoaffective disorder and bipolar disorder – since these diagnoses are by far the commonest among people in contact with specialist psychiatric rehabilitation services. However, an increasing minority of service users have other diagnoses, either as the primary problem or as a comorbidity. Chapter 12, 'Working with coexisting substance misuse', is new to this edition. Substance misuse is a common problem for rehabilitation services and their client group, and the topic's omission from the first edition has been rectified. Chapter 11, 'Working with challenging behaviour', draws on clinical experience of work in secure settings with people with borderline personality disorder.

Editors inevitably have to make decisions about what goes into a book but equally determine what is left out, either deliberately or by default. Our first edition included a brief chapter on the social context of mental illness, which discussed social factors implicated in the causation of schizophrenia, notably the experience of migration, and the social consequences of severe mental illness, including stigma and impaired self-image. Subsequent research has focused on other forms of psychosocial stress as possible causative factors for psychosis (Morgan *et al*, 2008; van Winkel *et al*, 2008), with, as noted in Chapter 5, 'Understanding madness', great interest in childhood trauma as a risk factor for schizophrenia in later life (Bebbington *et al*, 2011). Tackling the social consequences of psychosis at an individual level is a priority for rehabilitation services, although there are broader issues of discrimination and social exclusion that require a much larger-scale response (see Chapter 3, 'Rehabilitation as a values-led practice', and Thornicroft *et al*, 2010).

The content of any book reflects the interests and expertise of the editors and authors. Some may regret that this edition no longer has specific chapters on psychodynamic considerations in rehabilitation and gender-sensitive services (although our new chapter on 'Creative therapies and creativity', Chapter 13, is underpinned by psychodynamic thinking and both issues are discussed at length in the context of the assessment and management of challenging behaviour in Chapter 11). As editors, we did not feel it necessary to devote specific attention to issues of diversity, be it in terms of ethnicity, religious affiliation or sexual orientation, reflecting the fact that respect for diversity is firmly within the mainstream of practice (even being enshrined within the 'respect' principle that underpins the English and Welsh Mental Health Act).

One topic that is barely mentioned in the text is spirituality. Recovery narratives often emphasise the importance of specific religious belief and a more generalised spirituality (Davidson, 2003). There is much to be gained by supporting people to link in with their faith community, if that is their choice. NHS services have direct access to multi-faith chaplaincy, which is an important resource.

An issue that perhaps receives less attention than it deserves is that of intimate relationships and sexual expression, which are issues of deep concern to many service users. It is only relatively recently that psychiatrists have begun taking an interest in the sexual side-effects of psychotropic medication and these are still rarely enquired about during medication reviews. Inappropriate sexual expression, up to and including sexual offending, is a 'challenging behaviour' that can lead to a lengthy in-patient stay and will require specific therapeutic attention. Some patients are either on occasion or continually vulnerable to sexual exploitation and relationships may become the focus of 'adult safeguarding' concerns. Others are in stable and fulfilling relationships and may simply need advice on contraception and sexual health. The US literature advocates social skills training using a behavioural paradigm as a method of improving social networks, making friends and developing more intimate relationships (Liberman, 2008).

It is increasingly common in the era of deinstitutionalisation for people living with severe mental illness to be parents, a welcome sign of social inclusion. The parental role can be a source of fulfilment and purpose. Its enforced loss through separation or adoption can be a source of enormous sadness. Where a patient is involved in parenting this needs to be incorporated into the care plan. As Fadden notes in Chapter 10, 'Family interventions', services seem to have particular difficulties in addressing the needs of children living in families with a parent who is mentally ill. Children may find themselves in an age-inappropriate caring role.

Neither edition of *Enabling Recovery* has included specific discussion of the needs of elderly people with long-standing and disabling mental illness. As old-age mental health services are becoming increasingly dementia-only services, this brings new challenges to adult mental health and rehabilitation providers who need to be aware of physical comorbidities and the implications of ageing on psychopharmacology and the possibility of the onset of age-related cognitive impairment. Older people may have specific support needs for either domiciliary or residential care and mental health services need to be able to work effectively with the person and care providers.

One further important topic that has not been given a specific chapter is the philosophical and ethical aspects of rehabilitation practice. As we noted in the Preface, working in rehabilitation continually throws up ethical dilemmas. Throughout the book, authors have emphasised the importance of facilitating agency and autonomy: these are complex concepts that might be fruitfully explored at greater length than available to individual chapter authors. The process of assessment is strongly laden with value judgements (what to assess, whose perspective takes primacy and how the norms against which assessment is carried out are to be derived). Our authors have taken ethical stances but nowhere have we been able to reflect in depth on the differing approaches that are taken.

Part 4, 'Special topics in psychiatric rehabilitation', has allowed us to discuss in detail some aspects of contemporary practice that do not fit neatly within the first three parts of the book. Six topics are included, compared with three in the first edition.

The six topics

Rehabilitation and acquired brain injury – Chapter 24

Ryan Aguiar and Czarina Kirk remind us that acquired brain injury (ABI) is common and results in a great deal of disability. They provide a detailed description of the various forms of brain injury and emphasise the importance of post-traumatic amnesia as an indication of the severity of the injury. ABI often has psychiatric sequelae, including, albeit uncommonly, psychosis, which, importantly, may be a symptom of epilepsy. ABI is a risk factor for the subsequent development of schizophrenia. The authors provide guidelines for the treatment of post-ABI psychosis and a valuable description of the neuropsychological consequences of ABI, which are strikingly similar to the deficits encountered in some people with severe psychosis, as are the disabilities that may be experienced. Their discussion of rehabilitation in ABI provides valuable lessons to practitioners of psychiatric rehabilitation: a visit to a neuro-rehabilitation unit demonstrates the level of attention to detail required to support people who have developed severe behavioural problems following ABI.

Autism spectrum disorder – Chapter 25

It is still not uncommon to encounter in rehabilitation and continuing-care settings people with autism spectrum disorders who were, in the past, wrongly diagnosed as suffering from schizophrenia. Autism spectrum disorder and other neurodevelopmental disorders such as attention-deficit hyperactivity disorder are important comorbidities of schizophrenia, complicate the clinical picture and may well require treatment in their own right. Dene Robertson and Daniel de la Harpe Golden provide an up-to-date account of the autism spectrum, a term they adopt to avoid the negative associations of the word 'disorder'. They describe the familiar diagnostic triad of abnormalities in communication, abnormalities in social interaction and a restricted and repetitive repertoire of interests and activities. Less familiar are the difficulties that people with autism spectrum disorder have in sensory processing and insomnia, which are often linked, and 'stimming'. Typical 'stims' are hand-flapping, pacing and self-hitting. An important practical implication of a diagnosis of autism, be it primary or comorbid, is the need to provide an autism-friendly environment that is tailored to the person's specific profile of difficulties. Consistency of approach, appropriate levels of stimulation and clear communication are likely to be key.

Risk management in rehabilitation practice – Chapter 26

The first edition of *Enabling Recovery* included a chapter on forensic rehabilitation, at that time a relatively novel concept. The boundary between forensic and rehabilitation mental health services has become increasingly blurred and practitioners in both need a good understanding of the other discipline. In this edition we have substituted a chapter on risk management in rehabilitation practice. Shawn Mitchell addresses very difficult issues. There is a current obsession with risk assessment in mental healthcare, understandable given the fact that people in contact with mental health services commonly present risks to themselves or others. However, risk assessment has very serious limitations, largely for statistical reasons. The really bad outcomes in psychiatry – suicide, serious violence and homicide – are uncommon and at an individual level are essentially unpredictable, unless something really bad has happened before (by definition impossible for completed suicide). The limitations of risk assessment do not preclude effective risk management, however. Mitchell advocates involving service users in discussions about the risks they present to themselves and others under the rubric of the helpfully neutral rubric of 'safety management'. He also underlines the importance of developing a 'formulation … that explains the underlying mechanism for a risk behaviour and will propose hypotheses regarding action to facilitate change'.

Rehabilitation: an international perspective – Chapter 27

This new chapter seeks to provide an overview of the concepts and practices of psychiatric rehabilitation as understood internationally. There are significant consistencies – the core concepts underlying both rehabilitation and recovery as set out in this book are generally accepted, as is the relevance of 'values-based practice'. The evidence base is international and it is possible to identify best practice in longer-term mental healthcare (Taylor *et al*, 2009) despite subtle differences between what is accepted as best practice in different countries. All high-income countries, with the interesting exception of Japan, went through a process of deinstitutionalisation in the 50 years to 2000, albeit at different times and different rates. In Europe and the USA this process has involved 'trans-institutionalisation', with people moving from hospital-based care to other supported environments, which have the potential to adopt equally inappropriate practices as the traditional mental hospital.

Hospital bed numbers and highly supported community placements vary markedly between countries for reasons that we simply do not understand. The chapter ends with an account of an ambitious attempt to introduce patient-oriented recovery services (PROS) into the state-funded mental health services in New York. PROS has parallels with initiatives in other countries, for example the ImROC (Implementing Recovery through Organisational Change) programme in England (http://www.imroc.org).

Psychosocial rehabilitation across culture: the experience in low- and middle-income countries – Chapter 28

There is a very important dimension to our understanding of rehabilitation within mental health services that has not been discussed. R. Thara and Dinesh Bhugra write about the experience of implementing psychosocial rehabilitation in low- and middle-income countries (LMICs). They emphasise the importance of cultural values in shaping 'individual patients' idioms of distress, explanatory models and world view'. Traditionally, knowledge flowed from wealthy advanced countries to LMICs but, particularly in an era of austerity, lessons in developing effective psychosocial rehabilitation services at the lowest possible cost are universally relevant. Thara and Bhugra identify three core psychosocial interventions – medication management training, cognitive retraining (which needs to be tailored to a particular culture) and vocational rehabilitation. A significant volume of research into psychosocial interventions has now been carried out within LMICs, particularly in South East Asia and China.

Practical experience in LMICs suggests that effective and valued psychosocial interventions are most likely to be delivered by non-governmental organisations (NGOs), which are separate from the state. NGOs will have a variety of sources of funding and can be highly effective but, without careful support, do have significant limitations in terms of sustainability, accountability and geographical coverage – provision of all kinds tends to be located within the largest towns and cities, leaving other populations grossly underserved.

Expanding the evidence-base – Chapter 29

For our final special topic, Helen Killaspy and Steffan Davies look first at how we understand mental health services – 'imperfectly' is the answer! Although we know a fair amount about the elements of community-based services (see Chapter 8, 'Rehabilitation at the coalface'), in-patient care appears to have avoided good-quality evaluation both nationally and internationally. This is a striking finding, which deserves appropriate investment to clarify how scarce monies can best be protected for training, research and direct service provision. As one would expect, research requires a degree of standardisation that is at odds with the personalised approach to care that this book emphasises. In reality, a systematic approach to assessment and treatment is now expected by government, service commissioners, service users and their carers. Killaspy and Davies describe a potentially valuable assessment tool that looks at the quality of rehabilitation services, the QuIRC (http://www.quirc.eu) and an ongoing study (Rehabilitation Effectiveness for Activities for Life – REAL). There is an urgent need to develop similar tools to the QuIRC for other aspects of provision and to agree the outcome measures that are sensitive to both personal and clinical perspectives and should be used in daily practice.

References

Bebbington P, Jonas S, Kuipers E, *et al* (2011) Childhood sexual abuse and psychosis: data from a cross-sectional national psychiatric survey in England. *British Journal of Psychiatry*, **199**: 29–37.

Davidson L (2003) *Living Outside Mental Illness. Qualitative Studies of Recovery in Schizophrenia*. New York University Press.

Liberman RP (2008) *Recovery from Disability. Manual of Psychiatric Rehabilitation*. American Psychiatric Publishing.

Morgan C, McKenzie K, Fearon P (2008) *Society and Psychosis*. Cambridge University Press.

Taylor TL, Killaspy H, Wright C, *et al* (2009) A systematic review of the international published literature relating to quality of institutional care for people with longer term mental health problems. *BMC Psychiatry*, **9**: 55.

Thornicroft G, Rose D, Mehta N (2010) Discrimination against people with mental illness: what can psychiatrists do? *Advances in Psychiatric Treatment*, **16**: 53–9.

van Winkel R, Stefanis N, Myin-Germeys I (2008) Psychosocial stress and psychosis. A review of the neurobiological mechanisms and the evidence for gene–stress interaction. *Schizophrenia Bulletin*, **34**: 1095–105.

CHAPTER 24

Rehabilitation and acquired brain injury

Ryan Aguiar and Czarina Kirk

Introduction: the relevance of acquired brain injury

Acquired brain injury (ABI) is relevant to psychiatric rehabilitation for two reasons. First, it is common. Recent figures from the UK show that approximately 700 000 people attend accident and emergency departments each year with a head injury. Of those, approximately 90% will have minor injuries without life-altering consequences; however, the remainder will have a diagnosis of moderate or severe brain injury with life-altering effects. It is estimated that there are 500 000 individuals aged 16–74 in the UK who are living with long-term disabilities as a consequence of ABI (see the website of the brain injury association Headway UK, http://www.headway.org.uk). Second, ABI is associated with extensive psychiatric comorbidity. It is well recognised that the psychological sequelae of brain injury are more

---

Box 24.1 ICD-10 psychiatric diagnoses associated with acquired brain injury

- Organic hallucinosis
- Organic catatonic disorder
- Organic delusional (including schizophrenia-like) disorder
- Organic mood (affective) disorder
- Organic dissociative disorder
- Organic labile disorder
- Organic personality disorder
- Mild cognitive disorder
- Post-encephalitic syndrome
- Post-concussional syndrome
- Other organic personality and behaviour disorders due to brain damage
- Delirium, not induced by alcohol and other psychoactive substances
- Dementia in other specified diseases classified elsewhere
- Unspecified dementia
- Organic amnesic syndrome, not induced by alcohol and other psychoactive substances
- Other specified mental disorders due to brain damage

---

common than physical sequelae. Box 24.1 lists the psychiatric diagnoses associated with ABI. Depression, anxiety and sleep disorders are common; there is an increase in suicide rates compared with the general population; substance misuse and dependence rates are higher and there is also a significant link between schizophrenia and brain injury. Even if no formal psychiatric diagnosis can be made, there will often be cognitive, emotional and behavioural changes or changes in personality that result in breakdown of relationships and loss of occupation.

Understanding ABI

The most common classifications of ABI are:

- primary or secondary – referring to the cause of the injury
- according to severity (Table 24.1) – mild, moderate, severe, based on the duration of any post-traumatic amnesia
- according to location – focal parenchymal or diffuse axonal
- open or closed.

Primary acquired is the most common form of brain injury and includes: traumatic brain injury; vascular events – ischaemia or haemorrhage; space-occupying lesions – such as tumours or cysts; encephalitis or other infection; toxic injury – including from drugs or alcohol; and hypoxic or anoxic injury.

Causes of secondary acquired brain injury include hypoxia, haemorrhage (either from direct pressure effects or toxins from haemosiderin), infection (encephalitis, meningitis), post-traumatic epilepsy and the effects of medication. To illustrate a secondary brain injury, consider the case of a young man who presents unconscious with a focal, closed head injury. He had been drinking. A scan reveals a large subdural haematoma that requires evacuation. There is also some subarachnoid haemorrhage. While being anaesthetised he aspirates and his oxygen saturations drop. The haemorrhage is extensive. There is an increase in pressure and the neurosurgeon inserts an intracranial drain. The man is slow to recover and requires ventilation. His temperature spikes. He has a chest infection. His drain is infected and needs to be removed. When he is roused he is agitated and combative. He is sedated with benzodiazepines and neuroleptics. He has a seizure which lasts an hour, during which he becomes hypoxic. In this case, the subdural haematoma and the subarachnoid haemorrhage are primary injuries arising from the trauma to the head. The hypoxia, the secondary brain injury, arises much later.

Post-traumatic amnesia

Post-traumatic amnesia (PTA) is defined as the time from the moment of injury to the resumption of normal continuous memory (Russell & Smith, 1961). Duration of PTA is commonly used as a prognostic indicator

Table 24.1 Classification of the severity of traumatic brain injury

Severity	Score on the Glasgow Coma Scale	Post-traumatic amnesia
Mild	13–15	<1 hour
Moderate	9–12	30 minutes–24 hours
Severe	3–8	>1 day

in conjunction with score on the Glasgow Coma Scale (GCS; Teasdale & Jennett, 1974). Table 24.1 shows the classification of the severity of brain injury based on PTA and GCS score: severe brain injury is associated with a PTA of greater than 1 day.

While in PTA an individual is at the most vulnerable with regard to seizure threshold, sensitivity to medications and cognitions. It can be a period of confusion, agitation and occasionally aggression. The management of this agitation can be extremely difficult, owing to the vulnerability and sensitivity of the brain to medications and also the high-stimulus environment in which the individual finds himself or herself. A liaison psychiatrist will be very familiar with calls to neurosurgical wards with requests for advice on managing aggression and the use of the Mental Health Act or the Mental Capacity Act. There is evidence to link aggression during PTA with later development of psychosis.

The principles of managing PTA are similar to those employed when managing any confusional state, namely get the environment sorted (low stimulus, side room if possible, well lit, orientation aids for person and place), get the body sorted (infections, diabetes, withdrawal states, pain, seizures) and finally think about medication (Inouye, 1999). As for legal issues in England and Wales the Mental Capacity Act 2005 has clarified the 'best interests' procedures and should be used until the individual regains capacity.

Mental illness and ABI

As mentioned in the Introduction, psychological sequelae occur more frequently than physical sequelae after brain injury (Jennett et al, 1981). Of course, the relationship is complex and mental illness can be either comorbid or a consequence of the injury itself. The most common mental disorders seen in the general population are also those commonly encountered in a brain-injured population, although the symptoms can be different.

Depression

Depression (moderate to severe) occurs in approximately one-third of individuals who have had a brain injury (Jorge et al, 2004). It may present as an increase in irritability, sleep disturbance or cognitive impairment out of keeping with that expected for the severity of injury and so there is a potential for a delay in diagnosis and treatment. Even mild or moderate depressive disorders can have a significant impact on functioning and can delay recovery. At the other end of the spectrum, major depression is also common and there is an associated increased risk of suicide. It has been estimated from studies that the risk of suicide following severe brain injury is four times greater than found in the general population (Silver *et al*, 2001; Teasdale & Engberg, 2001). A brain injury can also lead to hugely significant changes in an individual's role and social functioning. Relationship breakdowns, unemployment and poverty are all commonly seen, as is substance misuse, all of which can be precipitating and maintaining factors for mental illness.

Anxiety disorders

This is often comorbid with depression and prolongs its course. Anxiety can present differently from in the general population and avoidance or social phobia can be misdiagnosed as poor motivation and obsessive–compulsive disorder as poor memory. Post-traumatic stress disorder is possibly more prevalent in those with mild traumatic brain injury, who present with flashbacks to the intensive care unit and false memories based on media coverage and their own reconstructions of the traumatic incident (Creamer *et al*, 2005; Bombardier *et al*, 2006). Panic disorder (9.2%), generalised anxiety disorder (9.1%) and obsessive–compulsive disorder (6.4%) are all more common in people with ABI (van Reekum *et al*, 2000).

Psychosis

Psychosis is relatively uncommon following a brain injury. However, it is more common in than in the general population: following a brain injury the risk of developing a schizophreniform psychosis over a 15- to 20-year period is between 0.7% and 9.8% (McAllister & Ferrell, 2002). Psychotic symptoms can occur immediately (delirium), early (confabulations, misidentification, lack of insight) or may be latent. Psychosis may also be a symptom of epilepsy.

There is an interesting and significant relationship between schizophrenia and ABI (David & Prince, 2005; Molloy *et al*, 2011). An individual with a diagnosis of schizophrenia is twice as likely to have had a brain injury. Early-onset psychosis is more common among people who had a brain injury in their childhood.

Is it possible to predict who will be at most risk of developing psychosis following an ABI? Location of injury certainly has a role to play. Several areas of the brain have been cited as being involved, including the orbitofrontal region, the dorsolateral prefrontal cortex, the temporal lobe and the hippocampus (which is particularly sensitive to anoxic damage and shows reduced volume following brain injury). There are conflicting reports about the hemispheric relationship. Taken together, the data suggest the involvement of several neural pathways and connectivity rather than a single region.

The type and severity of injury are not reliable predictors of post-ABI psychosis. Neither is gender or age. There is a correlation with underlying neurological/neurodevelopmental disorders such as intellectual disability, epilepsy and attention-deficit hyperactivity disorder (ADHD) and also an increasing risk with subsequent brain injuries. The best predictor of all, however, is genetic risk of schizophrenia. An individual with a brain injury *and* with a first-degree relative with schizophrenia has a 24% chance of developing psychosis following ABI (Molloy *et al*, 2011).

In common with depression and anxiety, psychosis can present differently following ABI. Formal thought disorder is uncommon, although dysphasias may be present, which can make this difficult to assess. Delusions may present as misinterpretation of normal stimuli and may relate to a neurological deficit (e.g. delusion that a paralysed limb is a under external control). Misidentification delusions (e.g. Capgras and Fregoli delusions) are more commonly seen. Paranoid and persecutory delusions, in particular nihilistic delusions, are also relatively common. Grandiose delusions, however, are no more common but can be confused with the disinhibition of frontal-lobe impairment. Hallucinations may be atypical, for example olfactory or somatic, and, like delusions, may relate to an impairment of neurological function.

None of the above symptoms is unique to psychosis following ABI and there are certainly many other common features between ABI psychosis and schizophrenia, including: changes in gait and speech; affect disturbance; and cognitive deficits (e.g. slowed speed of information processing, impaired recent memory, impairment of attention and concentration, in particular tracking and filtering of information, impaired executive function and apathy).

Individuals with ABI and psychosis or with comorbid schizophrenia have poorer outcomes than those with schizophrenia alone and it is important therefore to identify and diagnose these individuals and then offer appropriate treatment. They may present as having poor compliance or disengage from treatment, show frequent outbursts and low tolerance of frustration (impairment of executive function), and they may deteriorate despite treatment (brain vulnerability to medication) or be treatment resistant.

Treatment of psychosis after ABI

Careful attention should be paid to the management of psychosis in ABI. After establishing the diagnosis it is important to begin with improving and adapting the individual's environment to compensate for any cognitive deficits. This will include low-stimulus areas, opportunity for rest and a structured and predictable routine. This helps to minimise stress. It is also vital that comorbid conditions, such as diabetes (hypo- and hyperglycaemia can alter cognitive function), sleep cycle disturbance, withdrawal states or dependency, pain (headache is common and can persist for several years following ABI) and epilepsy, are adequately treated.

When antipsychotic medication is being considered for people who have psychosis and a known ABI the following approach is recommended:

1 Start with low doses (half the normal starting dose) and increase in smaller increments at a slower pace. This will give the clinician a better indication of the relationship between dose and side-effects and will allow the brain the opportunity to adapt to the new medications. The dose of depot medication is more difficult to control and therefore depot preparations should be used with caution.

2 Following a brain injury an individual is more susceptible to extra-pyramidal side-effects and therefore it is preferable to use atypical antipsychotics.

3 Try to avoid benzodiazepines as they impair cognitive functioning.

4 Be mindful of the seizure threshold, which may be reduced following brain injury. This is particularly in reference to clozapine. Prescribing an anti-eplileptic (e.g. sodium valproate or lamotrigine) can be considered.

5 Treat psychosis not aggression. This seems straightforward; however, often antipsychotics are prescribed for agitation or aggression rather than psychotic symptoms and there is little evidence to support their benefit when used in this way.

The use of medication in the management of agitation and aggression following ABI

The pharmacological management of challenging behaviours in the context of brain injury should be considered only as an adjunctive therapy. Fleminger *et al* (2006), in a Cochrane review which examined evidence of efficacy of medication for management of aggressive behaviours, concluded that:

> This review found no firm evidence that drug management of agitation and aggression in adults with acquired brain injury is effective. There was weak evidence, based on a few small randomized controlled trials, that beta blockers can improve aggression after acquired brain injury, but very large doses were used which would have been likely to produce significant adverse effects. For other classes of medication, reasonable size randomized controlled trials have not been published. Based on the lack of evidence, the review comes to no conclusion on the effectiveness of drugs. There is reasonable anecdotal evidence, for example in published cases series, that antipsychotics, mood stabilizers and antidepressants may be effective in the management of this situation.

With such a lack of evidence it will often therefore be left to individual clinical teams and service users to explore symptomatic management. For example, if mood swings predominate, consider prescribing a mood stabiliser; if sexual disinhibition is problematic to the extent that it causes harm, then anti-libidinal medications could be considered.

In these situations it is advisable to follow the advice for prescribing in psychosis as outlined above. It is also important to avoid polypharmacy and to be mindful of 'cognitive dulling', which may impair engagement in neurobehavioural therapies, a particular potential problem with benzodiazepines. Long-acting medications should be used with caution (particularly if there is a history of epilepsy).

Neuropsychological aspects of ABI

Behaviour, according to Lezak (1995), can be conceptualised in terms of three functional systems: *cognition*, the information processing and handling aspect of behaviour; *emotionality*, which pertains to feelings and motivation; and *executive functions*, which relates to how behaviour is expressed. To this we would add a fourth dimension, *awareness*. Damage to the brain from an ABI can be in the form of damage to a specific functional system from a circumscribed brain lesion (e.g. a visual agnosia caused by a posterior artery stroke) or it may involve multiple systems, as in the case of a high-velocity traumatic brain injury. Some neuropsychological impairments are more readily apparent and can be easily attributed to the effects of the brain injury. Disorders of memory, language and visual perceptual deficits are typical of this class of impairments. Others, however, are less apparent. Typical among this latter group of impairments are disorders of executive function, visuoconstructional disorders and disorders of praxis. These are inferred from the behaviour the person presents with. A comprehensive neuropsychological assessment is useful to identify cognitive, emotional and behavioural problems following an ABI.

Cognitive system

The assessment of cognitive impairment is set against the context of the person's general ability expressed in a neuropsychological assessment by an index such as the Full Scale IQ Index of the Wechsler Scales (Wechsler, 2008). This IQ measure must be interpreted with caution. A low Full Scale IQ score in the context of an ABI does not automatically indicate that the person is intellectually compromised or that his or her 'intelligence' has declined. Impairment of learning memory is probably the most ubiquitous of the cognitive impairments reported by individuals with an ABI (Tate *et al*, 1991; Levin, 1995). This can take the form of an amnesic syndrome such as that seen in Korsakoff's syndrome or following aneurysm of the anterior communicating artery (DeLuca & Diamond, 1995), where there is a profound impairment in the acquisition of new information. Alternatively, a specific process associated with memory such as encoding, consolidation and retrieval may be impaired following a traumatic brain injury (Curtiss *et al*, 2001; Vanderploeg *et al*, 2001). Impairments in attention, concentration, speed of information processing and working memory are common and may well account for the observed deficits in learning and memory. Classic aphasia syndromes are less likely than are problems with communication attributable to cognitive impairments. The person's communication may be tangential, fragmented, poorly thought out and devoid of content. Pragmatic aspects of speech may be affected, giving rise to difficulties in interpersonal communication (Sohlberg & Mateer, 2001; Dahlberg *et al*, 2006).

Executive function

Executive dysfunction is perhaps the most ubiquitous impairment encountered within rehabilitation settings. A range of cognitive (planning, problem-solving, abstract reasoning and cognitive flexibility) and behavioural (inhibition, self-monitoring, response initiation) skills make up the gamut of executive functions. It is inevitable that impairment to such a system will result in social disability, impaired day-to-day function and consequent stress within the family. Individuals with impaired executive function are less likely to engage in rehabilitation and are more likely to have lasting social disability. It is important that these individuals undergo thorough neuropsychological rehabilitation to address their social impairment and problems with their day-to-day function associated with their executive impairment.

Emotional functioning

Disturbance in this area can range from relatively straightforward adjustment reactions, such as a mood disorder, to more troubling disturbances of affect regulation characterised by restlessness, irritability and aggression. The person may present with the opposite extreme, with failure to initiate and maintain goal-directed activity. These disorders of diminished motivation arising out of damage to the medial frontal lobe and the cingulate cortex may present as abulia or in its milder form as apathy (Marin & Chakravorty, 2005). Impairment to this functional system is also linked to poor engagement in rehabilitation. These individuals are at great risk of neglect and will need considerable support and supervision in the community.

Awareness

There are two issues to bear in mind when considering a person's awareness of impairments, or lack of it, following a brain injury: one is that it falls on a spectrum and is not an absolute or a dichotic phenomenon, and the other is that it is dynamic.

Flashman & McAllister (2002) provide a useful framework for understanding the different dimensions that make up lack of awareness. First, does the person have knowledge of the difficulty or deficit he or she presents with? This can range from people having a vague feeling that they are not as able as before, to vehemently denying that there is any problem. The second dimension encompasses the emotional response of the person to the deficit or difficulty and this can range from complete indifference to intense distress. The third dimension is how the person construes the impact of the deficit on day-to-day function. Thus people who acknowledge their memory problem might yet not agree to use a diary as they do not recognise the need for it. Building on the above, at a functional level, does the person have *emergent awareness* that she or he is having difficulty while performing a task, for example cannot recall the list of items during a shopping trip? Does she or he show *anticipatory awareness* (Crosson *et al*, 1989) and predict that she or he will have difficulty remembering the shopping and therefore need to make a list? Lack of awareness is a major hurdle to engagement in rehabilitation and leads to poor outcomes. It often brings the person into conflict with others because she or he fails to appreciate the impact of particular behaviours on others. Impaired awareness can make the person vulnerable to neglect and abuse from others. It is imperative that the clinician seeks the view of family and others involved in the brain-injured person's care as the person's subjective account of problems can be unreliable.

ABI and disability

To fully appreciate the effects of a brain injury one has to consider the impact that it has on the person's everyday life. The World Health Organization (WHO) provides a useful model for conceptualising and understanding such disability. The WHO framework (World Health Organization, 1980) discusses disability in the context of three dimensions: *impairment to physical structures or mental functions* (e.g. damage to the frontal lobe or impairment of executive function); *disability* arising out of the impairment (e.g. impaired executive function in the form of poor planning and problem-solving); and *handicap*, defined as the disadvantage the person faces (e.g. being unable to continue in previous employment). In its most recent iteration – the *International Classification of Functioning, Disability and Health* (ICF; World Health Organization, 2001, 2002 – disability is seen as arising out of an interaction between the person's health condition and the context in which the person lives. Table 24.2 provides a description of the main components of the WHO model.

Disability is conceptualised at various levels. At the basic level is the impairment to body function or structure (e.g. damage to the frontal lobe). At the next level up it considers the activities the person is unable to undertake or needs support to undertake. The next level is the life situations the person is unable to participate in (e.g. not being able to attend a day centre because of challenging behaviour). The ICF also identifies contextual factors, which include the person's social and physical environment as well as premorbid and current personality traits that come to play a part in the disability. Fig. 24.1 illustrates the WHO model of

Table 24.2 Components of the International Classification of Functioning, Disability and Health model (World Health Organization, 2002)

No.	WHO model term	Description
1	Body function and structures	Refers to the physiological functions of the human body such as heart rate, vision, brain function etc. It also includes psychological and cognitive functions
2	Impairments (to body functions and structures)	Reflect a significant deviation or loss of functioning arising as a result of damage to a body function or structure
3	Activity and activity limitations	Difficulties that an individual may have in executing or undertaking specific activities
4	Participation and participation restriction	Problems the person may experience in becoming involved or engaging in life situations such as accessing a community, accessing therapeutic groups, accessing work or even accessing a particular part of the physical environment
5	Contextual factors	Environmental and personal factors. Environmental factors make up the physical and social attitudinal environment in which the person lives and the personal factors refer to current and premorbid characteristics of the individual

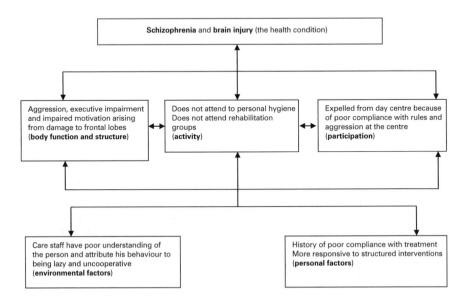

Fig. 24.1 The WHO model of disability

disability as it applies to a person who is living with schizophrenia and an acquired brain injury.

Various factors act in unison to confer disability. The chances of a successful outcome will be greatly reduced if the rehabilitation effort is wholly directed at the individual and, for example, the training needs of the residential and the day centre staff who are involved in the care of a service user are neglected. The WHO disability model provides the clinical team with a very useful tool with which to develop a comprehensive formulation of the person's problems. The framework also lends itself to developing targeted interventions to minimise disability. An effective intervention for a case of behavioural difficulties following traumatic brain injury would be to provide staff with training on the cognitive, emotional and behavioural consequences of brain injury. The rehabilitation care plan should aim to maximise the individual's overall functioning.

Rehabilitation following ABI

At the outset, clinical teams need to be clear and agree on what it is that needs to be rehabilitated. Wilson (2004: p. 345) suggests that 'it is not an impairment identified by a theoretically informed model, but a real life problem identified by the patient and his or her family' that should be the focus of rehabilitation. Rehabilitation should seek to reduce disability and enable the person to participate in life activities that are meaningful and enriching. Rehabilitation should enable the person to reintegrate into the community and function as independently as possible. Full independence may not always be possible, depending on the nature and extent of the person's disability, but should still remain an aspiration. Thus, a starting point for the clinical team would be the disability the person presents with. The WHO's ICF model provides a valuable framework for the formulation of a care plan that targets intervention at all levels that are pertinent to the needs of the individual and the context in which she or he lives.

Ideally, rehabilitation following an ABI should be provided within specialist ABI rehabilitation services. However, because of the limited availability of specialist brain injury or neurorehabilitation services, many individuals with ABI (especially those with minimal physical impairments) will be treated within mainstream mental health services. It is hard to justify the absence of such access to specialist brain injury rehabilitation in the face of evidence of its cost-effectiveness in reducing disability and enhancing psychosocial and other outcomes (Turner-Stokes, 2008). The nature and type of rehabilitation following an ABI falls on a spectrum and is determined by a number of variables, including injury severity, nature and extent of physical impairments, and the severity of cognitive, emotional and behavioural impairment.

Rehabilitation is usually delivered by a multidisciplinary team but the composition of the team will depend on the setting in which the rehabilitation is delivered. For example, most ABI rehabilitation teams in district hospitals have limited input available from a clinical neuropsychologist or a psychiatrist. They are more likely to have intensive input from a consultant in rehabilitation medicine, an occupational therapist and a physiotherapist, with the emphasis being on improving physical function. Rehabilitation of cognitive, emotional and behavioural impairments and associated social disability follows post-acute care with greater input from clinical neuropsychologists and neuropsychiatrists.

Cognitive rehabilitation

At its heart, cognitive rehabilitation involves the application of techniques and procedures and implementing support that will serve to reduce the person's disability and enable him or her to live as safe, productive and independent a life as possible (Sohlberg & Mateer, 2001). Cognitive rehabilitation is a collaborative endeavour between the person with brain injury and the rehabilitation team. It begins with a comprehensive assessment of cognitive function, emotional response and behaviour regulation. Careful attention is paid to the person's environment and the context the person will be returning to after rehabilitation so that appropriate interventions can be targeted to maximise reintegration to the environment. The intervention strategies used in cognitive rehabilitation can vary widely and will depend on the needs of the person and the resources available to meet that need. Box 24.2 provides a brief list of intervention strategies commonly employed under a cognitive rehabilitation paradigm.

Box 24.2 Intervention strategies used within cognitive and neurobehavioural rehabilitation

- Modification or management of the environment to minimise cognitive demand on the individual
- Use of compensatory strategies or external aids (e.g. planners, diaries, electronic systems)
- Restorative techniques (e.g. memory practice drills, teaching task-specific skills)
- Specialised instruction (e.g. errorless learning, expanded rehearsal, direct instruction)
- Metacognitive strategies (e.g. self-instructional training)
- Awareness-enhancement interventions
- Education of service user, family and carers
- Cognitive–behavioural and other psychological interventions to address emotional and adjustment issues
- Vocational and occupational rehabilitation

Neurobehavioural rehabilitation

Neurobehavioural rehabilitation shares much in common with cognitive rehabilitation but has as its main focus an emphasis on severe challenging behaviours and social handicap. Neurobehavioural rehabilitation is generally provided within specialist residential brain injury rehabilitation centres. It is provided after post-acute care as a clearer picture emerges about the persisting personality and behavioural problems the person is left with. Neurobehavioral rehabilitation is an intervention paradigm informed by cognitive and behavioural psychology theories and is aimed at the acquisition of functional and social skills. It provides an optimal learning environment to promote recovery of functional skills, cognitive abilities and social behaviours that have been disrupted by the brain injury (Wood & Worthington, 2001).

While some of the techniques of neurobehavioural rehabilitation can be applied in less specialist settings, a specialist environment allows for these techniques to be applied systematically, consistently and intensively. This promotes most effective learning and generalisation of that learning to the person's community. Neurobehavioural rehabilitation should be offered to those presenting with severe behavioural problems (e.g. sexual disinhibition, anger and violence), those with disorders of drive and motivation, and those with significant executive impairment affecting their social judgement and puts them at risk in their community (Wood & Worthington, 2001). Box 24.3 provides a brief list of commonly used strategies in neurobehavioural rehabilitation.

Box 24.3 Intervention strategies used in neurobehavioural rehabilitation

- Assessment and identification of target behaviours
- Awareness enhancement and education
- Learning and reinforcement principles (DRO, DRI, positive and negative reinforcements, TOOTS)
- Verbal mediation and direct instruction
- Regular feedback (incidental, structured and programmed)
- Habit formation through repeated practice and procedural learning
- Executive skills training
- Cognitive–behavioural and other psychological interventions to address emotional and adjustment issues
- Vocational and occupational rehabilitation

DRO is 'Differential Reinforcement of Other' behaviour, providing positive reinforcement for behaviour other than the identified target behaviour
DRI is 'Differential Reinforcement of Incompatible' behaviour, providing positive reinforcement for behaviour that is incompatible with target behaviour (e.g. polite request instead of shouting)
TOOTS is 'Time Out On The Spot'.

Resources

- The United Kingdom Acquired Brain Injury Forum (UKABIF). Brain injury forum providing information and supports and knowledge of brain injury. http://www.ukabif.org.uk
- Headway. The national brain injury charity provides information and support. http://www.headway.org.uk
- The Neurological Alliance. An organisation that aims to drive forward the implementation of the National Service Framework for long-term conditions, to increase understanding of neurological conditions and to speak for the neurological community with an authoritative voice. http://www.neural.org
- World Federation for NeuroRehabilitation (WFNR). This is a multidisciplinary organisation open to any professional with an interest in neurological rehabilitation. It exists to act as a forum of communication between those with an interest in the subject. The WFNR produces a twice-yearly newsletter (*WFNR Update*). http://www.wfnr.co.uk

References

Bombardier CH, Fann JR, Temkin N, *et al* (2006) Posttraumatic stress disorder symptoms during the first six months after traumatic brain injury. *Journal of Neuropsychiatry and Clinical Neuroscience*, **18**: 501–8.

Creamer M, O'Donnell ML, Pattison P (2005) Amnesia, traumatic brain injury, and posttraumatic stress disorder: a methodological inquiry. *Behaviour Research and Therapy*, **43**: 1383–9.

Crosson C, Barco PP, Velozo C, *et al* (1989) Awareness and compensation in postacute head injury rehabilitation. *Journal of Head Trauma Rehabilitation*, **4**: 46–54.

Curtiss G, Vanderploeg RD, Spencer J, *et al* (2001) Patterns of verbal learning and memory in traumatic brain injury. *Journal of the International Neuropsychological Society*, **7**: 574–85.

Dahlberg C, Hawley L, Morey C, *et al* (2006) Social communication skills in persons with post-acute traumatic brain injury: three perspectives. *Brain Injury*, **20**: 425–35.

David AS, Prince M (2005) Psychosis following head injury: a critical review. *Journal of Neurology, Neurosurgery and Psychiatry*, **76** (suppl 1): i53–i60.

DeLuca J, Diamond BJ (1995) Aneurysm of the anterior communicating artery: a review of the neuroanatomical and neuropsychological sequelae. *Journal of Clinical and Experimental Neuropsychology*, **17**: 100–21.

Flashman LA, McAllister TW (2002) Lack of awareness and its impact in traumatic brain injury. *NeuroRehabilitation*, **17**: 285–96.

Fleminger S, Greenwood RRJ, Oliver DL (2006) Pharmacological management for agitation and aggression in people with acquired brain injury. *Cochrane Database of Systematic Reviews*, **4**: CD003299.

Inouye SK, Bogardus ST, Charpentier PA, *et al* (1999) A multicomponent intervention to prevent delirium in hospitalised older patients. *New England Journal of Medicine*, **340**: 669–76.

Jennett B, Snoek J, Bond MR, *et al* (1981) Disability after severe head injury: observations on the use of the Glasgow Outcome Scale. *Journal of Neurology, Neurosurgery, and Psychiatry*, **44**: 285–93.

Jorge RE, Robinson RG, Moser D, *et al* (2004) Major depression following traumatic brain injury. *Archives of General Psychiatry*, **61**: 42–50.

Levin HS (1995) Neurobehavioral outcome of closed head injury: implications for clinical trials. *Journal of Neurotrauma*, **12**: 601–10.

Lezak MD (1995) *Neuropsychological Assessment (3rd edn)*. Oxford University Press.

Marin RS, Chakravorty S (2005) Disorders of diminished motivation. In *Textbook of Traumatic Brain Injury* (eds JM Silver, TW McAllister, SC Yudofsky): 337–52. American Psychiatric Publishing.

McAllister TW, Ferrell RB (2002) Evaluation and treatment of psychosis after traumatic brain injury. *NeuroRehabilitation*, **17**: 357–68.

Molloy C, Conroy M, Cotter DR, *et al* (2011) Is traumatic brain injury a risk factor for schizophrenia? A meta-analysis of case-controlled population-based studies. *Schizophrenia Bulletin*, **37**: 1104–10.

Russell WR, Smith, A (1961) Post-traumatic amnesia in closed head injury. *Archives of Neurology*, **5**: 4–7.

Silver JM, Kramer R, Greenwald S, *et al* (2001) The association between head injuries and psychiatric disorders: findings from the New Haven NIMH Epidemiologic Catchment Area Study. *Brain Injury*, **15**: 935–45.

Sohlberg MM, Mateer CA (2001) *Cognitive Rehabilitation: An Integrative Neuropsychological Approach*. Guilford Press.

Tate RL, Fenelon B, Manning ML, *et al* (1991) Patterns of neuropsychological impairment after sever blunt head injury. *Journal of Nervous and Mental Disease*, **179**: 117–26.

Teasdale G, Jennett B (1974) Assessment of coma and impaired consciousness: A practical scale. *Lancet*, **13**: 81–4.

Teasdale TW, Engberg AW (2001) Suicide after traumatic brain injury: a population study. *Journal of Neurology, Neurosurgery and Psychiatry*, **71**: 436–40.

Turner-Stokes L (2008) Evidence for the effectiveness of multi-disciplinary rehabilitation following acquired brain injury: a synthesis of two systematic approaches. *Journal of Rehabilitation Medicine*, **40**: 691–701.

Vanderploeg RD, Crowell TA, Curtiss G (2001) Verbal learning and memory deficits in traumatic brain injury: encoding, consolidation and retrieval. *Journal of Clinical and Experimental Neuropsychology*, **23**: 185–95.

van Reekum R, Cohen T, Wong J (2000) Can traumatic brain injury cause psychiatric disorders? *Journal of Neuropsychiatry and Clinical Neurosciences*, **12**: 316–27.

Wechsler D (2008) *Wechsler Adult Intelligence Scale, 4th edition (WAIS-IV)*. The Psychological Corporation.

Wilson BA (2004) Theoretical approaches to cognitive rehabilitation. In *Clinical Neuropsychology: A Practical Guide to Assessment and Management for Clinicians* (eds LH Goldstein, JE McNeil): 345–66. Wiley.

Wood RLI, Worthington AD (2001) Neurobehavioural rehabilitation: a conceptual paradigm. In *Neurobehavioural Disability and Social Handicap Following Traumatic Brain Injury* (eds RLI Wood, T McMillan): 108–31. Psychology Press.

World Health Organization (1980) *The International Classification of Impairments, Disabilities and Handicaps: A Manual of Classification Relating to the Consequence of Disease*. WHO.

World Health Organization (2001) *The International Classification of Functioning, Disability and Health (ICF)*. WHO.

World Health Organization (2002) *Towards a Common Language of Functioning, Disability and Health. ICF*. WHO.

CHAPTER 25

Autism spectrum disorder

Dene Robertson and Daniel De La Harpe Golden

Introduction

The autism spectrum disorders comprise a set of neurodevelopmental disorders characterised by a 'diagnostic triad' of impairments that manifest in early life and continue into adulthood:

- qualitative abnormalities in communication
- qualitative abnormalities in reciprocal social interaction
- a restricted and repetitive repertoire of interests and activities.

Many more or less synonymous terms are used to describe membership of the autism spectrum; this is a product of both medical legacy and of the sociopolitical agenda of people with autism and their supporters. Such terms include autism spectrum disorder, pervasive developmental disorder and autism spectrum condition. To avoid the negative connotations of the word 'disorder', this chapter refers to 'autism' unless a specific diagnosis within the spectrum is considered. People with autism will often emphasise the notion of 'difference' as opposed to 'disorder' by contrasting their way of being to that of people without autism, whom they may refer to as 'neurotypical'.

Approximately 1% of adults meet diagnostic criteria for autism of one form or another, and approximately half of these also have an intellectual disability. While some people with autism are highly dependent, many others live independently but at significant social disadvantage (Brugha *et al*, 2011). Recognition that people with autism include an invisible minority with significant unmet health and social needs has led to an increasing amount of clinical guidance and legislative attention over recent years. The National Institute for Health and Care Excellence (NICE, 2011, 2012) has published guidelines on autism in children and young people and on autism in adults. The Autism Act 2009 was the first disability-specific legislation to be passed in the UK and resulted in a national strategy for adults with autism in England and Wales, 'Fulfilling and Rewarding Lives'. This sets out recommendations for central government, local authorities, health services and other social agencies.

This chapter presents the clinical features of autism, describes its assessment and treatment, and considers recovery in autism.

The clinical features of autism

The autism spectrum

The current version of the World Health Organization's *International Classification of Diseases* (ICD-10) identifies a number of diagnoses within its chapter on pervasive developmental disorders (F84), of which the most familiar to adult mental health practitioners is Asperger syndrome (World Health Organization, 1992). The latest version of the *Diagnostic and Statistical Manual* of the American Psychiatric Association (DSM-5) replaces subtypes with a single category of 'autism spectrum disorder', which is somewhat more diagnostically restrictive than F84, and adds a new diagnosis of 'social communication disorder', for which the criterion 'restricted interests' does not apply (American Psychiatric Association, 2013).

The symptoms of autism

The features of autism typically become apparent before the age of 3 and include impairments in social interaction, problems with communication and restricted, repetitive and stereotyped patterns of behaviour, interests and activities. Childhood autism is associated with language delay, while Asperger syndrome is not associated with delay in language or general cognitive development. The behavioural manifestations are pervasive, appearing across all activities of life, and are lifelong, although they may ameliorate with increasing age.

Impairments in social interactions arise from inadequate appreciation of socio-emotional cues. There may be difficulties with 'theory of mind' (the ability to infer the mental states of others), leading to empathic difficulties. Low levels of socio-emotional reciprocity may first become apparent when eye contact is poor or when use of gestures to call attention is limited. In adults these difficulties typically lead to a severe restriction in social repertoire, occupational ability, romantic relationships and family life.

Communication difficulties are most noticeable with regard to language skills, which may be affected to widely differing degrees. Difficulties range from profound lack of language to problems with the 'pragmatics' of language, evidenced by unusual cadence[1] during speech or poor turn-taking during conversation. There may be an inability to use language creatively, with exchanges relying on concrete interpretations of other people's speech.

---

1. The deficit here is in 'prosody' – with people having an inability to appropriately modulate the pitch, loudness, intonation and rhythm of word formation. It is both subtle and obvious to a native language speaker.

The third domain, in which there is a restriction of interests and activities, may present as a consuming interest in a particular field, often to the exclusion of socially relevant material. For example, someone who has a disproportionate interest in cars may know the minutiae of the models and manufacture dates, and may talk about these to the exclusion of almost everything else. Repetitive movements, mannerisms, rigid adherence to timetables and ritualistic ways of performing tasks are also included within this diagnostic domain.

The difficulties associated with autism frequently lead to loneliness and social isolation, resulting in considerable distress. Some people reject interaction, even when deficits in reciprocal social interaction are mild. People with autism who have a high level of general intelligence may appear superficially to function well, but employment, education and home life may be profoundly affected. Carers may find the rigid adherence to sameness and routine difficult or impossible to manage.

The assessment of autism

Autism commonly presents in childhood because of parental or teacher concern or in the context of an assessment by intellectual disability services (also known as learning disability in UK health services). However, it presents increasingly in adulthood, typically when people request assessment because they have always felt 'different', or when it comes to attention as a result of comorbidity.

Psychiatric services in the UK may maintain that they are 'not commissioned' for autism, which can lead to a missed diagnosis of autism and of treatable mental health comorbidity. However, as a result of increasing recognition of the problem and the current policy and legislative framework, many local services are developing autism teams that include diagnostic expertise, thresholds for onward referral in subtle or complex cases and assessment of wider social needs.

Diagnosis

Autism is diagnosed on the basis of conformity to a behavioural phenotype, since there are currently no definitive biological markers for the condition. A number of screening tools are available for use with adults, including the Autism Spectrum Quotient (AQ; Baron-Cohen *et al*, 2001). The AQ is a free 50-item self-report forced-choice questionnaire that is available online; a 10-item version (the AQ-10; Allison *et al*, 2012) is recommended (NICE, 2012) for use by general practitioners with adults of normal intelligence. By definition, any screening tool gives rise to some 'false negative' results, so failure to achieve a 'threshold score' should not lead to refusal of assessment where clinical suspicion of subtle difficulties remains.

With adults, a focused developmental history, if at all possible including an account from the person's childhood carers, should then be taken. This is likely, when taken together with the patient's report of current difficulties, to provide sufficient information to include or exclude an autism diagnosis in a straightforward case. The Royal College of Psychiatrists has produced a *Diagnostic Interview Guide for the Assessment of Adults with Autistic Spectrum Disorder* (Berney *et al*, 2011). This allows clinicians not trained in formal diagnostic tools to collate the necessary information.

In subtle or complex cases, specific diagnostic tools should be employed. These require specialist training and will be used by tertiary services. The Autism-Diagnostic Interview – Revised (ADI-R; Lord *et al*, 1994), which includes a developmental interview conducted with a parent or carer, is often used. Where there is no childhood informant, the Autism Diagnostic Observation Schedule (ADOS; Lord *et al*, 2000) includes a suite of tasks that enables rating of current behaviours such as idiosyncratic use of words, unusual eye contact, reciprocal social communication, and mannerisms. Another instrument is the Diagnostic Interview for Social and Communication Disorders (DISCO; Wing *et al*, 2002).

Identifying needs

Once a diagnosis has been made, the heterogeneous nature of autism means that careful consideration should be given to individual needs (NICE, 2012). As well as the needs commonly encountered within rehabilitation practice, specific issues emerge in autism: sensory hypo- and hypersensitivities, assessment for hereditable genetic disorder and intellectual ability and neuropsychological functioning.

Recovery in autism

As with any condition with early childhood onset and persistent course, the notion of recovery from autism does not sit easily with a model that frames recovery as remission from disease. A person with autism has never been otherwise, and the core features of autism are stubbornly difficult to ameliorate with traditional treatment, whether biological or psychological. Moreover, the language of recovery is often explicitly rejected by people with autism, who may prefer to be seen as different rather than disordered. It is perhaps not surprising that some people with autism say that society should adapt to the needs of a person with autism, rather than expecting adaptation by a person without the resources to change.

Current understanding of recovery emphasises that a person is one part of a system, and that adjustments are likely to be required throughout that system in order for people to obtain higher levels of fulfilment. From this perspective, recovery can be seen as a process that includes instilling: hope and empowerment; personal growth and safety; satisfaction with social networks and active inclusion; and symptom control. This model lends itself well to autism because it aspires to attainable goals even when autism is uncomplicated by psychiatric comorbidity. Throughout the focus is on maximising quality of life.

The instillation of hope

The process of diagnosis itself may provide great relief to a person who has previously felt alone, different and misunderstood. The provision of psychoeducation is an important step: learning that your social difficulties are appreciated, have a neurobiological underpinning, that you have relative strengths, and that many others are in a similar position often improves self-esteem and encourages an optimistic stance. A diagnosis frequently helps a person reframe a difficult past, supports current identity, and provides a realistic framework for making choices about the future. Those with a new diagnosis may be empowered by understanding that the diagnosis is theirs, and that they can either use it or not in different circumstances, depending upon its likely utility. Some people may wish to embrace the diagnosis by joining the 'Aspie' community.

To build hope, it is important that the patient succeeds quickly in reaching attainable goals. 'Quick wins' – such as getting in touch with an autism-related support group online or enlisting appropriate support at work – may kick-start the recovery journey and promote motivation. It is often helpful to frame the existence of related mental health problems such as social anxiety as amenable to independent treatment, and to observe that treatment for this has become possible as a result of the process of acquiring a diagnosis of autism.

It is important to offer hope without offering false hope. The promotion of pseudoscientific ideas is rife within the autism field, and there is a large range of treatments and interventions that are lacking in evidence. Box 25.1 identifies treatments that should *not* be used for core symptoms of autism (NICE, 2012), although some may be useful when targeting comorbidities or associated features.

Box 25.1 Treatments that should *not* be used for the core symptoms of autism

- Anticonvulsants
- Chelation therapy
- Exclusion diets (such as gluten- or casein-free and ketogenic diets)
- Mineral and vitamin supplements
- Oxytocin
- Secretin
- Hyperbaric oxygen therapy
- Nootropics (such as cholinesterase inhibitors)
- Testosterone regulation therapies
- Antipsychotic medication
- Antidepressant medication

Adapted from National Institute for Health and Clinical Excellence (2012)

Personal growth and empowerment

Personal growth includes attaining maximum possible independence and developing enjoyable social networks. Milestones such as graduating from school or university, getting a job, developing intimate relationships and caring for children are representative of these. However, people with autism are more likely to rely on others for support in living, employment and relationships (Howlin *et al*, 2004; Eaves & Ho, 2008). It is therefore important to assess current function in these areas in order to enlist appropriate support in helping people to achieve their goals.

Education

Autism is associated with lower rates of completion at every educational level. The intellectual and social demands of primary, secondary and tertiary education differ widely, so it is important to regularly reassess the nature and quantity of support (Schall *et al*, 2012), especially at times of transition. Transition services are currently rudimentary, although there has been a considerable increase in autism awareness within tertiary education, and support services are in some cases excellent. Even for those of high intelligence, transition from school to further education or employment may be difficult owing to cognitive rigidity, a failure to understand social structures, and social anxiety. Ultimately, only a minority go on to live and work independently (Howlin *et al*, 2004).

Independence and employment

At one end of the spectrum of disability due to autism, a person may need assistance with all aspects of daily living, including physical healthcare, feeding and toileting. At the other, support needs may be minimal or non-existent and some people with autism function to a very high level in 'expert environments', where a consuming interest in a particular field which is in line with the demands of the job or career may be advantageous. People with autism may benefit from support in developing work-related skills and accessing employment (see the National Autistic Society, http://www.autism.org.uk, as a resource for such skills). Sheltered and supported employment programmes may be useful (Taylor *et al*, 2012).

Satisfaction with social networks

Friendships

Both children and adults with autism typically value friendship. Help in accessing structured leisure activities such as interest clubs or sporting activities (whether autism-specific or not) may support social engagement without leading to intolerable levels of anxiety. The growth of online communities has provided an opportunity for social communication without the need for potentially stressful face-to-face contact. Moreover, online

'Aspie' communities such as Wrong Planet (http://www.wrongplanet.net) and Autism Network International (http://www.autreat.com) normalise autism and promote coping and community inclusion.

Romantic and sexual relationships

Difficulties with sexual expression may give rise to particular distress. The sexual desires and fantasies of people with autism are similar to those of the general population, though rates of non-heterosexual identities, including asexuality, may be higher (Hellemans *et al*, 2007). Primary social skills deficits interact together with decreased peer-to-peer learning about sexual and romantic relationships, and may lead to naïve and inappropriate attempts to initiate romantic relationships. Therefore, sexual and relationship education are important in helping a person with autism stay safe and acquire the tools to develop fulfilled romantic attachments (Stokes *et al*, 2007). Group educational sessions and individual work can be useful (Stokes & Kaur, 2005).

Many people with autism are vulnerable to exploitation, whether sexual or other, by the more socially adept (Barnhill, 2007). Where exploitation is identified the UK has procedures surrounding safeguarding adults that must be followed (see http://www.scie.org.uk/adults/safeguarding).

Professional relationships

The vast majority of the ordinary needs of most people with autism are met by non-specialist services (e.g. a trip to the general practitioner). When mental health services are involved in care and support, it is important to identify a consistent contact person. Lists of local and national services suitable for people with autism together with contact details are invaluable and should be freely available in medical, social, police and educational environments. The National Autistic Society (http://www.autism.org.uk) provides people with autism and their families with valuable support in relation to the diagnosis of autism, benefits, accommodation, advocacy and social groups.

Reducing symptom interference

Autism is highly variable in presentation and is often associated with related problems and psychiatric comorbidities, so characterising individual needs is important. Roughly half of people with autism have an intellectual disability, which is associated with a worse outcome in adulthood. While it is predominantly comorbidity that leads to people with autism using rehabilitation services, much can be offered for the relief of core symptoms.

Core symptoms

No pharmacological treatment has been shown to be beneficial in treating the core symptoms of autism (NICE, 2012). In the absence of comorbidity, psychosocial interventions are first line in maximising quality of life.

Social skills deficits can be addressed through group or individually tailored social learning programmes, and it is common clinical experience that some adults with autism have already consciously learned social skills that are learned intuitively by those without autism. Behaviourally based training programmes are usually overseen by a clinical psychologist or nurse behaviour therapist and can be tailored to any ability or intellectual level. Target behaviours to be reinforced or extinguished may be related to shopping, laundry, personal hygiene and others, as well as social skills (Barnhill, 2007). Skills training programmes should be structured, predictable and consistent and should take account of neuropsychological strengths and weaknesses.

Cognitive–behavioural therapy delivered by practitioners experienced in working with autism, whether group or individual, may provide an appropriate framework for exploring the impact and meaning of a diagnosis of autism and provide strategies for improving self-esteem and confidence (NICE, 2012). Adults with autism who have limited social contacts may benefit from organised and structured leisure activities. These may be arranged by people with autism, charitable organisations or statutory services.

Sensory processing difficulties

Sensory difficulties are reported to occur in over 90% of people with autism and are considered core features in the DSM-5 diagnostic criteria for autism spectrum disorder:

> Hyper- or hyporeactivity to sensory input or unusual interests in sensory aspects of the environment (e.g. apparent indifference to pain/temperature, adverse response to specific sounds or textures, excessive smelling or touching of objects, visual fascination with lights or movement).

Sensory processing difficulties affect stress and arousal levels, leading to difficulties with attention and with remaining calm; these in turn interfere with the ability to engage in day-to-day activities. Interventions include modifying the environment to match a person's sensory profile (Brown & Dunn, 2002), practising sensory integration through multisensory activities, or task practice to increase comfort with a task avoided owing to sensory problems (Suarez, 2012). A wide range of aids has been designed to assist with these (e.g. heavy blankets) as part of a 'sensory diet'. While a number of professional groups can perform assessments of sensory function, the 'best bet' referral is to an occupational therapist if the index of suspicion is high.

Sleep problems

Around 50–80% of people with autism have sleep problems. Insomnia with prolonged sleep latency, bedtime resistance and decreased sleep efficiency with frequent awakenings are common. The aetiology of sleep disturbance in autism is likely to be multifactorial, although probably includes a primary abnormality of melatonin production and the sleep–wake cycle (for a recent review, see Rossignol & Frye, 2014).

Common comorbid mental health problems may also lead to abnormalities of the quantity and quality of sleep. Sleep disturbance increases generic stress levels and irritability, and can worsen challenging behaviour and symptoms of comorbid psychiatric illness. Shifted sleep patterns, seen in people with marked social phobia, are not compatible with employment and opportunities for social interaction (Reynolds & Malow, 2011).

Managing sleep problems follows generic approaches to sleep hygiene, with additional attention to the bed covering, which should suit the person's individual sensory profile. In people with sleep phase and sleep initiation problems, melatonin may be helpful (Richdale & Schreck, 2009). Night-time administration of melatonin has been associated with better daytime behaviours.

Challenging behaviour

A 'challenging behaviour' is by definition culturally abnormal, of such intensity, frequency or duration that the physical safety of the person or others is placed in serious jeopardy, and is likely to limit or deny access to ordinary community facilities, social networks and employment. Heterogeneous definitions of challenging behaviour mean that its frequency among people with autism is uncertain. Although much more common in people with comorbid intellectual disability, challenging behaviour also occurs in high-functioning individuals with severe autism, particularly those with comorbid psychopathology (Matson & Nebel-Schwalm, 2007).

Common types of challenging behaviour include aggression, self-injurious behaviour, sexually inappropriate behaviour and pica (eating inappropriate substances). Sexually inappropriate behaviour can have very serious consequences for the individual, including lengthy disposal into a hospital setting for treatment.

'Stimming' is stereotypical behaviour, usually involving repetitive movement (though sometimes involving vocalisation) that is assumed to lead to self-soothing. It can be construed as a disproportionate extension of the foot-tapping or nail-biting engaged in by people without autism, and may be related to sensory dysfunction. Typical 'stims' include hand-flapping, pacing and self-hitting, and may or may not be sufficiently serious to constitute 'challenging behaviour'. They may occur in people with autism and normal intelligence as well as those with intellectual disability.

The assessment and management of challenging behaviour in people with autism follows the same principles as described in Chapter 11, 'Working with challenging behaviour'. It is important to establish what

---

Case example 25.1 Carl

Carl had lived in residential care since he was young. He had moderate intellectual disability, autism and a number of challenging behaviours. He communicated through picture exchange, although also used some spoken language. The staff at his residential care home were well versed in techniques to manage his challenging behaviour, which included head-banging and attempting to hit others. There was predictable worsening of his behaviour whenever there were changes of staff, but with careful preparation and planning these were minimised. A sheltered-employment organisation offered Carl a placement, but he reacted negatively to when he began to attend, with an acute and serious worsening of aggression. Despite support from the residential staff this did not ameliorate sufficiently to keep Carl and others safe. A careful risk–benefit analysis demonstrated that there was more to gain from a short course of antipsychotic medication to facilitate the transition and ensure a successful placement. The trial was successful. Carl now spends 3 days a week at the sheltered workplace and no longer takes antipsychotic medication.

---

aspects of the environment reinforce a problematic behaviour by an examination of its antecedents, the behaviour itself and its consequences (the 'ABC' approach). Analysis of the data leads to hypothesis formation and opportunities for environmental intervention. Specific interventions include differential reinforcement of alternative behaviours, social skills training and contingency programmes, including token economies. Where behavioural interventions fail, antipsychotic and antidepressant drugs may be considered (see case example 25.1). Both may be effective at reducing challenging behaviour (see NICE, 2012). However, off-licence drug treatment should be thought of as a therapeutic trial. It is easy to start a drug but much more difficult to withdraw it, so an active and continuous balancing of benefits and risks is necessary to avoid an unnecessary side-effect burden (Matson *et al*, 2011; NICE, 2012).

Intellectual disability

Intellectual disability occurs in roughly half of all people with autism. It is much more common in people with childhood autism than in those with Asperger syndrome (which is not associated with general cognitive delay), and the severity of symptoms of autism tends to increase as the degree of intellectual disability increases (Matson & Nebel-Schwalm, 2007). People with autism and intellectual disability have poorer adult outcomes than those with autism alone (Howlin *et al*, 2004) and, conversely, people with intellectual disability who have autism have poorer social skills (Smith & Matson, 2010) and more psychiatric comorbidity than those with intellectual disability alone (Matson & Shoemaker, 2009).

Speech and language difficulties

Communication difficulties are very frequent in people with autism. When problems cause distress or significant impairment, a referral to a speech and language therapist is essential. Motor problems (dyspraxia or apraxia) are also common. Some patients also have specific intellectual disability (dyslexia or dyscalculia). In adults, autism has also been associated with catatonia of uncertain aetiology (Billstedt *et al*, 2005).

Physical health problems

Autism is associated with a range of physical health problems, notably seizure disorders. The presentation of physical health problems in people with autism may be modified by social avoidance, sensory integration difficulties (e.g. insensitivity to pain or cold), communication difficulties and low general intelligence. Unidentified and untreated physical health problems may contribute to or be the sole cause of behavioural difficulties, so a systematic medical history and physical examination are mandatory in all patients with autism and challenging behaviour.

Comorbid mental illness

Patients with autism in contact with rehabilitation services will have a psychiatric comorbidity. Attention-deficit hyperactivity disorder (ADHD), depression, anxiety, obsessive–compulsive disorder, psychosis, self-injury, tic disorders and eating disorders (Gillberg & Billstedt, 2000; Hofvander *et al*, 2009) are all common. The ICD-10 diagnostic criteria for autism exclude the possibility of some comorbid diagnoses: autism 'trumps' the diagnosis of ADHD in a person with childhood autism, for instance. Slavish adherence to a hierarchical diagnostic approach may lead to a failure to identify helpful treatment (e.g. stimulants and psychotherapy for comorbid ADHD).

The presence of multiple comorbidity is clinically challenging and a pragmatic approach to intervention may be appropriate. For example, an antidepressant may simultaneously address anxiety, compulsions and anger outbursts, and cognitive–behavioural therapy may simultaneously address mood, anxiety and social skills deficits. When initial interventions do not lead to problem resolution, the acquisition of objective data may allow a series of hypotheses to be tested sequentially to determine the most effective intervention.

In general, biological treatments appropriate for people with autism do not differ from those used in people without autism, and recourse should be made to the relevant guidelines from the National Institute for Health and Care Excellence. People with early-onset neurodevelopmental disorders are particularly vulnerable to the side-effects of psychotropic medication (these might affect seizure threshold, for example), so doses should be increased slowly. Cognitive–behavioural therapy for people with autism usually requires modification to take account of the core features of autism and associated neuropsychological difficulties.

Anxiety disorders

The prevalence of comorbid anxiety disorder of one form or another probably exceeds 50%, although community prevalence studies are lacking. Many people with autism meet criteria for multiple anxiety disorders.

People with autism who are aware of their social difficulties routinely experience anxiety in expectation of negative social feedback, leading to avoidance of peers and contributing to undesired social isolation (White & Roberson-Nay, 2009). This may become extreme and lead to total avoidance. Interventions may include social skills training, cognitive–behavioural therapy (to challenge unhelpful beliefs and to improve motivation and self-esteem), support with finding non-threatening social environments with like-minded people, and graded exposure where motivation is sufficient.

Obsessive–compulsive disorder

According to current psychiatric nosology, stereotypical thoughts and behaviours due to autism are ego-syntonic and unresisted, but the obsessions and compulsions of classical obsessive–compulsive disorder (OCD) are ego-dystonic and resisted. However, long-standing repetitive behaviours due to OCD (especially of childhood onset) may lose these qualities, so there is a phenomenological overlap between repetitive behaviours in autism and some cases of OCD that may make differential diagnosis difficult or impossible. Moreover, people with autism may be unable to explain links between thoughts and behaviours as a result of difficulties with theory of mind and communication. It is therefore difficult to estimate the true prevalence of OCD in people with autism, although rates are probably around 20%. Typically, repetitive behaviours consistent with OCD in people with autism are more likely to involve imposing order, hoarding, touching, tapping, rubbing and self-mutilating, while OCD in people without autism is characteristically associated with cleaning, checking and counting (McDougle et al, 1995). Overall, selective serotonin reuptake inhibitors appear to be only moderately effective, and some trials do not show efficacy in reducing repetitive behaviours (King et al, 2009). Modified cognitive–behavioural therapy and behavioural interventions may be effective.

While some repetitive behaviour exhibited by people with autism is highly resistant to intervention (and may or may not be 'true' OCD), it is clear that 'classical' OCD is also more common in people with autism than in people without. There is no evidence that OCD of this type responds less well to standard treatment than in people without autism, and outcomes are in some cases excellent. Therefore, repetitive behaviours that lead to social interference should never be ascribed to autism alone without in-depth investigation (see case example 25.2).

385

Case example 25.2 Betty

Betty was diagnosed with autism before she was 5. Soon after starting school a diagnosis of inattentive subtype attention-deficit hyperactivity disorder was made and she started methylphenidate, which helped her to focus. Nevertheless, she was also dyslexic and so received a high level of support throughout school, but ultimately passed examinations in two subjects at age 16. At home, she involved her family in complicated rituals around washing and cooking, which took up considerable amounts of everybody's time. If they refused, Betty would assault her mother and refuse to eat. Betty was mugged at age 19 and started refusing to leave the house. By her mid-20s she was still living in the family home and had not been outside for 3 years. Her parents had not had a holiday for 6 years, and her father had missed his own father's funeral because Betty would not allow him to go. After an assessment by secondary care psychiatric services, Betty was admitted to a specialist unit for people with 'high functioning' autism. Betty was hypothesised to suffer from severe obsessive–compulsive disorder. Selective serotonin reuptake inhibitors did not help, although ultimately she responded to a combination of clomipramine 'augmented' by an antipsychotic. Betty received cognitive–behavioural therapy (CBT) for post-traumatic symptoms relating to her mugging and started to use the hospital grounds. CBT for her compulsions was initially unsuccessful because Betty did not think that her rituals were a problem, and she was unable to gain insight with motivational interviewing. A behavioural programme was devised in which Betty was rewarded for the time that she did not spend in ritualistic behaviour. An ever-increasing occupational therapy programme facilitated a daily routine which led to volunteer work in the community. Betty came to realise that she would not be able to do the work that she enjoyed so much if she spent so much time on her 'rituals'. Support was provided to her parents, who learned the limits of reasonable behaviour and how they had unwittingly re-inforced Betty's behaviour. Betty was discharged from hospital after 11 months. She continued going to work after her return home. Her parents supported her recovery and improved their quality of life by refusing to engage in rituals. They are helping social services to find Betty supported accommodation.

Depressive disorder

Depression is reported to be the most frequent comorbid psychiatric illness in people with autism (Ghaziuddin *et al*, 2002) but assessment is difficult. Worthlessness, guilt, diminished concentration and thoughts of suicide are said to be less commonly reported. Particular care should be taken not to assume that because suicidal ideation is not articulated it is not present.

In people with autism who are depressed, social withdrawal and poverty of speech may be mistaken for core symptoms of autism. Biological symptoms may not be observed to the same degree as in people without autism, and their absence may lead to missed diagnosis. On the other hand, flat or diminished range of affect, decreased gesture and vocal monotony are core features of autism and may lead to a false positive diagnosis. In general, the index of suspicion for presence of depressive disorder should increase when there is worsening of pre-existing core symptoms, at periods of transition or other environmental change, and if the person is subject to bullying. There is minimal treatment response data for either pharmacological or psychological interventions for depressive disorder in people with autism, and treatment of mood disorder in people with autism should reflect clinical guidelines from the National Institute for Health and Care Excellence.

Schizophrenia and other psychoses

In 1911 Eugen Bleuler proposed that profound social withdrawal was a core feature of schizophrenia and he called such withdrawal autism (from the Greek 'autos', meaning self). However, over the past 50 years it has become clear that enduring autism of early childhood onset is not characteristically associated with positive psychotic symptoms and has a different lifetime course. As a result (childhood) autism has come to be accepted as a diagnostic entity in its own right.

However, some evidence suggests that the prevalence of schizophrenia is increased among people with autism, although the evidence base is poor. For example, Mouridsen *et al* (2008) reported that 34% of people with 'atypical autism' had been previously diagnosed with a schizophrenia spectrum disorder. Neurodevelopmental psychiatrists regularly meet patients with autism who evidence (non-delusional) overvalued ideas, typically persecutory in nature. While these are assumed to be due to theory-of-mind deficits that contribute to the misinterpretations of others' mental states and intentions, it has been argued that such overvalued ideas have been misinterpreted by psychiatrists and are responsible for false-positive diagnoses of schizophrenia. Other reasons for a false-positive diagnosis of psychotic disorders include the presence of rigid idiosyncratic beliefs or unusual ways of describing personal experiences. For example, difficulties with theory of mind may make it more likely that a person with autism will report a thought as alien; a similar phenomenon is sometimes seen in people with an intellectual disability.

Overall, the clinical lessons are that it is important to examine the phenomenology carefully and consider alternative (including neuropsychological) explanations before concluding that psychotic disorder is present, but that psychotic disorder should not be assumed to be absent. Antipsychotic drugs form the mainstay of treatment, and reference should be made to the relevant guidelines from the National Institute for Health and Care Excellence (NICE, 2014).

Tic disorders

Tic disorders are reported to be more common in Asperger syndrome than in childhood autism (Gillberg & Billstedt, 2000). Tourette syndrome has been reported to affect 4–8% of young people with autism in the UK

(Baron-Cohen *et al*, 1999). Where possible, tics should be differentiated from the stereotypies and repetitive behaviours of autism (including 'stimming') and the compulsive behaviour of OCD – this may require repeated observations (including by carers) and mental state examination.

Eating disorders

Obsessionality, food fads, rituals around the order of eating food (including the separation of food on the plate) and pica are common in people with autism. It is therefore no surprise that people with autism may be over-represented in patients with eating disorders (Treasure *et al*, 2010). Autistic traits may impede and complicate treatment and worsen prognosis (Wentz *et al*, 2005), so it is important to identify people with eating disorder who have autism in order to target treatment appropriately. This is an active area of research.

Conclusions

Despite increasing awareness of autism, barriers to receiving an accurate diagnosis of autism remain. Once a person has a diagnosis, obstacles to recovery continue. These include the challenge inherent in coordinating a recovery programme that potentially spans social care, health, charitable organisations and a number of other areas. In addition, there is frequently institutional reluctance to take responsibility for meeting the needs of people who have previously been invisible to services, and who have not given rise to direct costs to these services, although there has been a significant cost burden at an individual and societal level. From the perspective of psychiatric care, additional difficulties may stem from:

- boundary disputes between social care and health agencies, and between mental health in intellectual disability and general adult psychiatrists
- difficulty overcoming the cultural hurdles necessary for organisational change
- unfamiliarity with the manifestations of autism and uncertainty about the identification of comorbidity
- overlap between the manifestations of autism and the symptoms of mental illness, such that it is possible to assert that a person does not have secondary healthcare needs
- lack of suitable treatment environments for people with autism within secondary care services.

This chapter has attempted to provide a framework for those working to support the recovery of people with autism. Effective support in enabling a currently disenfranchised group will incorporate recognition of the complex needs of both the person with autism as well as the range of services required. The effective clinician will need to possess the motivation, hope and imagination to play his or her part in effecting a change that is of benefit to people with autism and that is also of benefit to wider society.

References

Allison C, Auyeung B, Baron-Cohen S (2012) Toward brief 'red flags' for autism screening: the Short Autism Spectrum Quotient and the Short Quantitative Checklist for Autism in toddlers in 1,000 cases and 3,000 controls [corrected]. *Journal of the American Academy of Child and Adolescent Psychiatry*, **51**: 202–12.

American Psychiatric Association (2013) *Diagnostic and Statistical Manual of Mental Disorders* (5th edn) (DSM-5). APA.

Barnhill GP (2007) Outcomes in adults with Asperger syndrome. *Focus on Autism and Other Developmental Disabilities*, **22**: 116–26.

Baron-Cohen S, Scahill VL, Izaguirre J, *et al* (1999) The prevalence of Gilles de la Tourette syndrome in children and adolescents with autism: a large scale study. *Psychological Medicine*, **29**: 1151–9.

Baron-Cohen S, Wheelwright S, Skinner R, *et al* (2001) The Autism-Spectrum Quotient (AQ): evidence from Asperger syndrome/high-functioning autism, males and females, scientists and mathematicians. *Journal of Autism and Developmental Disorders*, **31**: 5–17.

Berney T, Brugha T, Carpenter P (2011) *Royal College of Psychiatrists Diagnostic Interview Guide for the Assessment of Adults with Autism Spectrum Disorder (ASD)*. At http://www.rcpsych.ac.uk/PDF/Asperger_interview_USE_THIS_ONE.pdf (accessed December 2014).

Billstedt E, Gillberg IC, Gillberg C (2005) Autism after adolescence: population-based 13- to 22-year follow-up study of 120 individuals with autism diagnosed in childhood. *Journal of Autism and Developmental Disorders*, **35**: 351–60.

Brown C, Dunn W (2002) *Adolescent/Adult Sensory Profile*. Pearson.

Brugha TS, McManus S, Bankart J, *et al* (2011) Epidemiology of autism spectrum disorders in adults in the community in England. *Archives of General Psychiatry*, **68**: 459–65.

Eaves LC, Ho HH (2008) Young adult outcome of autism spectrum disorders. *Journal of Autism and Developmental Disorders*, **38**: 739–47.

Ghaziuddin M, Ghaziuddin N, Greden J (2002) Depression in persons with autism: implications for research and clinical care. *Journal of Autism and Developmental Disorders*, **32**: 299–306.

Gillberg C, Billstedt E (2000) Autism and Asperger syndrome: coexistence with other clinical disorders. *Acta Psychiatrica Scandinavica*, **102**: 321–30.

Hellemans H, Colson K, Verbraeken C, *et al* (2007) Sexual behavior in high-functioning male adolescents and young adults with autism spectrum disorder. *Journal of Autism and Developmental Disorders*, **37**: 260–9.

Hofvander B, Delorme R, Chaste P, *et al* (2009) Psychiatric and psychosocial problems in adults with normal-intelligence autism spectrum disorders. *BMC Psychiatry*, **9**: 35.

Howlin P, Goode S, Hutton J, *et al* (2004) Adult outcome for children with autism. *Journal of Child Psychology and Psychiatry*, **45**: 212–29.

King BH, Hollander E, Sikich L, *et al* (2009) Lack of efficacy of citalopram in children with autism spectrum disorders and high levels of repetitive behavior: citalopram ineffective in children with autism. *Archives of General Psychiatry*, **66**: 583–90.

Lord C, Rutter M, Le Couteur A (1994) Autism Diagnostic Interview – Revised: a revised version of a diagnostic interview for caregivers of individuals with possible pervasive developmental disorders. *Journal of Autism and Developmental Disorders*, **24**: 659–85.

Lord C, Risi S, Lambrecht L, *et al* (2000) The Autism Diagnostic Observation Schedule – Generic: a standard measure of social and communication deficits associated with the spectrum of autism. *Journal of Autism and Developmental Disorders*, **30**: 205–23.

Matson JL, Nebel-Schwalm M (2007) Assessing challenging behaviors in children with autism spectrum disorders: a review. *Research in Developmental Disabilities*, **28**: 567–79.

Matson JL, Shoemaker M (2009) Intellectual disability and its relationship to autism spectrum disorders. *Research in Developmental Disabilities*, **30**: 1107–14.

Matson JL, Sipes M, Fodstad JC, *et al* (2011) Issues in the management of challenging behaviours of adults with autism spectrum disorder. *CNS Drugs*, **25**: 597–606.

McDougle CJ, Kresch LE, Goodman WK, *et al* (1995) A case-controlled study of repetitive thoughts and behavior in adults with autistic disorder and obsessive-compulsive disorder. *American Journal of Psychiatry*, **152**: 772–7.

Mouridsen SE, Rich B, Isager T (2008) Psychiatric disorders in adults diagnosed as children with atypical autism. A case control study. *Journal of Neural Transmission*, **115**: 135–8.

National Institute for Health and Clinical Excellence (2011) *Autism Diagnosis in Children and Young People* (CG 128). NICE.

National Institute for Health and Clinical Excellence (2012) *Autism: Recognition, Referral, Diagnosis and Management of Adults on the Autism Spectrum in Adults* (CG 142). NICE.

National Institute for Health and Care Excellence (2014) *Psychosis and Schizophrenia in Adults: Treatment and Management* (CG 178). NICE.

Reynolds AM, Malow BA (2011) Sleep and autism spectrum disorders. *Pediatric Clinics of North America*, **58**: 685–98.

Richdale AL, Schreck KA (2009) Sleep problems in autism spectrum disorders: prevalence, nature, and possible biopsychosocial aetiologies. *Sleep Medicine Review*, **13**: 403–11.

Rossignol DA, Frye RE (2014) Melatonin in autism spectrum disorders. *Current Clinical Pharmacology*, **9**: 326–3.

Schall C, Wehman P, McDonough JL (2012) Transition from school to work for students with autism spectrum disorders: understanding the process and achieving better outcomes. *Pediatric Clinics of North America*, **59**: 189–202.

Smith KR, Matson JL (2010) Social skills: differences among adults with intellectual disabilities, co-morbid autism spectrum disorders and epilepsy. *Research in Developmental Disabilities*, **31**: 1366–72.

Stokes MA, Kaur A (2005) High-functioning autism and sexuality: a parental perspective. *Autism*, **9**: 266–89.

Stokes M, Newton N, Kaur A (2007) Stalking, and social and romantic functioning among adolescents and adults with autism spectrum disorder. *Journal of Autism and Developmental Disorders*, **37**: 1969–86.

Suarez MA (2012) Sensory processing in children with autism spectrum disorders and impact on functioning. *Pediatric Clinics of North America*, **59**: 203–14.

Taylor JL, McPheeters ML, Sathe NA, et al (2012) A systematic review of vocational interventions for young adults with autism spectrum disorders. *Pediatrics*, **130**: 531–8.

Treasure J, Claudino AM, Zucker N (2010) Eating disorders. *Lancet*, **375**: 583–93.

Wentz E, Lacey JH, Waller G, *et al* (2005) Childhood onset neuropsychiatric disorders in adult eating disorder patients. A pilot study. *European Child and Adolescent Psychiatry*, **14**: 431–7.

White SW, Roberson-Nay R (2009) Anxiety, social deficits, and loneliness in youth with autism spectrum disorders. *Journal of Autism and Developmental Disorders*, **39**: 1006–13.

Wing L, Leekam SR, Libby SJ, *et al* (2002) The Diagnostic Interview for Social and Communication Disorders: background, inter-rater reliability and clinical use. *Journal of Child Psychology and Psychiatry*, **43**: 307–25.

World Health Organization (1992) *The ICD-10 Classification of Mental and Behavioural Disorders* (10th revision) (ICD-10). WHO.

CHAPTER 26

Risk management in rehabilitation practice

Shawn Mitchell

Introduction

'Risk', as a noun, implies a danger of 'loss, injury or other adverse circumstances' or 'commercial loss' (*Shorter Oxford English Dictionary*). In mental healthcare the 'injury' or 'loss' clearly applies to the service user or to others, or to both, caused by the service user, or inflicted upon the service user owing to that user's vulnerability. For professionals and healthcare organisations, risk has an additional element: the financial and reputational consequences of something being perceived as having gone wrong. Risk management involves attempts at both minimising the harms experienced by service users and others and the potential for reputational risk or blame. Our focus is on how to minimise harm, but it has to be acknowledged that many of the risk management practices, policies and procedures adopted by mental health services primarily work to decrease the potential for blame.

While media attention is skewed towards concerns about the risks that service users might pose to others, the reality remains that users are more likely to pose a risk to themselves or be the victim of violence and aggression than to engage in serious violence. Rehabilitation practitioners will be aware of the risks of vulnerability and of service users being exploited by others. Risk, in the sense of trying things out, is part of everyday living and inherent in every life choice and decision. Learning from experience reinforces self-confidence, capacity and coping skills, all necessary components of rehabilitation, and consequently supported risk-taking can foster recovery and personal development. It follows that the focus of risk assessment and management should be on safety enhancement rather than risk reduction (Morgan, 2007).

Service users are referred to rehabilitation services not only because of treatment resistance, chronicity or their complex needs (many patients in contact with generic services and living in the community have these characteristics) but also because of concerns about safety/risk as a consequence of these factors. Safety is a key issue when considering admission to or discharge from rehabilitation services and deciding what support a service user requires in the community.

A significant proportion of people receiving long-term in-patient care are, at least at some stage, detained under the mental health legislation. Admission for treatment under the Mental Health Act 1983 (section 3), which applies to England and Wales, must be 'necessary for the health or safety of the patient or for the protection of others'. The decision to detain (and treat compulsorily if necessary) is therefore partially risk-based but importantly includes consideration of improving the person's mental health.

Risk and recovery: collaborative approaches

The Department of Health's (2007a) *Best Practice in Managing Risk* sets out 'principles and evidence base for best practice in the assessment of risk to self or others'. It attempts to 'balance care needs with risk needs' (implying that they are in some form of tension). The executive summary (p. 4) identifies four important issues that are often lost in discussions about risk: positive risk management; collaboration with the service user and others involved in care; the importance of recognising and building on the service user's strengths; and the organisation's role in risk management alongside the individual practitioner's. These sentiments were echoed in the *Twelfth Biennial Report* of the Mental Health Act Commission (whose function is now undertaken by the Care Quality Commission), which stated that: 'Services should ensure that risk assessment of detained patients takes account of "positive risk management" and is undertaken in collaboration with patients and, where appropriate, carers and relatives' (Mental Health Act Commission, 2007: p. 35). *Best Practice in Managing Risk* brings together

---

Box 26.1 Principles to guide risk assessment and risk management

- Accurate risk prediction is never possible at an individual level; however, the systematic use of structured risk assessment can enhance clinical judgement
- Risk assessment informs risk management and the two processes should be integral to one another
- Risk assessment can be considered to be a vital element of the clinical risk assessment process, and inform clinical interventions for risk factors that are amenable to treatment
- Risk management must recognise and promote the patient's strengths and should support recovery
- Needs assessment and risk assessment should inform one another, and be considered together
- Positive risk management is part of a carefully constructed plan and is a required competence for all mental health practitioners
- Risk management requires an organisational strategy as well as competent efforts by individual practitioners

Adapted from *Best Practice in Managing Risk* (Department of Health, 2007a)

Box 26.2 Management of violence on an in-patient ward: involving the patient after the incident

- Engage in positive conversations soon as possible after the incident to establish whether the patient understands why interventions were used
- Provide opportunities for the patient to write about the incident
- Continue with patient choice regarding rapid tranquillisation and environments in which he or she is to be nursed
- Involve the patient in all debriefs, where possible
- Offer debriefing, looking at antecedents and impact of the behaviour on others

From: College Centre for Quality Improvement (2007)

a wealth of information on assessing and managing risk, from which a number of key principles emerge (see Box 26.1).

It is important to ensure that the responsibility and ownership for maintaining safety are shared between the service provider and the service user, with the service user taking on increasing responsibility as circumstances allow, and this can be done only through collaborative working. A concrete example of this emerged from a national audit of violence on in-patient units, which looked at how services responded to episodes of violence and aggression (College Centre for Quality Improvement, 2007). The audit identified potential changes to post-incident clinical management, including specific actions around involving the patient or other perpetrator of violence (see Box 26.2).

The increasing public and political emphasis on risk, particularly on risk to others, has resulted in concerns expressed by service users, mental health professionals and even regulatory bodies. The dilemma is well summarised by Morgan (2007: p. 12):

> Risk taking on the part of clinicians is a necessary component of rehabilitation, and a risk-averse psychiatric culture can only be to the detriment of this process. This perspective has been deeply criticised within the Media and other public agencies.... The politics of risk management are not always related to its science.

A focus on risk alone, without considering protective factors, can encourage stigma and pessimism in both professionals and service users. In a Department of Health (2006) consultation document, *Reviewing the Care Programme Approach*, service users expressed their concern at the lack of attention to their wider social care needs. They felt that the focus was on problems and risks rather than building on their strengths towards recovery. Further issues raised by service users about the risk assessment process are summarised in Box 26.3.

Langan & Lindow (2004) carried out a detailed qualitative study of the processes surrounding risk assessment and management of people leaving

---

Box 26.3 Service user experience of the risk assessment and risk management process

- Risk assessment being undertaken without any input by the service user or explanation by the clinicians
- Lack of dialogue when understanding and formulations of risk issues are different between service user and clinicians
- Blanket risk assessment decisions, rather than decisions based on the individual service user and circumstances
- A possible over-reliance on basing the risk management decision on historical risk
- Lapses being viewed as relapses, and not seen in proportion to the circumstances

---

hospital as described by the service user and staff. They identified particular difficulties in fully involving service users presenting a risk to others, who are often not informed by professionals that they are considered to be a risk to others. The reasons given by staff for non-disclosure included problems with insight, perceived risk of disengagement from services, concerns about stigma and fears for the professionals' own safety. Professionals may also worry that they may be seen as primarily concerned with risk management rather than support and care, and as 'the arm of the state' rather than as therapeutic agents.

Historically, there has been limited guidance on how to involve service users in risk assessment and management. Other sources of guidance can be used. These include tools for user-oriented care planning processes that incorporate relapse management planning and crisis management plans, which are key to maintaining safety. Langan & Lindow (2004) found that discontinuing medication, substance misuse and lack of support from services were seen as important triggers for relapse of mental illness. Motivating factors for staying well included suitable accommodation, financial security, employment or constructive activity, social networks and supportive relationships, which are generally accepted as increasing the likelihood of service users staying well and reducing risk. However, Langan & Lindow noted that professionals were likely to focus on trigger factors such as discontinuing medication, while service users were likely to focus on stresses related to social circumstances as precipitants of relapse. In practice both are important and the dialogue between the professional and service user should encompass social as well as clinical issues.

The Department of Health strategy for mental health, *No Health Without Mental Health* (2011), puts recovery at the centre of delivery of mental health services. However, there is potential tension between managing risk and working in a recovery-oriented fashion. Psychiatrists working in South London concluded:

Risk is inherent in all mental health services and in recovery orientated services risk will remain. A recovery orientated service will require a change in our emphasis from risk avoidance to constructive and creative risk taking. (South London and Maudsley NHS Foundation Trust & South West London and St George's Mental Health NHS Trust, 2010)

This is perhaps easier said than done in a risk-averse climate.

Risk assessment

The limitations of risk assessment

With the benefit of hindsight, examination of a case of homicide or suicide can readily produce a very compelling narrative involving previous worrying behaviour and warnings from concerned others that leads inevitably to the terrible outcome (Szmukler et al, 2013). An obvious question is why were these outcomes not predicted? The reason is simply put: 'Risk … cannot be eliminated. Accurate prediction is never possible for individual patients' (Royal College of Psychiatrists, 2008: p. 9).

Practitioners (and the courts) tend to have a poor understanding of the statistical basis for statements about risk (Gigerenzer, 2002). The essential problem is that of the base rate for a particular adverse outcome – where the base rate is very low (as it is for the suicide of an in-patient or homicide) even robust predictive factors or good tools simply cannot result in accurate prediction at an individual level because of the numbers of false positives and false negatives. The National Confidential Inquiry into Suicide and Homicide by People with a Mental Illness (2013) reported that in England in 2010 there were 184 suicides by patients in contact with services with a diagnosis of schizophrenia. We do not have accurate base-rate data on the number of people with schizophrenia in current contact with services but at a low estimate of 100000, suicides represent less than 0.2% of patients. We do have data on adult in-patient admissions per year in England, approximately 120000. There were 75 suicides by in-patients in 2010 (0.06%).

It is therefore unsurprising that prediction of both in-patient and post-discharge suicide has been shown to be very poor indeed (Powell et al, 2000; Large et al, 2011). This robustly evidence-based statement has not deterred the UK Supreme Court in the Rabone case from confirming an 'operational duty' under the Human Rights Act on services to prevent the suicide of an informal patient sent home on leave. The Supreme Court did, however, have to take as fact the expert testimony given to a lower court that provided estimates of risk of suicide that were surprisingly high and do not match experience from services that routinely admit people because of suicidality (Szmukler et al, 2013).

One of the challenges for clinicians is the lack of a validated comprehensive assessment schedule that assesses risk to self, risk to others and other potential risks, such as vulnerability. The available validated tools that facilitate 'structured professional judgement' are specific to particular risk issues.

Risk assessment in practice

Despite the limitations on the prediction of severe adverse outcomes it is clear that risk assessment and (perhaps more importantly) risk management need to be integral to the care delivered by services. Discussions about risk will often be a significant part of the therapeutic relationship between the clinician and the service user. The emphasis should be on openness, honesty and transparency. To facilitate this, clinicians should make the discussion, assessment and management of risk explicit when describing the key components of their clinical contact with service users. Services should make the need for, and the focus on, safety explicit in any literature detailing their work.

There are two obvious and basic points about risk assessment that are often overlooked. First, future risks are strongly associated with past risk. Second, accurate documentation of risk behaviours is vital, both for the assessment of risk at some future date and for clear and honest discussion with service users. 'Tick-box' risk assessment tools, while both required and reassuring, have less practical utility than good-quality documentation of risk behaviours.

Despite the importance of past behaviour, risk is dynamic and therefore risk assessment needs to take account of the person's varying and changeable circumstances. Clinicians need to be aware that risk assessment is merely the start of the process: risk assessment and risk management are integrally linked. Steps taken to enhance safety management will alter the assessment of current risk.

Rethinking Risk to Others in Mental Health Services (Royal College of Psychiatrists, 2008) provided some general principles surrounding the

---

Box 26.4 Principles surrounding risk assessment

- Risk assessment should inform risk management and contribute to the clinical care and meeting the needs of patients
- Structured risk assessment should involve clearly defined factors derived from research
- Risk assessment should include the clinical experience and knowledge of the service user, and the service user's own view of his or her experience
- The role of unpaid carers in making judgements of risk should be recognised and valued
- Risk assessment should be proportionate to the perceived level of risk
- Risk assessment should be carried out within the multidisciplinary team, allowing sharing of information and application of different perspectives
- Risk cannot be eliminated
- Risk is dynamic, can alter over time, and must be regularly reviewed
- Risk assessments should be linked with needs assessments

From Royal College of Psychiatrists (2008)

---

development of local risk assessment frameworks. These are set out in Box 26.4. At its best, risk assessment combines statistical data with clinical information that integrates historical variables, current crucial variables and contextual or environmental factors. Some of these are potential areas of need and therefore needs assessment may both inform and be a response to the risk assessment process. Better-quality care can be provided if there are established links between the assessment of patients' needs and their risk assessment.

Risk to self

The epidemiological background

For the purposes of this discussion, self-harm and suicide will be considered together, irrespective of the motivation. People who self-harm and attempt suicide are at risk not only of death but also of long-term health problems, such as liver damage from paracetamol overdose and permanent damage to tendons and nerves from cutting. The assessment of risk of self-harm and suicide needs to take into consideration biopsychosocial factors that lead to increased risk. People at increased risk of self-harm include asylum-seekers, some minority ethnic groups, people in various forms of institutional care, sexual minorities, former members of the armed forces and people bereaved by suicide (Royal College of Psychiatrists, 2010).

There is extremely robust epidemiological evidence that alcohol and substance misuse, being unemployed and having a diagnosed mental illness increase the risk of self-harm and suicide, and both are associated with 'loss events' such as relationship breakdown. Self-harm is commoner in women and completed suicide commoner in men. In rehabilitation services, clinicians will be aware of the high rate of suicide in schizophrenia, although in contemporary assessments the suicide rate is lower than previously believed, at roughly 5% (Hor & Taylor, 2010). Risk factors include being young, male, well educated and, rather worryingly for clinicians, a higher level of insight into the condition. A history of suicide attempts, the severity of illness, comorbid depression (which can be difficult to diagnose), post-psychosis depression, substance misuse and social isolation have also been identified as risk factors. Hor & Taylor (2010) noted that the only protective factor for suicide was delivery of and adherence to effective treatment. Risk of suicide is somewhat higher overall in bipolar disorder than in schizophrenia (7.8% for men, 4.8% for women) (Nordentoft et al, 2011). The risk of suicide for all patient groups is greatest immediately after discharge from hospital.

Assessment

A through assessment of the immediate risk to self requires a detailed psychiatric history and mental state examination (Royal College of Psychiatrists, 2010). A history of serious self-harm with suicidal intent

---

Box 26.5 Issues to consider in assessing risk for people who engage in self-harm

- Methods and frequency of current and past self-harm
- Current and past suicidal intent
- Depressive symptoms and their relationship to self-harm
- Any psychiatric illness and its relationship to self-harm
- Comorbid alcohol and substance misuse (including misuse of over-the-counter medicines)
- Co-occurring risky behaviours (e.g. unprotected sex)
- The personal and social context and any other specific factors preceding self-harm, such as specific unpleasant affective states or emotions and changes in relationships
- Specific risk factors and protective factors (social, psychological, pharmaco-logical and motivational) that may increase or decrease the risks associated with self-harm
- Coping strategies that the person has used either to limit or to avert self-harm or to contain the impact of personal, social or other factors preceding episodes of self-harm
- Significant relationships that may either be supportive or represent a threat (such as abuse or neglect) and may lead to changes in the level of risk
- Immediate and longer-term risks
- Access to means of self-harm (e.g. family members' medications)
- Age: self-harm in the elderly is associated with a higher risk of subsequent suicide

Adapted from National Institute for Health and Clinical Excellence (2011)

---

remains relevant to suicide risk even decades later. There are guidelines from the National Institute for Health and Clinical Excellence (2004, 2011) on both the immediate and the longer-term management of self-harm; one striking observation is how poor the evidence base is for making recommendations. The latter guideline makes helpful specific recommendations on the risk assessment process (see Box 26.5).

Thoughts of suicide are a question in self-assessment scales such the Beck Depression Inventory (Beck *et al*, 1996). There are specific assessment schedules for hopelessness (Beck *et al*, 1990) and suicide, for example the Scale for Suicidal Ideation (Beck *et al*, 1979) and the Suicide Intent Scale (Beck *et al*, 1974). Although hopelessness has been identified as a predictor of suicide (Beck *et al*, 1990) this has not been consistently replicated in studies of people who have self-harmed. One study found that scores on the Suicide Intent Scale significantly predicted death by suicide at 12-year follow-up of people who were assessed after an episode of self-harm (Suominen *et al*, 2004). This appears impressive until one looks at the odds ratio for high scores predicting subsequent suicide (1.18:1 – very statistically significant but not that useful at an individual level).

The National Institute for Health and Clinical Excellence (2011: p. 21) notes that risk assessment tools (checklists) and scales can be helpful in structuring completed risk assessments but specifically states that these should not be used 'to predict future suicide or repetition of self-harm' and not be used 'to determine who should or should not be offered treatment or who should be discharged'.

Risk to others

The epidemiological background

Six per cent of people committing a homicide in England between 1997 and 2011 were assessed as having been psychotic at the time of the offence (National Confidential Inquiry into Suicide and Homicide by People with a Mental Illness, 2013). This does need to be put into context. The epidemiological data suggest that at any one time less than 1% of the population are living with a psychotic illness, so psychosis is a definite risk factor for homicide. In 2010, 24 people committed a homicide while psychotic (in the region of one in 20000 people living with psychosis). Ten people with a diagnosis of schizophrenia who were in contact with psychiatric services (out of 100000 or more) committed a homicide (0.01% or less).

Homicide by a service user living with a psychotic illness is a rare and statistically unpredictable occurrence – although lesser degrees of violence and aggression are not rare (Walsh et al, 2002). The relationship between violence and psychosis is complex. The victims of aggression perpetrated by mental health service users are most likely to be family members or carers. Much of the violence risk is associated with the factors that are associated with violence in the general community (male sex, younger age and alcohol, stimulant and cannabis misuse).

A recent systematic review and meta-analysis found a number of 'static' risk factors for violence (i.e. those that one cannot change), of which the most significant are a history of violent behaviour and a criminal history (Witt et al, 2013). Potentially modifiable risk factors include hostile behaviour, recent drug and alcohol misuse, lack of impulse control, non-adherence with psychological treatment and medication and active psychotic symptoms. Negative symptoms are not associated with risk of violence. There is some suggestion that clozapine has 'anti-aggressive' effects (similar to its impact on substance misuse). Although risk factors have differing effects on serious violence, less serious violence and violence in in-patient settings, studies always identify the same risk factors.

Assessment of the risk of violence

Given the importance of a history of violence on the risk of future violence, it follows that a good history of offending behaviour and violence is a vital starting point. Clinically, during an assessment it is important to seek clarification from service users regarding their responses to identified psychotic symptoms, particularly persecutory ideation and passivity phenomena. It is always important to take threats to others seriously. Where violence has previously occurred the practitioner needs to develop a good understanding of the incident(s), the service user's perception of what happened and the extent to which factors contributing to what happened have been or could be modified.

Structured professional judgement

Over the past two decades, a variety of risk assessment tools have been developed that provide 'structured professional judgement' of violence risk. These combine 'actuarial' data on risk factors with clinical assessment (Webster & Hucker, 2007) and include the Short Term Assessment of Risk and Treatability (START; Webster *et al*, 2009) and the Structured Assessment of PROtective factors for violence risk (SAPROF; de Vogel *et al*, 2011). Other structured risk assessment tools include: the Sexual Violence Assault Risk – 20; the Spousal Assault Risk Assessment; the Hare Psychopathy Checklist (strictly an item within the HCR, discussed below, which is rarely completed because of the training requirements to use the instrument); the SAFARI (St Andrew's Fire and Arson Risk Instrument); and the HCR-20 FAM (Female Additional Manual).

START considers strengths as well as risks and SAPROF looks at protective factors; in both, the focus has moved from attempting to predict risk to active risk management in a more constructive framework that seeks to reduce risk. The most familiar and influential instrument is the HCR-20, which is now in its third version (Douglas *et al*, 2013). HCR stands for 'Historical', 'Clinical' and 'Risk management' – the historical items reflecting those issues that cannot be altered by services, while the other items are potentially amenable to intervention. The focus of the latest version of HCR-20 is on formulating plans to manage and reduce risks to others, given the current situation and future scenarios.

Strengths-based risk assessment tools have the potential to be much less stigmatising and to prompt discussion of how strengths may be increased, thereby reducing risk further, providing increased hope for change.

Self-neglect and vulnerability

The impact of self-neglect and vulnerability among people living with severe mental illness has received minimal academic attention. Nonetheless, experienced practitioners will be well aware of the potential risks of self-neglect. It is not rare for service users to be admitted to hospital with marked weight loss and dehydration. Some people live in squalor for months or years before coming to the attention of services. Others, in the context of their illness, engage in dangerous behaviours like tampering with the electricity or gas supply. Vulnerability includes vulnerability to financial and sexual exploitation.

As with all kinds of risk, previous episodes of self-neglect or vulnerability predict future risk. In England and Wales these risks may be used as justification for the continued use of statutory powers for detention in hospital or supervised community treatment.

Factors increasing the risk of self-neglect and vulnerability

Cognitive deficits and chronic psychosis can predispose people with schizophrenia to exploitation. Otherwise there is little guidance as to factors that increase the risk of self-neglect and vulnerability in users of mental health rehabilitation services. However, evidence from studies of older people with mental health difficulties can be extrapolated to users of rehabilitation services. Factors intrinsic to the person that increase risk in the elderly include substance misuse and medical comorbidity (Culo, 2011). An unwillingness to accept help can also increase the risk of self-neglect and exploitation. 'External' factors, those that are potentially modifiable, include lack of social support, living alone, lack of community resources, inadequate housing, unsanitary living conditions, high-crime neighbourhoods, adverse life events and poverty.

Assessment

While service users themselves or other informants might volunteer information about self-neglect or vulnerability, identification requires the vigilance of staff. Vulnerability issues are assessed in structured risk assessments such as the START and in local 'tick-box' risk tools. Assessment of capacity is essential for a service user who appears vulnerable to exploitation and self-neglect, in order to determine whether poor self-care, neglect of the environment and questionable social contacts reflect capacitous choices. The parameters of what is acceptable and unacceptable can be difficult to delineate clearly and depends to a degree on the values of the assessor and therefore it is important that complex issues are reviewed and discussed in a multidisciplinary setting. Adult safeguarding procedures need to be followed where appropriate.

Involving the service user in safety management

Safety management requires a delicate balance between ensuring that the service user remains safe and does not impact on the safety of others, while allowing a degree of therapeutic risk-taking. It should not be so restrictive that it does not allow the service user to take some risks as part of recovery and rehabilitation, which would enable the service user to learn from experience. Safety management should be conducted in a spirit of collaboration and be based on a relationship between the service user, carers and the service provider that is as trusting as possible. The aim of the process should be for the service user to take ownership of his or her

401

own safety and the safety of others, with appropriate support when needed. The process should be built on recognition of the service user's strengths and should emphasise recovery.

Independence, Choice and Risk (Department of Health, 2007*b*) provides a useful generic guide to the difficult balancing act that professionals (and carers) have to make when seeking to manage risk while fostering choice and independence. It starts from a general principle: 'People have the right to live their lives to the full as long as that does not stop others from doing the same'. Patricia Deegan (1996) describes the meeting point of risk management and recovery from a user perspective succinctly: 'Professionals must embrace the concept of the dignity of risk, and the right to failure if they are to be supportive of us'.

Positive risk-taking can be a challenge for clinicians. The crucial first step is therapeutic engagement. The relationship between the clinician and the service user must be based upon honesty on the part of the clinician, with the aim of building up trust. When risk issues are not openly discussed with service users, they may first come to learn of perceived risks and any resultant concerns in Care Programme Approach reviews or when reading the report of a mental health tribunal. This can lead to dispute about the facts, distress, denial and ongoing avoidance of risk issues.

Approaching risk in an honest and open way may initially lead to the service user experiencing a state of dissonance (Horstead & Cree, 2013), but can in the longer term result in a shared formulation and ultimately motivation to change. Once this has been achieved, the professional's role can be characterised as closer to that of a 'coach', who has professional knowledge and experience, working closely with the service users, acknowledging their expertise in their own experience, and maintaining hope and optimism for their future (Roberts & Wolfson, 2004).

However, it has to be acknowledged that clinicians have wider responsibilities for the health and safety of service users and the public (including staff and fellow service users within mental health services). Coercive actions (which should be within a legal framework) may be necessary to maintain safety. The reasons for coercion need to be discussed with the service user. We have already underlined the importance of a dialogue about safety and risk. Finding shared acceptable words and terminology is key to ensuring that discussions about risk assessment and management are collaborative. An example is using the word (and concept of) 'safety' instead of 'risk', which service users find pejorative. Other examples include finding words to describe an index offence, or other situations where safety was significantly compromised.

Discussion should include user-defined risks. In this way, risks can be identified that *should* be taken, for example trying to get a job or other attempts to be more included in the local community. The timing and pace of these discussions will need to be considered carefully. The service user's strengths in relation to maintaining safety and reducing potential risk must

---

Box 26.6 Actions to promote service users' involvement in safety management and therapeutic risk-taking

- Identifying with the service user what is likely to work
- Obtaining the views of carers and others around the service user when deciding a plan of action
- Weighing up the potential benefits and harms of choosing one action over another
- Being willing to take decisions that involve an element of risk because the potential benefits outweigh the risk
- Being clear to all involved about the potential benefits and the risks
- Developing plans and actions that support the positive potentials and priorities stated by the service user, and minimising the risks to the service user or others
- Ensuring that the service user, carer and others who might be affected are fully informed of the decision, the reasons for it, and associated plans. There is a duty on the clinician to warn anyone who may be at significant risk from a service user
- Using available resources and support to achieve a balance between a focus on achieving the desired outcomes and minimising a potential harmful outcome

---

be identified. Exploring service users' own priorities is far more likely to engage them and ensure that they take responsibility for their own safety.

The process of therapeutic risk-taking needs to be negotiated. This includes explicit discussion about boundaries to behaviours and the reasons for these. For example, a tenancy is likely to have conditions stated within the tenancy agreement, which set out the expectations of the tenant. Sensitive involvement of carers and advocates will often be helpful. They may have additional insights into the impact of risk behaviours, as well as providing a valuable resource for future safety management planning. However, this involvement may not always be appropriate: clinical judgement is key here, as therapeutic interactions cannot fit into rigid protocols.

Box 26.6 identifies some actions that the clinician can undertake to promote service user involvement in safety management and therapeutic risk-taking.

Supporting processes and documentation

Essential to safety assessment and management are processes to support decision-making and safety-planning and the clear recording of these processes. Recording is important in order to ensure that the safety assessment and management plan is shared with all, including family and carers and other involved professionals. Documentation is also important in order to demonstrate the decision-making process should there be an

403

adverse outcome of a decision involving safety and risk. Documentation should avoid the use of jargon and be understandable to people who will access the documentation.

Informing service users about risk and safety

The importance of the service user knowing about risk and safety issues and how these are to be managed has already been emphasised. Information about risk and safety may be included in information leaflets about a service that routinely works with 'high-risk' individuals. Where appropriate, clinicians must be explicit that addressing risk and maintaining safety are a core part of their work: obvious examples are discussions with service users about levels of in-patient observation and the granting of leave where the person is being detained in hospital under mental health legislation. Some forensic services offer a psychoeducational group specifically about risk and safety (Horstead & Cree, 2013). Once a service user has completed this group, rating of risk, using structured professional judgement tools, is undertaken with the person and the information is shared with her or him in a user-friendly format.

Formulation and risk management

'Formulation' is a key component of structured professional judgement tools such as the HCR-20. A good formulation can offer a narrative that explains the underlying mechanism for a risk behaviour and will propose hypotheses regarding action to facilitate change. The formulation can then be used to understand why the service user behaved in an unsafe manner and why he or she might do so again, which in turn will inform scenario planning, a process of identifying possible circumstances in the future when the service user could be unsafe, and using the scenarios to safety plan.

A formulation should describe the problem (the risk issue) and set out predisposing, precipitating, perpetuating and protective factors. Early-warning signs that risk may be escalating should also be identified. This information may lead to a risk management plan, which, in the words of the Department of Health (2007a: p. 5) in a counsel of perfection, 'should include a summary of all risks identified, formulations of the situations in which identified risks may occur, and actions to be taken by practitioners and the service user in response to crisis'.

Safety planning

Treatment (or rehabilitation) in the context of safety requires the development of strategies that moderate risk factors and enhance protective factors. The formulation can be helpful in identifying factors underpinning past safety concerns: these might, for example, include non-adherence to treatment resulting in rapid relapse or reinstatement of alcohol and substance misuse. Focusing on positive lifestyle factors such personal support, stable relationships, employment and reducing stress can reduce risk.

In England and Wales, the Mental Health Act allows services to exercise a great deal of control over the lives of detained patients and patients on leave from hospital. People with a mental disorder who have been identified by the courts as presenting serious risk to the public can be placed on a restriction order (under section 37 or 41), which will result in a lengthy in-patient stay for treatment and rehabilitation. Restricted patients will, on leaving hospital, generally be subject to conditional discharge. The conditions put in place are designed to minimise future risk and maintain wellness; breach of these conditions may result in recall to hospital. Supervised community treatment (under section 17A) allows for rather similar powers over people who have previously been detained under section 3 and section 37. For some service users with significant risks to others, support can include supervision, residential accommodation, monitoring of alcohol and drug use, and testing for this, and, in some circumstances, restrictions on contact with negative family and peer influences.

The Mental Capacity Act can also be used in circumstances where an individual lacks capacity and could be vulnerable to others. If someone has to live in a highly restrictive community setting, 'deprivation of liberty' safeguards may need to be put into place. Simple interventions such as responding quickly to missed appointments can be important; for instance, the 2011 annual report of the National Confidential Inquiry found that 28% of service users who committed suicide missed their last appointment. Addressing lifestyle in the form of activity, structure, boundaries and role expectations can all enhance protective factors.

Care Programme Approach and 'My Shared Pathway'

As readers working in England will be aware, *Refocusing the Care Programme Approach* (Department of Health, 2008) focused the Care Programme Approach (CPA) on those service users with complex needs who were likely to have more than one involved professional and to present with concerns surrounding risk and safety. Integral to the CPA process is care planning, key components of which include risk and safety management and crisis-planning and contingency-planning.

'My Shared Pathway' is an approach to care planning that was introduced in secure hospital settings (see http://www.networks.nhs.uk/nhs-networks/my-shared-pathway). It structures the process of care planning, requiring the development of clearly identified goals that are shared by the service user and professional staff and the setting out of actions needed to help the service user achieve these goals within a projected timescale. The aim is for the service user to be able to move to a lower level of security. Documentation has been developed that seeks to emphasise the centrality of the user rather than the service.

'My Shared Pathway' has five domains: (1) 'A shared understanding', which identifies patients' past difficulties and achievements; (2) 'Me and my recovery', which includes 'My mental health recovery' and 'Making feasible plans'; (3) 'My safety and risks', which includes 'Stopping my problem behaviours', 'Getting insight' and 'Recovery from drug and alcohol problems'; (4) 'My health'; and (5) 'My relationships'. While safety is most likely to be addressed within 'Stopping my problem behaviours', contributing factors may arise within the other domains. The elaboration of shared goals reinforces that the process is collaborative rather than undertaken by the care coordinator, which is something that tends to occur with care planning under the CPA. This structure is likely to be more facilitative of discussions regarding safety, thereby ensuring that risk and safety are integral to the care plan. 'My Shared Pathway' identifies specific outcomes, with the service user and staff rating these outcomes, thereby using the process as an outcome measure. There is also a focus on service users telling their story.

Tools developed by service users include the Wellness Recovery Action Plan® (http://www.mentalhealthrecovery.com), which covers early warning signs, coping strategies that the service user can use, as well as a detailed crisis plan, in which the service user can direct what others should or should not do. Integral to this would be plans for the service user to maintain his or her safety.

Safe environments

In in-patient rehabilitation settings safety can be enhanced through three aspects of security: relational, procedural and environmental. Procedural and environmental security increase with the level of security, and are defined within the standards used by the Royal College of Psychiatrists' Medium and Low Secure Quality Networks (see http://www.rcpsych.ac.uk/workinpsychiatry/qualityimprovement/qualityandaccreditation/forensic/forensicmentalhealth.aspx). The annual Ligature Audit undertaken by all services in England is another initiative to ensure that in-patient environments are safe and reduce the risk of suicide by ligature. The design of in-patient and residential facilities can contribute significantly to creating a calming and containing environment.

Relational security

Rehabilitation in-patient units may be locked, open or community-based. As the environmental security and procedural security become less, 'relational security' becomes the most important aspect of maintaining a safe environment. Relational security is 'the knowledge and understanding staff have of a patient and of the environment, and the translation of that information into appropriate responses and care' (Department of Health, 2010). Aspects of relational security include: what the team is offering (setting boundaries, offering therapies); the 'inside world' (understanding the user's personal world, managing the physical environment); the 'outside world' (making appropriate outward connections, managing visitors); and other patients (patient mix, patient dynamics). Enhancing relational security requires constant effort by the staff team.

Conclusions

Concerns about risk have come to dominate discourse within mental health services. Risk is a complex and contested construct, although it is clear that the assessment of risk is an empty exercise unless it results in plans to manage risk. Staff and service users may have radically different perceptions of risk issues and we have suggested that an emphasis on developing a shared understanding based on the concept of safety and an acknowledgement of the value of positive risk-taking may provide a fruitful approach. While it is necessary to acknowledge the realities of a risk-averse society that emphasises the duty of care that services owe to vulnerable individuals, the aim should always be to enhance people's ability to manage their own lives.

References

Beck AT, Schuyler D, Herman I (1974) Development of Suicidal Intent Scales. In *The Prediction of Suicide* (eds AT Beck, HLP Resnick, DJ Lettieri): 45–56. Charles Press.

Beck AT, Kovacs M, Weissman A (1979) Assessment of suicidal ideation: the Scale for Suicide Ideation. *Journal of Consulting and Clinical Psychology*, **47**: 343–52.

Beck AT, Brown G, Berchick RJ, et al (1990) Relationship between hopelessness and ultimate suicide: a replication with psychiatric outpatients. *American Journal of Psychiatry*, **147**: 190–5.

Beck AT, Steer RA, Brown GK (1996) *Manual for the Beck Depression Inventory – II*. Psychological Corporation.

College Centre for Quality Improvement (2007) *National Audit of Violence. Module 3a National Report*. CCQI.

Culo S (2011) Risk assessment and intervention for vulnerable older adults. *BC Medical Journal*, **53**: 421–5.

Deegan PE (1996) Recovery as a journey of the heart. *Psychiatric Rehabilitation Journal*, **19**: 91–7.

Department of Health (2006) *Reviewing the Care Programme Approach*. Department of Health.

Department of Health (2007a) *Best Practice in Managing Risk*. Department of Health.

Department of Health (2007b) *Independence, Choice and Risk: A Guide to Best Practice in Supported Decision-Making*. Department of Health.

Department of Health (2008) *Refocusing the Care Programme Approach: Policy and Positive Practice Guidance*. Department of Health.

Department of Health (2010) *Your Guide to Relational Security. See Think Act*. Department of Health.

Department of Health (2011) *No Health Without Mental Health*. Department of Health.

407

de Vogel V, de Vries RM, de Ruiter C, *et al* (2011) Assessing protective factors in forensic population practice: introducing the SAPROF. *International Journal of Forensic Mental Health*, **10**: 171–7.

Douglas KS, Hart SD, Webster CD, *et al* (2013) *HCR-20V3: Assessing Risk of Violence – User Guide*. Mental Health, Law, and Policy Institute, Simon Fraser University.

Gigerenzer G (2002) *Reckoning with Risk*. Penguin Books.

Hor K, Taylor M (2010) Suicide and schizophrenia: a systematic review of rates and risk factors. *Journal of Psychopharmacology*, **24** (suppl 4): 81–90.

Horstead A, Cree A (2013) Achieving transparency in forensic risk assessment: a multimodal approach. *Advances in Psychiatric Treatment*, **19**: 351–7.

Langan J, Lindow V (2004) *Living with Risk: Mental Health Service User Involvement in Risk Assessment and Management*. Policy Press/Joseph Rowntree Foundation.

Large M, Sharma S, Cannon E, *et al* (2011) Risk factors for suicide within a year of discharge from psychiatric hospital: a systematic meta-analysis. *Australia and New Zealand Journal of Psychiatry*, **45**: 619–28.

Mental Health Act Commission (2007) *Risk, Rights, Recovery. Mental Health Act Commission's Twelfth Biennial Report, 2005–2007*. TSO (The Stationery Office).

Morgan J (2007) *Giving Up the Culture of Blame. Risk Assessment and Risk Management in Psychiatric Practice* (Briefing Document for the Royal College of Psychiatrists). London: Royal College of Psychiatrists.

National Confidential Inquiry into Suicide and Homicide by People with a Mental Illness (2011) *Annual Report: England, Northern Ireland, Scotland and Wales*. NCISHPMI.

National Confidential Inquiry into Suicide and Homicide by People with a Mental Illness (2013) *Annual Report: England, Northern Ireland, Scotland and Wales*. NCISHPMI.

National Institute for Health and Clinical Excellence (2004) *Self-harm: The Short-Term Physical and Psychological Management and Secondary Prevention of Self-harm in Primary and Secondary Care* (CG 16). NICE.

National Institute for Health and Clinical Excellence (2011) *Self-harm: Longer-Term Management* (CG 133). NICE.

Nordentoft N, Mortensen PB, Pedersen CB (2011) Absolute risk of suicide after first hospital contact in mental disorder. *Archives of General Psychiatry*, **68**: 1058–64.

Powell J, Geddes J, Hawton K (2000) Suicide in psychiatric hospital inpatients. Risk factors and their predictive power. *British Journal of Psychiatry*, **176**: 266–72.

Roberts G, Wolfson P (2004) The rediscovery of recovery: open to all. *Advances in Psychiatric Treatment*, **10**: 37–49.

Royal College of Psychiatrists (2008) *Rethinking Risk to Others in Mental Health Services. Final Report of a Scoping Group* (CR 150). Royal College of Psychiatrists.

Royal College of Psychiatrists (2010) *Self-harm, Suicide and Risk: Helping People Who Self-harm* (CR 158). Royal College of Psychiatrists.

South London and Maudsley NHS Foundation Trust & South West London and St George's Mental Health NHS Trust (2010) *Recovery Is for All. Hope, Agency and Opportunity in Psychiatry: A Position Statement by Consultant Psychiatrists*. SLaM & SWLSTG.

Suominen K, Isometsa E, Astamo A, *et al* (2004) Level of suicide intent predicts overall mortality and suicide after attempted suicide: a 12 year follow-up study. *BMC Psychiatry*, **4**: 11.

Szmukler G, Richardson G, Owen G (2013) 'Rabone' and four unresolved problems in mental health law. *The Psychiatrist*, **37**: 297–301.

Walsh E, Buchanan A, Fahy T (2002) Violence and schizophrenia: examining the evidence. *British Journal of Psychiatry*, **180**: 490–5.

Webster CD, Hucker SJ (2007) *Violence Risk Assessment and Management*. Wiley.

Webster CD, Martin ML, Brink J, *et al* (2009) *Short-Term Assessment of Risk and Treatability (START), Version 1.1*. British Columbia, Mental Health and Addiction Services and St Joseph's Healthcare.

Witt K, van Dorn R, Fazel S (2013) Risk factors for violence in psychosis: systematic review and meta-regression analysis of 110 studies. *PLoS ONE*, **8**: 2.

CHAPTER 27

Rehabilitation: an international perspective

Frank Holloway, Matthew Erlich and Lloyd I. Sederer

Introduction

Psychiatric rehabilitation has global relevance (Rossler, 2006). Our aim in this chapter is to offer an account of key trends in policy and practice internationally. Providing a brief but accurate account of the literature is fraught with difficulty. The day-to-day working of mental health services is dependent on a host of country-specific factors relating to the funding and organisation of health and social care, mental health legislation and policy, and the social and cultural context. (The significance of culture is discussed in detail in Chapter 28, 'Psychosocial rehabilitation across culture', which focuses on rehabilitation in low- and middle-income countries.) The lack of reliable data makes comparison between countries very difficult, as does the enormous disparity in the resources available to mental health services, even within a generally wealthy region such as Europe (Muijen, 2008; World Health Organization Mental Health Europe, 2008).

Much of what is written about rehabilitation and recovery, particularly at the policy level, comes across as rather abstract – full of positive sentiments but short on practicalities. To counteract this we provide some comparative data on key components of rehabilitative mental healthcare and end with a description of a large-scale service change in New York State that two of us (LIS and ME) have been involved in.

Core concepts in rehabilitation and recovery

There is a general consensus that psychiatric or psychosocial rehabilitation has as its goal helping people experiencing persistent and severe mental illness to live good lives as independently as possible (Rossler, 2006). In the past, rehabilitation was often seen as a stand-alone process offering selected technical interventions to people, either living within the traditional mental hospital or in the community, who were 'rehabilitation ready'. A more contemporary understanding sees rehabilitation as embedded within the fabric of health and social care services that work with the individual, his or her social network and the wider social context, with an overarching aim

409

of promoting social inclusion (Barbato, 2006). Rehabilitation and recovery are, in this sense, the business of all mental healthcare, although in practice specific rehabilitation services tend to become involved when the patient's journey to social inclusion has become stuck.

A useful contemporary definition of psychiatric rehabilitation, which was based on responses to a survey of rehabilitation practitioners in the UK, is:

> A whole system approach to recovery from mental ill health which maximizes an individual's quality of life and social inclusion by encouraging their skills, promoting independence and autonomy in order to give them hope for the future and which leads to successful community living through appropriate support. (Killaspy *et al*, 2005: p. 163)

As Farkas (2006) observed, psychiatric rehabilitation involves both evidence-based practice and values-based practice, which she states 'starts with the notion that recovery, or the taking back/regaining of a meaningful life has become ... the relevant mission of services' (p. 161). Recovery is a complex and, to an extent, contested concept (see Chapter 3, 'Rehabilitation as a values-led practice', for a more detailed discussion). The recovery focus on hope, functional gains, rehabilitation, shared decision-making and wellness management is increasingly part of mainstream psychiatric practice in North America, Australasia, the UK and Ireland. However, defining recovery is challenging and the concept is both profound and paradoxical. There are significant potential tensions between consumer versus clinical definitions of need, individualised recovery goals versus system-wide policies of psychosocial rehabilitation and the need for personalised assessment as well as widespread measurement across a population (Whitley & Drake, 2010; Slade & Davidson, 2011).

Rehabilitation, recovery and treatment guidelines

Guidelines for the treatment of people living with severe mental illness have been developed in many countries: a review published in 2005 identified 27 practice guidelines for schizophrenia from 21 countries (Gaebel *et al*, 2005). These guidelines, which are being continually updated, offer a reasonable though incomplete degree of consensus on pharmacological and psychosocial treatments, at the time of writing best summarised in the schizophrenia guideline produced in the UK by the National Institute for Health and Care Excellence (NICE, 2009).

Guidelines are not infallible and need to be viewed within a cultural and service context. As an example, the latest version of the PORT treatment recommendations, which emanate from the USA, identify a number of recommended psychosocial treatments (Kreyenbuhl *et al*, 2010): assertive community treatment (ACT); supported employment; skills training; cognitive–behavioural therapy; token-economy interventions; family-based services; psychosocial interventions for alcohol and substance misuse disorder; and psychosocial interventions for weight management. PORT treatment recommendations contain elements that are generally accepted and others that are contested. ACT, to be pedantic not a treatment but a mode of service delivery, has not been shown to be effective in European contexts where there are reasonably well developed community mental health services. The meta-analytic reviews underpinning successive schizophrenia guidelines from NICE have not supported the specific social skills training programmes that are so enthusiastically promoted in the USA (see National Collaborating Centre for Mental Health, 2010: p. 322). Token-economy programmes for people with schizophrenia were explored in the UK during the 1980s and failed to find a place in clinical practice. Part 2 of this book provides updates on treatment approaches that take full account of the evidence base but, crucially, offers suggestions where the evidence base becomes tenuous.

Although clinical practice guidelines for schizophrenia provide some support for specific interventions that may be used within rehabilitation services, they offer scant help for those seeking to design and operate rehabilitation services. 'Recovery-focused' interventions have yet to find their way into practice guidelines. The word 'rehabilitation' is not mentioned at all in the most recent guidelines published in the UK and the USA (NICE, 2009; Kreyenbuhl et al, 2010).[1] The Australian and New Zealand guideline repeatedly emphasises the importance of vocational rehabilitation and refers to the potential value of 'cognitive rehabilitation' (more commonly described as cognitive remediation) (Royal Australian and New Zealand College of Psychiatrists, 2005), as does the Canadian guideline (Canadian Psychiatric Association, 2005). Interestingly, the Canadian guideline notes the potential value of assessing cognitive function to help design psychosocial rehabilitation strategies for an individual and stresses the importance of optimising pharmacological treatments to support psychosocial and rehabilitation interventions, which suggests that contributors to that guideline had a sophisticated understanding of psychiatric rehabilitation.

The failure of guidelines to address rehabilitation and recovery is in part due to the methodology of contemporary guideline development, with its understandable emphasis on high-quality research and the primacy of the randomised controlled trial (RCT). The complex interventions involved in a whole-system approach to an individual's rehabilitation and recovery are not readily amenable to the RCT, although attempts are now being made to distil elements of good rehabilitation practice that can be assessed through an RCT (see Chapter 29, 'Expanding the evidence base').

---

1. The full British guideline (National Collaborating Centre for Mental Health, 2010) does endorse supported employment, a form of vocational rehabilitation, as a 'service level intervention', as does PORT (Kreyenbuhl et al, 2010).

Practice: what the literature tells us

Textbooks can legitimately go beyond the tyranny of the meta-analytic review by incorporating practical wisdom, which can include views on the organisation of services. Given the level of disability, distress and financial cost associated with severe mental illness there are surprisingly few textbooks devoted to psychiatric rehabilitation. Three relatively recently published books from the USA provide a useful scope to the field (Pratt *et al*, 2007; Corrigan *et al*, 2008; Liberman, 2008). There is a clear overlap between these texts, but there are also important differences in emphasis. All three acknowledge the power of the recovery narrative, underline the importance of actively involving the family in care (a rather obvious point in most cultures but clearly problematic for professionals in the USA and the UK) and the relevance of vocational rehabilitation and education. Liberman (2008) focuses on the fruits of a lifetime working in the field and provides a detailed discussion of the skills-based behavioural interventions he and his group have developed. Both Liberman (2008) and Corrigan *et al* (2008) describe at length ways of enhancing the person's illness self-management and touch on the issue of managing the cognitive impairment that is often associated with severe psychotic illness.

Pratt *et al* (2007) and Corrigan *et al* (2008) discuss the importance of peer support services, case management and assertive community treatment and housing options. Corrigan *et al* (2008) provide rather startling data that an estimated 5% of people with schizophrenia in the USA are living in shelters or on the streets, 6% are in prison, 8% in nursing homes and 18% in supported housing. A high but undetermined proportion of people in contact with public mental health services in the USA are living in supported housing (largely 'board-and-care homes'), which suggests that a significant degree of 'trans-institutionalisation' has taken place.

Day care has long been a central element of rehabilitation in the USA and is particularly associated with the Clubhouse movement, although its stock is currently falling in the face of support for vocational rehabilitation and individualised case management (Pratt *et al*, 2007). A day-care setting could offer a base for the provision of evidence-based psychosocial treatments, such as those advocated by Liberman (2008), but many authorities now doubt the efficacy of daily attendance at a centre for 'milieu therapy'.

Deinstitutionalisation

High-income countries, with the notable exception of Japan, have experienced a marked decline in psychiatric in-patient bed numbers (Holloway & Sederer, 2011). This decline started in the USA and the UK, which had a very large numbers of beds, in 1955. The timing, extent and pace of decline have varied, being very steep and beginning early in Australia and New Zealand (Whiteford & Buckingham, 2005) but starting later and proceeding much more gently in the Netherlands (van der Gaag, 2011), Belgium (de Hert *et al*, 2010) and Germany (Salize *et al*, 2007), which have at least equally advanced systems of health and social care. Deinstitutionalisation has been associated in many countries with the closure of large mental hospitals (asylums) and their replacement with in-patient care in smaller local psychiatric units, often within a general hospital setting. These are generalisations: in France the mental hospitals have not closed and remain the backbone of the mental healthcare system (Verdoux, 2007), while in Italy, following Law 180 passed in 1978, all the traditional mental hospitals have been closed (di Girolamo *et al*, 2007).

The striking failure of Japan to deinstitutionalise deserves brief comment. It appears to relate in part to the high levels of stigma associated with mental illness in Japan. This cannot be the only explanation, since stigma remains a serious problem for people living with mental illness throughout the world. One additional explanation is professional attitude: we know that the decline in bed numbers in the USA and the UK long predated changes in policy because professionals were keen to facilitate discharge, even at a time when community support after discharge was often inadequate. Another is the way that mental health services are provided and funded in Japan – funding is from the state but provision largely lies in the private sector, which at least until recently has had strong incentives to retain patients in hospital.

Trans-institutionalisation

Although in many countries the mental hospitals have closed, this has not meant that 'institutional' care for people living with severe mental illness has been abolished. For many people it means, rather, that the location of their institutional care has changed. Trans-institutionalisation is:

> A process whereby individuals, supposedly deinstitutionalized as a result of community care policies, in practice end up in different institutions, rather than their own homes. For example, the mentally ill who are discharged from, or no longer admitted to, mental hospitals are frequently found in prisons, boarding-houses, nursing-homes, and homes for the elderly. (Scott & Marshall, 2009)

In some countries, for example Germany and Italy, for many people 'deinstitutionalisation' meant not a move from a hospital to a community setting but the redesignation of the hospital unit as a residential or nursing care facility (Salize *et al*, 2007). As time has gone on, such units have taken in younger people with severe and intractable mental illness (Franz *et al*, 2010).

Much has been written about the displacement of people with a mental illness into the criminal justice system, particularly in the USA. More significant in numerical terms has been the development of nursing and residential care homes, which have the potential to be just as, if not more, institutionalised than in-patient mental health services. In some European countries the decline in in-patient psychiatric beds since the 1980s has been matched bed for bed by alternative forms of residential care and dedicated forensic psychiatric provision (Priebe *et al*, 2005, 2008).

Mental health policy

All wealthy countries have laws and policies surrounding the care and treatment of people with a mental illness. The World Health Organization (WHO) has identified the elaboration of a legal and policy framework as an essential first step in the development of effective mental health services. A WHO European Ministerial Conference on Mental Health, held in Helsinki in 2005, agreed a Mental Health Declaration for Europe, which set out a number of priorities and actions (reproduced in WHO, 2008).[2] In its preamble, which is clearly influenced by the tenets of psychosocial rehabilitation, it states: 'We believe that the primary aim of mental health activity is to enhance people's well-being and functioning by focusing on their strengths and resources, reinforcing resilience and enhancing protective external factors'. One of the five priorities for reform and modernisation of mental healthcare that the ministers endorsed is to 'design and implement comprehensive, integrated and efficient mental health systems that cover promotion, prevention, treatment and rehabilitation, care and recovery'. Health ministers acknowledged a need for 'comprehensive evidence-based mental health policies ... aimed at achieving [the] mental well-being and social inclusion of people with mental health problems'. Although high-level policy in Europe strongly supports deinstitutionalisation and the development of rehabilitation services, its very patchy implementation was demonstrated in a survey of policy and practice undertaken by the WHO (2008).

The development and implementation of policy is likely to be more complex in countries with a devolved or federal constitution than in unitary states: there is no national mental health policy *per se* in, for example, Germany, Spain and the UK, where responsibility for healthcare is devolved. Australia, which is a commonwealth of states, each with its own department of health, has produced a National Mental Health Plan, now in its fourth iteration (Australian Health Ministers, 2009); leverage into the Australian states is partly intellectual and partly financial, since central government finances are available to reimburse particular programmes. Despite this leverage, and the generally rapid and profound deinstitutionalisation that occurred in Australia, the extent of deinstitutionalisation and the development of community support services are very variable between states and territories (Department of Health and Ageing, 2010), Similar variability, in terms of both bed reductions and the development of

---

2. The WHO European Region includes 53 countries, stretching from Iceland to the Russian Federation.

alternative community-based services, is apparent between the Canadian provinces (Sealy & Whitehead, 2004).

The US healthcare system is highly complex, with a plethora of commissioners and providers and multiple funding sources, including private (usually employment-based) insurance. Public funding is focused on people with more severe illnesses, who would not otherwise receive treatment (Patel & Wells, 2009). The Federal Government in the USA has leverage on state mental health policies through reimbursement of Medicare and Medicaid, together with Federal funding streams for vocational rehabilitation, housing and disability income support (Corrigan *et al*, 2008: ch. 21), but provision varies enormously across the country (National Alliance on Mental Illness, 2009).

The Australian Mental Health Plan (Australian Health Ministers, 2009) offers little detail about rehabilitation services (they are mentioned only three times in an 89-page document). In contrast, the Plan discusses recovery at great length (it is mentioned 55 times) and makes 'Recovery and Social Inclusion' its first priority. With the notable exception of Ireland (Department of Health and Children, 2006), this failure to describe rehabilitation services is typical of policy in Anglophone countries. The 2010 mental health policy produced by the UK government mentions rehabilitation only three times in the text (in the context of the rehabilitation of offenders, vocational rehabilitation for people with minor mental disorders and care of the elderly) (Department of Health, 2010) but English policy documents on recovery abound.

Policy documents that draw together rehabilitation psychiatry and the recovery paradigm are uncommon. One Australian state, South Australia, has developed an exemplary document that sets out a 'Framework for recovery-oriented rehabilitation in mental health care' (Mental Health and Substance Abuse Division, 2012). We describe below the process of introducing recovery-oriented rehabilitation practice into New York State's mental health system.

Israel is unique in having specific legislation supporting psychiatric rehabilitation (Homik-Lurie *et al*, 2012).[3] The law defines a 'basket' of rehabilitation services that 'attempts to address the key disadvantages consumers often face by providing them with services that focus on building skills, and support in the domains such as work, recreation, education, social life and housing'.

There is good evidence that legislation and policy can make a difference to provision. In England the NHS Plan, which was closely performance-managed by the Department of Health, led to an enormous expansion in specific services, such as assertive outreach and early intervention in psychosis (Mental Health Strategies, 2013). In Israel following the enactment of the 2001 law on psychiatric rehabilitation, the number of

---

3. The law has the less than politically correct title 'Rehabilitation of the Mentally Disabled in the Community Law of 2001'.

people in receipt of the defined rehabilitation services increased from 4600 in 2001 to 16 000 in 2008, with a marked decrease in the number of patients spending over a year in a psychiatric hospital (Homik-Lurie *et al*, 2012).

Mental health services and psychiatric rehabilitation

The concept of psychiatric rehabilitation is internationally recognised but is not commonly the subject of specific policy, let alone legislation. All high-income countries do provide rehabilitation services that, at a minimum, include long-term residential care and some form of day care. Only one country, Italy, has reported that it does not have any long-stay psychiatric beds. Community support services (often provided by a community mental health team or community mental health centre with a defined catchment area) are uniformly available but may or may not have an identifiable focus on rehabilitation and recovery. In some countries, particularly vulnerable people receive an enhanced level of community support through assertive community treatment (ACT), although the benefits of ACT are less apparent where the general level of community mental healthcare is better.

In-patient beds

The dominant narrative surrounding mental health services over the past 50 years is one of deinstitutionalisation. However, a significant proportion of in-patient beds is still taken up by people who are 'long stay' (over 1 year). Obtaining accurate data on the numbers of 'long stay' patients, who have become stuck within the mental health system, is difficult. Routinely available statistics do not provide specific information on the numbers of 'long stay' patients and the services that they receive.

In Germany, which has a large number of in-patient beds, an estimate of the proportion of 'long stay' beds, at 2.5% (Salize *et al*, 2007), is both implausibly low and artificially decreased by the redesignation of hospital beds as 'psychiatric homes' in the grounds of mental hospitals (Franz *et al*, 2010). Many residents in these homes are required to live there under guardianship legislation, which is equivalent to detention under mental health legislation in other countries. In France, which has a comparatively large number of beds, studies report between 25% and 41% of in-patients are 'long stay' (Chapireau, 2005; Verdoux, 2007).

In some countries designated 'long stay' beds are predominantly within forensic mental health services. Forensic beds may be administratively completely separate from mainstream mental health services, as is the case in Germany (Salize *et al*, 2007), which has the highest number of forensic beds in Europe. Italy has closed its public psychiatric hospitals other than its six forensic hospitals (Preti *et al*, 2008), but there remains a flourishing private hospital sector in Italy,

We do have detailed data on in-patient rehabilitation services in England (Killaspy *et al*, 2005, 2013) and Ireland (Ijaz *et al*, 2011; Lavelle *et al*, 2011) (see Chapter 17, 'Rehabilitation in hospital settings'). The Irish data include non-hospital high- and medium-support accommodation, which for historical reasons are provided by the Health Service, but these data do not allow for meaningful cross-national comparisons.

Supported and sheltered accommodation

There is a wide range of 'community' accommodation for people with a severe mental illness, from what are essentially rebadged psychiatric hospital wards to individual tenancies with 'floating' support (see Chapter 19, 'Housing: a place to live'). There is abundant evidence that high-support residential care is very significantly institutional in character; in Italy, Germany and Australia, there is a low probability of residents moving into less supported accommodation (di Girilamo *et al*, 2002; Franz *et al*, 2010; Meehan *et al*, 2011).

The need for supported housing will depend in part on the expectation that families will provide care and support for a family member with a mental illness or disability and societal aspirations for young people to achieve independent living, which are very high in wealthy Anglophone countries and northern Europe. In southern Europe people with schizophrenia are much more likely to live with families than alone, although this has been associated with increased difficulties and distress for families (Becker *et al*, 2002). Although in some countries, such as Ireland, supported accommodation is provided through the health service, in general it is provided by either local authorities or non-governmental organisations (NGOs).

Good practice in long-term mental healthcare

Taylor *et al* (2009) carried out a systematic review of what constitutes best practice in the institutional care of people with longer-term mental health problems. They identified a limited number of specific interventions (cognitive–behavioural therapy, family psychoeducation and supported employment) that should be available, as well as a range of characteristics of the setting, for example a flexible regime, decent accommodation and good working relationships between residents and staff. This review fed into the development of the Quality Indicator for Rehabilitative Care (QuIRC) (see Chapter 17, 'Rehabilitation in hospital settings'). QuIRC provides data on the quality of care for people living in very-high-support long-term care. Developed in a study funded by the European Union involving ten countries, it assesses seven quality domains (the built environment; the therapeutic environment; treatments and interventions; self-management and autonomy; social interface; human rights; and recovery-oriented practice). It offers the potential for benchmarking units against national norms (there are differences in QuIRC scores between countries). Institutional quality in the QuIRC domains is related to service users' experience of care and autonomy, with some evidence that patients in hospital-based units had poorer experiences of care (Killaspy *et al*, 2012). The same project also found substantial differences across European countries in the user experience, with users of long-term high-support care reporting the most positive experience of care in England and the Netherlands (White & Taylor, 2011).

A study of psychosocial rehabilitation in Belgium, which in common with many northern European countries has a relatively large number of psychiatric beds, provides detailed information on the services available to people with schizophrenia (de Hert *et al*, 2010). Access to the wide range of rehabilitation services and psychosocial treatments identified by the authors as representing best practice was found to be better in services based in psychiatric hospitals than in those based in general hospitals and ambulatory care settings. There was a much broader range of staff involved in rehabilitation based in the psychiatric hospitals, which had access to more community-based supported accommodation, offered more training in living skills and provided more specific psychosocial treatments.

A European Union publication (de Almeida & Killaspy, 2011) provides vignettes of exemplary services in particular catchment areas in Italy, Spain, Sweden and France. Each is unique, and indeed generally atypical of other areas in their respective countries. Common themes of good practice are ending reliance on traditional mental hospitals and developing local mental health services that have strong links to local communities and local government. Characteristically, there is a strong emphasis on providing access to occupational and vocational services, again usually provided by NGOs rather than the state sector.

Rehabilitation and recovery: lessons from New York State

The overall picture of mental health provision in the USA is one of fragmented care (and for some people no care at all) (Hogan, 2008). People with severe mental illness have, as in many countries, very poor employment opportunities, lack affordable housing and experience frighteningly high levels of physical comorbidity.

In common with the rest of the USA, deinstitutionalisation in New York State has been very marked: state hospital in-patient numbers decreased from 93 314 in 1955 to 11 717 in 1994. In 2011, the daily hospital census for people aged over 18 in receipt of public mental healthcare was 7167, of whom just under 3000 were in state psychiatric centres; almost all the rest were in psychiatric units in general hospitals (New York State Office of Mental Health, 2013*a*).

As the state hospital sector has declined, community-based services have expanded. The sheer complexity of mental healthcare is illustrated in the 'Program Definitions' listed by the Office of Mental Health of New York State (OMH). In all, 74 types of programme are included, covering emergency and crisis care, in-patient care, out-patient care (which includes a wide range of non-hospital services, such as assertive community treatment, case management teams and out-patient clinics), residential services, education, forensic services, self-help, general support, vocational services and care coordination (New York State Office of Mental Health, 2013b). These services are overseen by the OMH, which licenses, regulates and to an extent funds mental health services. Providers operate in a very complex contractual and financial environment.[4]

Up until the 1990s, a central element of the community care system was community day treatment (CDT). CDT programmes were funded through Federal Medicaid payments and ostensibly provided rehabilitation and clinical care in a 'partial hospitalisation' setting. Unfortunately CDT programmes were unable to demonstrate a capacity to return patients to independent functioning in the community (Becker *et al*, 2001). They also failed to show that they were using evidence-based practices or developing person-centred care plans.

Developing and implementing personalised recovery-oriented services

The OMH has used its regulatory and financial powers to introduce a programme that encourages recovery-oriented practice, aims to rationalise a fragmented out-patient landscape and prioritises best practices, within a new service model – personalised recovery-oriented services (PROS) (New York State Office of Mental Health, 2013c). PROS is the largest recovery-oriented programme of its kind with, at the time of writing, over 70 programmes across New York State serving over 10 000 consumers. These are large numbers, but need to be put in the context. In 2011, of 140 000 adults using public mental health services in New York per week, 29 000 were receiving residential services, 10 000 in-patient care, 93 000 out-patient services and 33 000 'support' (New York State Office of Mental Health, 2013d).

The PROS programme was developed after consideration by policy-makers of four questions. How can we incorporate individualised treatment goals and evidence-based practices that are attainable and measurable on a statewide level? How can economic incentives foster a statewide recovery-oriented programme? What is the best approach to disincentivise the underperforming, yet at the time profitable CDT programmes? Should recovery-oriented services of varying intensity (e.g. acute out-patient stabilisation versus employment training) be combined under 'one roof'?

---

4. Readers from outside the USA can experience this complexity by accessing the PROS website, http://www.omh.ny.gov/omhweb/pros, which includes detailed information on bidding, contracting and funding of services.

One essential element of PROS is the individualised recovery plan (IRP), within which consumers communicate their goals, strengths and barriers with a mental health counsellor to shape their own path towards recovery. Family members can be a part of this process. The first IRP must be made within the first 30 days of admission. The second IRP should be completed after the first 3 months and include a relapse-prevention plan with recovery goals. Throughout, shared decision-making is at the forefront of the IRP. PROS offers four pathways (see Box 27.1). In principle, consumers select their own pathway based upon the intensity of intervention needed to meet their goals. The components of PROS are influenced by statements of best practice in psychosocial rehabilitation as identified within a US context (see for example Farkas & Anthony, 2010).

Box 27.1 The four components of PROS

(1) Intensive rehabilitation (IR)

This component is a time-sensitive 'immediate need' service for a consumer with acute stabilisation requirements. Interventions are provided within the PROS programme at an individual and/or group level that focus upon relapse prevention, short-term intensive goal acquisition, and emergent needs. This is the PROS' highest level of care, similar in ethos to the original community day treatment, but it is time-limited and only a small proportion of the PROS consumers are allowed into this component.

(2) Community rehabilitation and support (CRS)

These individualised and/or group services are designed to help individuals re-acclimatise into the community (i.e. developing or re-establishing supports, financial management skills, restoring wellness-promoting skills, and assisting individuals to manage their mental health conditions). This component builds upon the Clubhouse model, with the primacy of person-centred care and peer supports. Evidence-based practices are delivered (integrated dual-disorder treatment, wellness self-management programmes, cognitive–behavioural therapy, peer support programmes, to name but a few). The length of stay in this component is longer than with IR, but also time-limited. Also, in this component, a consumer may train to become a compensated peer provider.

(3) Ongoing rehabilitation and support (ORS)

This component is primarily off-site and the consumer receives on-site assistance with skills training and support centred upon maintaining a job and promoting positive relationships with co-workers, friends and family, and the larger community.

(4) Clinical treatment (CT)

Clinical treatment is an optional component in PROS programme design. All PROS are licensed, but not all PROS have intensive rehabilitation and clinical treatment services. Consumers have the option to pursue clinical treatment and symptom management with supervised credentialed staff as well as physical health integration at the PROS, or they may use an out-patient provider outside of the PROS.

The PROS programmes must be financially viable and consequentially were designed to receive Medicaid reimbursements for the evidence-based services that are required within the service definition. The OMH, through its ability to license PROS, seeks to ensure the provision of quality recovery-oriented mental health services. Former CDT programmes that could not offer the range of services expected within PROS faced closure.

There are limitations to PROS. While vocational support is integral to PROS, supported housing is not, though referral resources to supported housing are robust. Consumers with severe mental illness who require services beyond intensive rehabilitation cannot remain in a PROS programme: they must be referred to day hospital programmes, an ACT team, intensive case management programmes or in-patient care. There is also a limited requirement for involvement of a psychiatrist (or nurse practitioner) within a PROS programme: the licensed clinical treatment team must include one full-time psychiatrist or nurse practitioner per 320 patients.

At the time of writing there is no published academic description or study regarding the implementation or the effectiveness of PROS. It remains unclear whether PROS will significantly reduce rehospitalisations, improve consumer satisfaction, lead to increased gains in functional status (i.e. employment, social skills, relationships) and improve engagement in self-care and wellness. However, in New York State the pendulum has swung – the state mental health authority has shifted its priorities from custodial to recovery-oriented care. In summary, we see recovery as an integrated approach that fulfils the goals of the consumer, clinician and mental health policy-maker alike. Recovery is the means to 'wellness management', where living *well* means a manageable illness compatible with a life filled with hope and aspirations, manageable pain and suffering, and opportunities for work, school and relationships (Sederer, 2013). The PROS programme is centralised but not prescriptive, it is individually tailored to the consumer's needs and preferences, and it embodies hope. Implementing person-centred care, recovery-oriented programmes and accountability in a large public health arena takes will, time and hard work. However, we anticipate that PROS signals the next chapter in recovery-oriented programmes and mental health policy in 21st-century America.

Conclusions

In this chapter we have provided a very brief overview of international trends in policy and practice relating to rehabilitation and recovery. Deinstitutionalisation is universally supported, although in some countries at least the process has involved a significant degree of 'trans-institutionalisation'. Although policy supports psychiatric or psychosocial rehabilitation, these concepts are often not clearly articulated in policy documents. There is a clear trend towards the development of 'recovery-oriented' services for people living with severe mental illness in Anglophone countries; however, there is less evidence of the penetration of the tenets of recovery into other countries with advanced health and social care systems.

References

Australian Health Ministers (2009) *Fourth National Mental Health Plan: An Agenda for Collaborative Government Action in Mental Health 2009–2014*. Commonwealth of Australia. At http://www.health.gov.au/internet/main/publishing.nsf/Content/mental-pubs-f-plan09 (accessed December 2014).

Barbato A (2006) Psychosocial rehabilitation and severe mental disorders: a public health approach. *World Psychiatry*, **5**: 162–3.

Becker DR, Bond GR, McCarthy D, *et al* (2001) Converting day treatment centers to supported employment programs in Rhode Island. *Psychiatric Services*, **52**: 351–7.

Becker T, Knapp M, Knudsen HC, *et al* (2002) The EPSILON Study – a study of care for people with schizophrenia in five European countries. *World Psychiatry*, **1**: 45–7.

Canadian Psychiatric Association (2005) Clinical Practice guidelines. Treatment of schizophrenia. *Canadian Journal of Psychiatry*, **50** (suppl 1).

Chapireau F (2005) Les nouveaux longs séjours en établissements de soins spécialisés en psychiatrie: résultats d'une enquête nationale sur un échantillon représentatif (1998–2000) [Old and new long-stay patients in French psychiatric institutions: results from a national random survey with two-year follow-up.] *Encephale*, **31**: 466–76.

Corrigan P, Mueser K, Bond G, *et al* (2008) *Principles and Practice of Psychiatric Rehabilitation: An Empirical Approach*. Guilford Press.

de Almeida JMC, Killaspy H (2011) *Long-Term Mental Health Care for People with Severe Mental Disorders*. European Union. At http://ec.europa.eu/health/mental_health/docs/healthcare_mental_disorders_en.pdf (accessed December 2014).

de Hert M, Detraux J, Peuskens J (2010) Practice of and services for psychosocial rehabilitation of people with schizophrenia in Belgium. *Journal of Psychopathology*, **16**: 255–65.

Department of Health (2010) *No Health Without Mental Health*. Department of Health.

Department of Health and Ageing (2010) *National Mental Health Report 2010: Summary of 15 Years of reform in Australia's Mental Health Services under the National Mental Health Strategy 1993–2008*. Commonwealth of Australia.

Department of Health and Children (2006) *A Vision for Change. Report of the Expert Group on Mental Health Services*. TSO (The Stationery Office).

di Girilamo G, Picardi A, Micciolo R, *et al* (2002) Residential care in Italy. National survey of non-hospital facilities. *British Journal of Psychiatry*, **181**: 220–8.

di Girilamo G, Bassi M, Neri G, *et al* (2007) The current state of mental health care in Italy: problems, perspectives and lessons to learn. *European Archives of Psychiatry and Clinical Neuroscience*, **257**: 83–91.

Farkas M (2006) Identifying psychosocial rehabilitation interventions: an evidence and value based practice. *World Psychiatry*, **5**: 161–2.

Farkas M, Anthony WA (2010) Psychiatric rehabilitation interventions: a review. *International Review of Psychiatry*, **22**: 114–29.

Franz M, Meyer T, Dubowy M, *et al* (2010) Accumulation of 'new' long-stay patients in homes being part of psychiatric hospitals: a challenge for psychiatric care. *Psychiatrische Praxis*, **37**: 240–7.

Gaebel W, Weinmann S, Sartorius N, *et al* (2005) Schizophrenia practice guidelines: international survey and comparison. *British Journal of Psychiatry*, **187**: 248–55.

Hogan M (2008) Transforming mental health care: realities, priorities and prospects. *Psychiatric Clinics of North America*, **31**: 1–9.

Holloway F, Sederer LI (2011) Inpatient treatment. In *Textbook of Community Mental Health* (eds G Thornicroft, *et al*): 167–77. Oxford University Press.

Homik-Lurie T, Zilber N, Lerner Y (2012) Trends in the use of rehabilitation services in the community by people with mental disabilities in Israel; the factors involved. *Israel Journal of Health Policy Research*, **1**: 24.

Ijaz A, Killaspy H, Holloway F, *et al* (2011) Mental health rehabilitation services in Ireland: vision and reality. *Irish Journal of Psychological Medicine*, **28** (2): 69–75.

Killaspy H, Harden C, Holloway F, *et al* (2005) What do mental health rehabilitation services do and what are they for? A national survey in England. *Journal of Mental Health*, **14**: 157–65.

Killaspy H, White S, Wright C, *et al* (2012) Quality of longer term mental health facilities in Europe: validation of the Quality Indicator for Rehabilitative Care against service users' views. *PLoS ONE*, **7** (6): e38070.

Killaspy H, Marston L, Omar RZ, *et al* (2013) Service quality and clinical outcomes: an example from mental health rehabilitation services in England. *British Journal of Psychiatry*, **202**: 28–34.

Kreyenbuhl J, Buchanan RW, Dickerson FB, *et al* (2010) The Schizophrenia Patient Outcomes Research Team (PORT): updated treatment recommendations 2009. *Schizophrenia Bulletin*, **36**: 94–103.

Lavelle E, Ijaz A, Killaspy H, *et al* (2011) *Mental Health Rehabilitation and Recovery Services in Ireland: A Multicentre Study of Current Service Provision, Characteristics of Service Users and Outcomes for Those With and Without Access to These Services. Final Report.* Mental Health Commission of Ireland.

Liberman RP (2008) *Recovery From Disability: Manual of Psychiatric Rehabilitation.* American Psychiatric Publishing.

Meehan T, Stedman T, Robertson S, *et al* (2011) Does supported accommodation improve clinical and social outcomes for people with severe psychiatric disability? The Project 300 Experience. *Australian and New Zealand Journal of Psychiatry*, **45**: 586–92.

Mental Health Strategies (2013) *2011/12 National Survey of Investment in Adult Mental Health Services.* At https://www.gov.uk/government/publications/investment-in-mental-health-in-2011-to-2012-working-age-adults-and-older-adults (accessed 8 September 2014).

Mental Health and Substance Abuse Division (2012) *The Framework for Recovery-Oriented Rehabilitation in Mental Health Care.* SA Health.

Muijen M (2008) Mental health services in Europe: an overview. *Psychiatric Services*, **59**: 479–82.

National Alliance on Mental Illness (2009) *Grading the States 2009. A Report on America's Health Care System for Adults with Serious Mental Illness.* National Alliance on Mental Illness.

National Collaborating Centre for Mental Health (2010) *Schizophrenia* (National Clinical Guideline Number 82). British Psychological Association.

National Institute for Health and Clinical Excellence (2009) *Schizophrenia: Core Interventions in the Treatment and Management of Schizophrenia in Adults in Primary and Secondary Care* (Clinical Guideline 82). NICE.

New York State Office of Mental Health (2013*a*) County Mental Health Profile. MH Inpatient Use. At http://bi.omh.ny.gov/cmhp/dashboard#tab4 (accessed 12 September 2013).

New York State Office of Mental Health (2013*b*) Mental Health Program Directory. At: http://bi.omh.ny.gov/bridges/definitions (accessed 12 September 2013).

New York State Office of Mental Health (2013*c*) Personalized Recovery Oriented Services. At http://www.omh.ny.gov/omhweb/pros (accessed 12 September 2013).

New York State Office of Mental Health (2013*d*) County Mental Health Profiles. Mental Health Service Use. At http://bi.omh.ny.gov/cmhp/dashboard#tab2 (accessed December 2014).

Patel K, Wells K (2009) Applying health care reform principles to mental health and substance abuse services. *JAMA*, **302**: 1463–72.

Pratt C W, Gill K, Barrett NM, *et al* (2007) *Psychiatric Rehabilitation* (2nd edn). Academic Press.

Preti A, Picardi A, Fioritti A, *et al* (2008) A comparison between former forensic and non-forensic patients living in psychiatric residential facilities. A national survey in Italy. *Journal of Forensic Psychiatry and Psychology*, **19**: 108–28.

Priebe S, Badesconyi A, Fioritti A, *et al* (2005) Reinstitutionalisation in mental health care: comparison of data on service provision from six European countries. *BMJ*, **330**: 123–6.

Priebe S, Frottier P, Gaddini A, *et al* (2008) Mental health care institutions in nine European countries, 2002–2006. *Psychiatric Services*, **59**: 570–3.

Rossler W (2006) Psychiatric rehabilitation today: an overview. *World Psychiatry*, **5**: 151–7.

Royal Australian and New Zealand College of Psychiatrists (2005) Royal Australian and New Zealand College of Psychiatrists clinical practice guidelines for the treatment of schizophrenia and related disorders. *Australian and New Zealand Journal of Psychiatry*, **39**: 1–30.

Salize HJ, Rossler W, Becker T (2007) Mental health care in Germany. Current state and trends. *European Archives of Psychiatry and Clinical Neurology*, **257**: 92–103.

Scott J, Marshall G (2009) *A Dictionary of Sociology*. Oxford University Press.

Sealy P, Whitehead PC (2004) Forty years of deinstitutionalization of psychiatric services in Canada: an empirical assessment. *Canadian Journal of Psychiatry*, **49**: 249–57.

Sederer LI (2013) *The Family Guide to Mental Health Care*. WW Norton.

Slade M, Davidson L (2011) Recovery as an integrative paradigm in mental health. In *The Oxford Textbook of Community Mental Health* (eds G Thornicroft, G Szmukler, KT Mueser, *et al*): 26–33. Oxford University Press.

Taylor TL, Killaspy H, Wright C, *et al* (2009) A systematic review of the international published literature relating to quality of institutional care for people with longer term mental health problems. *BMC Psychiatry*, **9**: 55.

van der Gaag RJ (2011) Mental health 'cure and care' in the Netherlands: risks and opportunities. *International Review of Psychiatry*, **23**: 113–17.

Verdoux H (2007) The current state of adult mental health care in France. *European Archives of Psychiatry and Clinical Neuroscience*, **257**: 64–70.

White S, Taylor, T (2011) Service users in longer term rehabilitative care across Europe: what are their experiences of care? *Psychiatrische Praxis*, **38**: S08-3-EC.

Whiteford HA, Buckingham WJ (2005) Ten years of mental health service reform in Australia: are we getting it right? *Medical Journal of Australia*, **182**: 396–400.

Whitley R, Drake RE (2010) Recovery: a dimensional approach. *Psychiatric Services*, **61**: 1248–50.

WHO (2008) *Policies and Practices for Mental Health in Europe – Meeting Challenges*. World Health Organization Mental Health Europe.

CHAPTER 28

Psychosocial rehabilitation across culture: the experience in low- and middle-income countries

Rangaswamy Thara and Dinesh Bhugra

Introduction

Access to and delivery of mental healthcare in the professional sector has major problems in low- and middle-income countries (LMICs). There are a number of reasons for this, and a lack of human and financial resources is only one of many problems. Specialist services are often not available or are difficult to set up, which may be related to a shortage of specialists and the stigma surrounding mental ill-health. Psychosocial rehabilitation (PSR), which is resource-intensive, often does not feature high on the healthcare agenda. Other factors may include a lack of understanding of the role that rehabilitation plays in recovery and integration within the larger society. An understanding of serious mental illness and its ramifications may also affect the establishment of services. In many LMICs clear mental health policies may not be available, and this makes accessing resources more difficult. Consequently, patients and their families may be discouraged from seeking help and clinicians may find it difficult to engage with people who are severely mentally ill. Patients and their families may focus on expectations of cure rather than living with disability. These expectations may discourage some individuals and their carers from seeking rehabilitation and from providing the required long-term engagement. Mental health and mental illness are strongly underpinned by biological substrate but also by cultural and social factors. Psychosocial rehabilitation has widespread psychological, social, cultural, behavioural, spiritual and even physical health ramifications.

Cultures are common shared heritages and belief systems which give meaning to an individual. Cultural values inevitably influence an individual's world view and also cognitions. Cultures also mould an individual's inner world, thereby influencing responses to the external world. Hence it is essential for clinicians to understand individual patients' idioms of distress, explanatory models and world view if they are to be engaged successfully in any therapeutic endeavour. Beliefs about sickness, behaviours exhibited by those who are sick and the expectations of their treatment, and the responses to such individuals by families and societies are all aspects of the social reality within which we all live. A major aspect of any understanding of the healthcare system depends upon a clear understanding of a culture's chief sources of power (social, political, mythological, religious, technological, etc.). This knowledge will ensure that clinicians are aware of what models of illness are likely to be more common and will enable them to recognise beliefs about the causes of illness and how cultures deal with illness and those affected. This social reality needs to be differentiated from the psychological, biological and physical realities of the culture. Culture plays a key role in defining deviance, where help is sought from and who is the first port of call, and subsequent sources of help. These depend upon available health resources, which are dictated by cultures and societies. The way culture responds to certain behaviours will also influence whether patients and their families are willing to engage in rehabilitation.

Culture teaches other members of the community (at large or those around the patient) about acceptable emotional outlets and cathartic strategies. Dealing with sick members is part of the process and the cultural environment affects whether people who are sick or ill are isolated, marginalised or treated with respect. Cultures may allow sick individuals to shed stresses associated with their social roles and may create a gratifying environment in which ill individuals and their families can cope. There are key stakeholders at the policy and governmental levels who must be involved. These stakeholders include those working not only in health but also in social welfare, education, labour, employment agencies and law. Therefore, it is critical that all stakeholders are involved in the process of determining resources and healthcare policies, and that there is joined-up thinking regarding policy development.

In Western and high-income countries, psychiatric rehabilitation has acquired prominence in the past couple of decades from both clinical and academic perspectives, whereas the data from LMICs are still scant. In this chapter we draw largely on experience and evidence from Asian LMICs. It is clear that across different cultural settings and even within the same country there are variations in the understanding and delivery of rehabilitation services. The very diverse methods and processes of intervention have few principles in common. Many non-governmental organisations (NGOs) provide psychosocial rehabilitation.

It is apparent that in this field the countries of the southern hemisphere have, for a variety of reasons, not kept pace with their northern counterparts. These differences can be attributed to both cultural and resource variations. Inevitably, these factors affect the attitudes of clinicians as well as of other stakeholders, as rehabilitation is not seen as sufficiently exciting or rewarding. Often, rehabilitation is seen simply as a part of occupational therapy, where such facilities are available. In spite of being free of the effects of institutionalisation, in south Asian LMICs psychiatric rehabilitation is still not considered attractive enough to merit the attention of mental health professionals. Consequently, in healthcare policy itself psychosocial rehabilitation is not given the prominence it deserves. In LMICs, therefore,

PSR is often provided by NGOs. We illustrate this below with some examples.

The nature and principles of PSR interventions

Psychosocial rehabilitation is about facilitating the adequate performance of the social roles expected of a person with a disability in the areas of self-care, marital and parental roles, extended social roles and occupational role. Integrated and standardised programmes exist that provide interventions so that the disabling impact of severe mental disorders on the sufferer can be reduced. Many of these well researched programmes (Test & Stein, 1977; Anthony & Farkas, 1982; Anthony et al, 1988a, 1988b) are also reflections of local healthcare systems and therefore are often not easily applicable elsewhere. However, some common features can be modified and these components include: medication management training, cognitive retraining, and vocational rehabilitation and support.

Medication management training (MMT) is usually done in a personalised setting on a one-on-one basis, but it is not unusual to find more didactic forms of instruction being used as well to increase adherence. Different cultures see the role of medicine differently and ethnopsychopharmacology will guide the clinicians. It is well known that different ethnic and racial groups will respond in different ways to medication dosages and sociocultural models of what medicine does to people. For example, individuals in many cultures believe in the notion that hot or cold medicines have different actions on different organs in the body. In order to counter these effects, patients also expect dietary restrictions while on medication.

Cognitive retraining is usually one of the first-level PSR interventions. This includes giving information to patients, challenging any misconceptions they may have of their symptoms, illness or potential therapeutic interventions. It is basic information provided in very simple language. In addition, according to the cultural perspective, patients may be given specific information about their social roles and role expectations and how they might be able to deal with their functioning in social, personal and occupational domains. The strategy includes behavioural interventions which are more likely to be acceptable culturally. These skills need to be culturally appropriate and culturally sensitive.

Vocational rehabilitation is a critical element of PSR in many LMICs, where there may be no significant disability welfare benefits available for people who are severely mentally ill and a substantial part of treatment costs will be borne by the families. However, much vocational rehabilitation is confined to work in sheltered conditions to foster a work habit rather than skill acquisition. The process of job placement and support is not well organised. The possibilities of supported employment are often limited in these countries.

Locations for PSR

There have been local initiatives in many countries to manage the gap between the need for and the delivery of mental health services. PSR programmes have been organised in state-run hospitals and centres, at home, in the community and most effectively by NGOs. In this chapter we aim to provide an overview of the special factors and issues that may affect psychosocial rehabilitation as well as the role the NGOs play in LMICs.

Mental health services in the south Asian region include large very old mental hospitals, many of which need constant upgrading of their infrastructure and services, psychiatry departments in general hospitals with a large out-patient turnover, and smaller private clinics, which use predominantly psychopharmacological interventions. Some mental hospitals in India do offer limited rehabilitation programmes, according to a report by the National Human Rights Commission (1999); there appears to have been little change since that report. These programmes are further hampered by the fact that they are isolated geographically and have little or no contact with outside communities.

Non-governmental organisations have filled the gap in PSR by delivering a plethora of services, including care, treatment, rehabilitation, education, awareness, community outreach, advocacy and human rights (Thara & John, 2012). Some of these NGOs have deservedly gained international recognition for their work and have acted as good role models. Intense and focused work, credibility, closeness to the communities they serve, and the capacity to innovate and network are the some of the positive aspects of these NGOs. They are also closer to the local culture and communities, thereby being aware of subtle cultural nuances and expectations. Although there are many documented NGOs providing PSR, there has been little evaluation of their effectiveness (Thara & John, 2012). Some NGOs do not last long, owing to a lack of sustainability and transparency, high staff turnover and burnout. There has been a recent worrying trend in the development of small unregistered and unmonitored facilities delivering poor-quality care.

Community care and PSR

In most countries of the south Asian region, community care centres for people who are severely mentally ill are meager (Thara & Padmavati, 2013). In fact, the absence of such services in the community has been a deterrent to the closure of large mental hospitals. Families and not the state are still the major carers for such people in many LMICs.

In the past few years, studies have attempted to look at community-based interventions for this group. One such, the Community Care for People with Schizophrenia in India (COPSI), was a multisite, parallel-group, randomised controlled trial in three centres in India which compared a facility-based intervention with one involving trained community health workers. A 1-year follow-up revealed that lay workers were able to offer simple rehabilitation measures aimed at patients and families that were marginally more effective than those offered by a psychiatrist alone (Chatterjee et al, 2011; Balaji et al, 2012).

The MANAS intervention, another study that tested the effectiveness of an intervention led by lay health counsellors in primary care settings, looked at outcomes for people with common mental disorders in 24 primary care facilities (12 public, 12 private) in Goa (India). This also concluded that trained lay counsellors working within a collaborative care model can reduce the prevalence of common mental disorders, suicidal behaviour, psychological morbidity and disability days among those attending public primary care facilities (Patel et al, 2010).

Home-based interventions

In the past few decades, a few studies have looked at home care for patients with schizophrenia. In one by Pai & Kapur (1983), 27 patients diagnosed with schizophrenia suffering their first episode of illness and who had not received any prior medical treatment for the present illness were treated in their own homes. The treatment was carried out by a visiting nurse trained in follow-up assessment and counselling. The outcome for this group was compared with that for a similar group of 27 patients who underwent initial mental hospital admission and subsequent out-patient follow-up. Both groups were followed up for 6 months. The home treatment through a visiting nurse resulted in better clinical outcomes, better social functioning of the patient and a greatly reduced burden on patients' families. This treatment modality was also noted to be more economical.

A more recent study used a randomised case-control design to evaluate the effectiveness of intervening at home. Patients who were diagnosed with chronic schizophrenia, but who were not compliant with centre-based rehabilitation, were recruited into the study. They were then randomly assigned to the experimental or control group. The patients in the experimental group received an intervention that was indigenous, 'home-friendly' and utilised existing, accessible resources. The control group did not receive any home-based intervention. Post-intervention evaluation indicated that patients receiving intervention at home did better than the group not receiving intervention. Areas pertaining to self-care, socialisation and work showed significant improvement. Coping by carers also improved (Padmavati, 2005).

Home-based care for persons with schizophrenia and other chronic mental illnesses is a feasible strategy, especially in resource-sparse countries. Strategies for home-based care are seen to be necessarily indigenous and contingent on available resources. The effectiveness of these strategies is seen in the reduced rates of hospitalisation for crisis management, social outcomes and reduction of carer burden. Patients who cannot or refuse to access services may get an opportunity to be exposed to some elements of PSR.

In China, a home care programme has been developed as a major community healthcare service, with outreach in several provinces, particularly in rural areas, and mostly as part of the primary care programme (Shan-Cheng, 1998). This programme has demonstrated a clear trend towards marked clinical improvement and diminished relapse rates.

Community-based rehabilitation in India

Community-based rehabilitation, essentially an offshoot of community-based medical care, was first initiated in the 1980s under the impetus provided by the National Mental Health Programme of India. Community care strategies involve operating mental health clinics in the community and a focus on mental health literacy in the general population. A critical strategy has been the use of lay community volunteers trained in the recognition, identification and referral of persons with mental disorders as the first level of rehabilitation. Thara *et al* (1998) suggest that rehabilitation can be further facilitated by networking with governmental and non-governmental organisations involved in social and developmental activities. NGO community-based programmes, although efficacious and cost-effective, have always been restricted by their dependency on time-limited funding (Thara *et al*, 1998). However, collaborations with NGOs are seen as an important approach to reach out to a wide geographical area, with a shared economic commitment to the collaboration (Padmavati, 2005).

Community-based programmes have suffered from poor allocation of resources, insensitivity to the needs of people with mental illness on the part of both professionals and policy-planners, and indifference to mental health in general. The sustainability and continuity of programmes, especially by NGOs, are largely limited as most are time-bound projects, contingent upon the funding resources.

The efforts of NGOs in delivering PSR

India

The NGO movement in India has been gradually building up its base and force over the past few decades as a result of commitment and drive. It is clear that NGOs cannot replace or compete with government agencies, but they are often more innovative and likely to think outside the box in order to deliver services (especially in PSR) that statutory services may not be able to provide.

Many mental health NGOs (MHNGOs) have been very successful despite a lack of resources. Their programmes are largely urban (although some are beginning to extend their services to urban conurbations and surrounding rural areas) and found in the southern states of India. These rural and urban differences are discussed further below. Most MHNGOs serve a defined community and may deal with only one condition; an example is the Alzheimer and Related Disorders Society of India (ARDSI), which started in Cochin, but which has now spread to more than a dozen centres in India. The Richmond Fellowship Society has three centres. The oldest MHNGOs in India are probably those working in the field of child mental health and, in particular, intellectual disabilities.

Many MHNGOs working with people with severe mental illness, such as the Schizophrenia Research Foundation (SCARF) in Chennai, the Medico-Pastoral Association (MPA) in Bangalore and Shristi in Madurai, were started by psychiatrists who already held full-time faculty positions in local medical schools. They sought to meet the need for a holistic approach to the management of severe mental disorders. These organisations provide family counselling as well as vocational rehabilitation, which are rarely available in out-patient clinics. Substance and alcohol abuse attracted considerable interest and led to the development of MHNGOs such as the TTK Hospital in Chennai, the TRADA in Kerala and Karnataka, Alcoholics Anonymous and the Samaritans in many parts of the country, and the National Addiction Research Centre in Mumbai. Some MHNGOs, such as ACMI (Bangalore) and Aasha (Chennai), are entirely run by and focus on the families of those affected by severe mental disorders. The perceived need of the community appears to have catalysed the MHNGOs as a result of personal histories, tragedies and first-hand experiences.

The activities of the MHNGOs can be one or more of the following, depending upon the purpose of the organisation: care and rehabilitation; other community-based activities; managing substance misuse; suicide prevention; dealing with specific vulnerable groups such as women, children, the elderly, lesbian, gay, bisexual and transgender individuals and prisoners; research and training; and advocacy and lobbying (Thara & Patel, 2010).

In the past few decades, private centres offering treatment, rehabilitation and long-term, even lifetime care have sprung up across India. There are potential problems with these settings. The quality control and licensing of these facilities can vary tremendously. They require close monitoring to ensure that human rights and medical needs are met.

Sri Lanka

Although voluntary organisations have been around in Sri Lanka for a considerable period, there was a clear upsurge in their numbers after the Asian tsunami of 2004 (Vijayakumar et al, 2006). The UK-based organisation Voluntary Service Overseas (VSO) worked with government and other NGOs to strengthen the delivery of community-based mental health services. Their activities included developing training curricula for new mental health staff, strengthening the liaison with government departments and supporting the expansion of successful rehabilitative projects, such as a gardening project run by VSO partner Basic Needs.

Sahanaya, or the National Council for Mental Health, is a prominent NGO in Sri Lanka which works to develop mental health and mental healthcare in the country. Established in 1982 and incorporated by an Act of Parliament in 1986, its objective is to develop a centre of excellence with expertise and the necessary competence to respond to emerging mental health needs and issues. It runs two resource centres.

Navajeevana, meaning 'new life', is an NGO based in the Hambantota district of southern Sri Lanka. While beginning to work with persons with disabilities, since 2002 Navajeevana has provided community mental health services in partnership with Basic Needs. In 2008 Basic Needs moved away from the project area and Navajeevana officially became the implementing body on mental health in collaboration with the Health Ministry. The programme provides community mental health, along with sustainable livelihoods, as well as building capacity and resources.

Pakistan

Since its inception in 1971, Fountain House in Lahore has been providing state-of-the-art PSR facilities to persons with mental disorders not only from Pakistan but also for Pakistani families living abroad. This has been described as a model for LMICs. Another big NGO, the Pakistan Association for Mental Health, was established in 1965. Its mission is to involve communities and families in a cost-effective (affordable) and culturally relevant (acceptable) programme of treatment and aftercare for people who are mentally ill. The provision of out-patient care and support along with a telephone helpline offers an interesting example of community engagement.

Nepal

The small country of Nepal has several NGOs working in mental health. Of these, the Centre for Mental Health and Counselling (CMC-Nepal) was established in 2003 and works on preventive, promotional and curative aspects of mental health, aiming to provide mental health services in the community. It supports other organisations in their psychosocial programmes. It takes on the responsibility of capacity-building, with the aim of increasing access and psychosocial support at the community level. The Transcultural Psychosocial Organisation is one of Nepal's leading psychosocial organisations; it promotes psychosocial well-being and the mental health of children and families in conflict-affected and other vulnerable communities, through the development of sustainable, culturally appropriate, community-based psychosocial support systems. Another organisation, Maryknoll Nepal, established in 1991, aims for all those with chronic mental illness who are detained in prisons to be released, and to be provided with treatment and rehabilitation within the community.

Bangladesh

The Bangladeshi Mental Health Association was established in 1992 and works in both the UK and Bangladesh to promote and provide a culturally appropriate community-based mental health service to the people of Bangladesh as well as to counter violence and its consequences.

Afghanistan

The structures and delivery of mental health services in Afghanistan are at a difficult stage of development because of the political situation. There are some interesting developments, such as transcultural teaching using medical anthropologists and the delivery of interventions using patients' traditional beliefs about mental illness. Traditional practices of chaining people who are severely mentally ill at home or at Sufi shrines are still rife, but with the recent introduction of some UK psychiatrists of Afghan origin, matters are beginning to change.

Limitations of NGOs

Mental health NGOs have played a leading role in the provision of PSR in the South Asian countries reviewed. However, they are subject to limitations which include difficulties in the sustainability of programmes (most of which are funded by donor agencies), lack of accountability in some cases and limited geographical scope. NGOs should work to establish models of PSR that can be generally replicated.

Rural–urban differences

There are inevitable differences between rural and urban areas. Accessibility of services and availability of resources are likely to be greater in urban areas, although family support among migrants to the cities may be lacking. In South Asia, rural–urban differences are dramatic in terms of quality of life and expectations of the population. Educational and economic differences will affect the way individuals seek help and engage with services. For the most part, rural areas in the region remain substantially underdeveloped and have access to minimal services, if any. The largely agrarian rural population continues to operate around sets of beliefs and attitudes which may be seen as more traditional than their urban counterparts. Thara et al (1998) showed that, in spite of geographical proximity to a large metropolitan city, people living in rural areas held more traditional, medico-religious views in explaining the causation of mental illness. While this did not seem to impact too much on their acceptance of Western methods of medical intervention, it certainly reflected the way they viewed family members with a mental disability. This dichotomy needs to be explored and understood further so that interventions are appropriate and acceptable culturally.

There exist tensions between proven models and their introduction to the communities where different explanatory models and different value systems exist and where cultural factors in cognitions vary. It is important that service providers carry out exploration before setting up services. This is illustrated by Coleridge (2000), who points out that in Afghanistan the concept of 'empowerment' has poor acceptance but its equivalent 'enablement' is easily understood and accepted.

Conclusions

Rehabilitation of patients with chronic and severe mental illness is a critical aspect of psychiatric services. Countries may have out-of-date policies in place. Policies may lack an adequate framework for translation and implementation, thus creating a tension within the healthcare system. Also, there do not seem to be significant research findings from studies in LMICs that could feed into their PSR programmes. The ongoing struggle to find appropriate professionals to work in PSR is yet another challenge.

In countries with poor resources, rehabilitation services may be more reliant on NGOs than on statutory delivery. PSR training is also deficient in many countries and lack of trained personnel often exacerbates this. Finally, the implementation of PSR strategies should consider community attitudes, explanatory models and community expectations of service providers. When services are being planned, the first thing to identify is a community's cultural values and attitudes, which will influence their models of illness. Then the expectations of the community can be explored so that the services can be appropriate and accessible – both emotionally and geographically.

References

Anthony WA, Farkas M (1982) A client outcome planning model for assessing psychiatric rehabilitation interventions. *Schizophrenia Bulletin*, **8**: 13–38.

Anthony WA, Cohen M, Farkas M (1988a) Professional pre-service training for working with the long term mentally ill. *Community Mental Health Journal*, **24**: 258–69.

Anthony WA, Cohen M, Farkas M, *et al* (1988b) The chronically ill case management. *Community Mental Health Journal*, **24**: 219–28.

Balaji M, Chatterjee S, Koschorke M, *et al* (2012) The development of a lay health worker delivered collaborative community based intervention for people with schizophrenia in India. *BMC Health Service Research*, **12**: 42.

Chatterjee S, Leese M, Korschorke M, *et al* (2011) Collaborative community based care for people and their families living with schizophrenia in India: protocol for a randomized controlled trial. *Trials*, **12**: 12–18.

Coleridge P (2000) Disability and culture. In *Selected Readings in Community Based Rehabilitation, Series 1 – CBR in Transition* (eds M Thomas, M J Thomas): 21–38. National Printing Press.

National Human Rights Commission (NHRC) (1999) *Quality Assurance in Mental Health.* NHRC.

Padmavati R (2005) Community mental health care in India. *International Review of Psychiatry,* **17**: 103–7.

Pai S, Kapur RL (1983) Evaluation of home care treatment for schizophrenia patients. *Acta Psychiatrica Scandinavica,* **67**: 80–8.

Patel V, Weiss HA, Chowdhary N, *et al* (2010) Effectiveness of an intervention led by lay health counselors for depressive and anxiety disorders in primary care in Goa, India (MANAS): a cluster randomized controlled trial. *Lancet,* **377**: 2086–95.

Shan-Cheng W (1998) Family management of schizophrenia. *Hong Kong Journal of Psychiatry,* **8**: 17–19.

Test MA, Stein LI (1977) A community approach to the chronically disabled patients. *Social Policy,* **8**: 8–16.

Thara R, John S (2012) PSR in developing countries. *International Review of Psychiatry,* **24**: 499–503.

Thara R, Padmavati R (2013) Community health care in South Asia. *World Psychiatry,* **12**: 176–7.

Thara R, Patel V (2010) Role of non-governmental organizations in mental health in India. *Indian Journal of Psychiatry,* **52** (suppl 1): S389–95.

Thara R, Islam A, Padmavati R (1998) Beliefs about mental illness – a study of rural south Indian community. *International Journal of Mental Health,* **21**: 70–85.

Vijayakumar L, Thara R, John S, *et al* (2006) Psychosocial interventions after tsunami in Tamil Nadu, India. *International Review of Psychiatry,* **18**: 225–31.

CHAPTER 29

Expanding the evidence base

Helen Killaspy and Steffan Davies

Introduction

Tuke's (1813) *Description of The Retreat* (see Chapter 17, 'Rehabilitation in hospital settings') compares outcomes for 'moral treatment' favourably with the less progressive Leeds Asylum and Bethlem Hospital. Moral treatment has many parallels with modern rehabilitation (see below) and emphasised: strengthening and assisting the patient to control the disorder; coercion being employed only when absolutely necessary; and promoting the general comfort of the insane, including occupation and physical health. While attempts were made to provide evidence for programmes of treatment aimed at 'rehabilitation', the first high-quality evidence for their effectiveness probably came from the highly influential Three Hospitals Study (Wing & Brown, 1970), which compared the characteristics of long-stay patients with a diagnosis of schizophrenia and the clinical culture of the wards in which they were receiving treatment. The study was carried out over an 8-year period and its cohort design allowed for investigation of the 'direction of causality'. One of the three hospitals had a good reputation for the care of long-stay patients, including a focus on occupation and rehabilitation. The main finding was a positive association between the degree of stimulation of the therapeutic environment and the severity of patients' 'clinical poverty syndrome' (characterised by social withdrawal, poverty of thought and blunted affect). Patients at the hospital that provided better-quality rehabilitation also showed less clinical disturbance and more autonomy than those in the comparison hospitals, and staff had greater optimism regarding their recovery. The Three Hospitals Study highlighted the negative consequences of 'institutionalism', a concept now very familiar to us, eloquently described by Erving Goffman in his book *Asylums: Essays on the Social Situation of Mental Patients and Other Inmates*, published in 1961.

The social and political desire to 'deinstitutionalise' mental healthcare was one of the major drivers in the development of community-based services that took place in the latter half of the 20th century in the UK and other countries. Rehabilitation practitioners were very involved in this process and in the development of community-based supported accommodation that provided an alternative to long-term hospitalisation for many of those leaving the asylum. As described in Chapter 19, 'Housing: a place to live', a large cohort study carried out in the 1990s by the Team for the Assessment of Psychiatric Services (TAPS) investigated outcomes for 700 long-stay patients discharged to the community after the closure of the two large asylums in north London. Most did well, with only a minority requiring readmission to hospital and most experiencing improvements in their quality of life over the subsequent 5 years (Leff & Trieman, 2000). Positive outcomes were also evident for those with the highest levels of need and challenging behaviours, 40% of whom were able to progress from a community-based or hospital-based in-patient unit to less supported settings (Trieman & Leff, 2002). Residents in these units showed improvements in functioning and reductions in challenging behaviours. Trieman and Leff concluded that 'a high proportion of patients with severe disabilities, designated as *"difficult to place"* in the community, could benefit from slow-stream rehabilitation within specialised facilities, enabling them to move into ordinary community homes' (2002: p. 428).

Outcomes for people with a diagnosis of schizophrenia

In order to understand whether mental health rehabilitation services really provide 'added value', it is important to interpret the findings from the TAPs studies in the context of cohort studies that have investigated outcomes for people with a diagnosis of schizophrenia and other psychoses. However, although there have been numerous such studies, the heterogeneity of design, duration of follow-up and definition of what is meant by 'recovery' has made it difficult to draw definite conclusions. A review of 114 cohort studies carried out since 1801, with follow-up assessments between 2 and 25 years, concluded that around 20% of people diagnosed with schizophrenia show complete recovery and 40% partial recovery over the longer term (Warner, 2004).

One large international cohort study attempted to improve on the methodology of earlier research by using stringent diagnostic and recovery criteria. The International Study of Schizophrenia (Harrison *et al*, 2001) involved 14 countries and 1633 people diagnosed with a psychotic illness who had participated in earlier cohort studies. Of these, 1171 were newly diagnosed ('incidence') cases and the remainder were 'prevalence' cases. Because of the different time frames of the cohorts included, follow-up data were gathered at 15 and 25 years for different cohorts. At follow-up, 14% had died. Over half of those still alive were rated as 'recovered' using a standardised assessment tool (56% of incidence cases and 60% of prevalence cases), with no psychotic episodes being recorded during at least the previous 2 years for 49% of incidence and 48% of prevalence cases.

The recovery rates were slightly worse for those with a clear diagnosis of schizophrenia (48% for incidence cases, 53% for prevalence cases, with 43% and 41% experiencing no psychotic episodes within the previous 2 years, respectively). It is important to note that despite these relatively positive outcomes, 11.6% of those in the schizophrenia incidence case group had been living in some form of 'institutional' setting for the previous 2 years and one-third of those with schizophrenia were rated as having been continuously ill. When stricter criteria were used to define 'recovered' (including a Global Assessment of Functioning rating of over 60 and no treatment episodes within the previous 2 years) the rate fell to 36% for the whole incidence case sample and 13% for the schizophrenia incidence cases. Of note, 16% of the schizophrenia incidence case group were assessed as having a 'late recovery effect', in that although rated as recovered at 15-year follow-up, they had been rated as continuously unwell at earlier time points. The authors concluded that these data supported the case for maintaining therapeutic optimism and rehabilitation programmes for people who had not responded well to treatment at earlier stages.

The Vermont longitudinal study of schizophrenia (Harding et al, 1987a,b), which is widely quoted in the recovery literature, also provides evidence for the effectiveness of rehabilitation for those with longer-term psychoses. A cohort of 269 'long stay' patients discharged from the Vermont State Hospital at the time of its closure, between 1955 and 1960, were referred to a community rehabilitation programme delivered by a multidisciplinary team. Those referred had been unwell for an average of 16 years and had been hospitalised for an average of 6 years before discharge. They were selected for the rehabilitation programme on the basis of the chronicity of their problems and attended for an average of 10 years. The programme included finding participants suitable community housing, vocational rehabilitation to facilitate their access to work and education, social activities, individualised care planning and social skills training. Harding and her colleagues interviewed all but seven of the original cohort an average of 32 years after their last admission to Vermont State Hospital. Around two-thirds (62–68%) were assessed as having improved clinically or recovered completely and around half were not taking psychotropic medication.

For some populations with severe enduring mental illness, particularly those treated in forensic psychiatric services, outcomes remain very poor. A long-term follow-up (mean 9.5 years) of 600 patients discharged from a medium-secure unit (Davies et al, 2007), the majority with psychotic illnesses, found 10% had died, almost half had been convicted and over 60% had been readmitted at some time, with almost 40% being readmitted to medium-secure or high-secure services (Clarke et al, 2013). This is an important subgroup within rehabilitation services; around 20% of patients at in-patient mental health rehabilitation services in England have previously been treated within a forensic psychiatric unit (see the section below on the REAL study).

Investigating the effectiveness of contemporary mental health rehabilitation services

It is generally accepted that long-term hospitalisation is best avoided, and that alternatives to hospital admission during an episode of acute mental illness are both clinically effective and cost-effective (Johnson *et al*, 2009). However, there remains a group of people with particularly complex mental health problems, often associated with risk to themselves and others, whose needs are such that they cannot return home immediately from an acute admission ward and who require extended in-patient treatment to maximise their chances of a successful and sustained community discharge. This is the group that mental health rehabilitation services in the UK focus on. As we have seen in Chapter 2, 'What is psychiatric rehabilitation?', it is estimated that around 10% of people newly diagnosed with psychosis will have complex needs and require mental health rehabilitation services (Craig *et al*, 2004). These complex needs include severe 'negative' symptoms, ongoing 'positive' symptoms, other coexisting mental and physical health problems, substance misuse problems and challenging behaviours (Holloway, 2005). Although they are relatively small in number, this high-needs group absorbs between 25% and 50% of mental health resources (Mental Health Strategies, 2010) yet, until recently, there had been little focus on research into the effectiveness of contemporary mental health rehabilitation services.

Part of the difficulty in producing evidence for the effectiveness of mental health rehabilitation is that it is a highly complex intervention. In Chapter 2 we saw that the definition of rehabilitation has evolved over time, reflecting the changing culture within which mental health services are delivered, including the adoption of recovery-oriented approaches. The specific interventions delivered by rehabilitation services have also, necessarily, varied over time in response to the expansion of the evidence base for treatments for schizophrenia. This evidence base is detailed in Part 2 of this book, 'Treatment approaches', and is summarised in national treatment guidelines such as those for schizophrenia published by the National Institute for Health and Care Excellence (NICE, 2011). The interventions used in mental health rehabilitation are, ideally, delivered through care plans drawn up in collaboration with service users and their carers that are individually tailored to address their specific needs. The reality, therefore, is that rehabilitation will constitute different treatments, approaches and support delivered for variable amounts of time to different people by different staff. This type of complex intervention does not lend itself to straightforward evaluation through a simple randomised controlled trial. Furthermore, the remit of rehabilitation services, the characteristics of those receiving these services, the treatment settings in which they are delivered and the resources available all vary across countries, with heterogeneity of socioeconomic and political contexts, making it difficult

439

to generalise from the results of international studies. Despite these difficulties, there has been an increasing focus on the evaluation of mental health rehabilitation services in the UK and elsewhere in recent years.

Building an evidence base for mental health rehabilitation services in England and Ireland

In 1999 the UK government published the *National Service Framework for Mental Health* (Department of Health, 1999). This was followed by a *Policy Implementation Guide*, which described the implementation of specialist community mental health teams, including crisis resolution, early intervention and assertive outreach (Department of Health, 2001). Rehabilitation services received no specific mention. In 2002, the National Institute for Clinical Excellence (now known as the National Institute for Health and Care Excellence) published its first treatment guideline, which focused on people with a diagnosis of schizophrenia. The guideline made no specific reference to mental health rehabilitation services. The lack of representation in policy and treatment guidelines may well have reflected something of an identity crisis for rehabilitation services and certainly there was little in the way of robust evidence available at the time to make a strong case to service planners and commissioners to support investment in them.

In order to begin to address this evidence gap, Killaspy *et al* (2005) carried out a survey of all mental health rehabilitation services in England. Telephone interviews were carried out with service managers and rehabilitation psychiatrists who provided descriptive data on their services and were asked to answer the question 'what is rehabilitation psychiatry?'

Of the National Health Service (NHS) mental health organisations (trusts) in operation at the time in England, a total of 89% responded. The majority (77%) provided short-term in-patient rehabilitation units with a length of stay of up to 12 months and a mean of 13 beds. Over half also provided long-term units, with a mean of 11 beds. There were no differences between urban and rural services in bed numbers. Most services had input from all members of a multidisciplinary team, and where services had short-term and longer-term units, staff tended to cover both. The majority of services (79%) had specific referral criteria, 42% had exclusion criteria and 85% carried out a pre-admission assessment. Over half (56%) had a community rehabilitation team. A consensus definition of 'rehabilitation' was formulated from respondents' answers:

> A whole system approach to recovery from mental ill health which maximizes an individual's quality of life and social inclusion by encouraging their skills, promoting independence and autonomy in order to give them hope for the future and which leads to successful community living through appropriate support. (Killaspy *et al*, 2005: p. 163)

This definition has been drawn on by many contributors to this book.

The national survey was followed by a descriptive study detailing characteristics of all users of the mental health rehabilitation services of one NHS trust in north London in 2005 (Killaspy *et al*, 2008). Rehabilitation services provided comprised two short-term in-patient rehabilitation units, one longer-term 'complex care' in-patient unit, three community rehabilitation units and four community residential care units. Service users were assessed using staff-rated standardised measures of needs, challenging behaviours, social functioning and substance misuse. Two-thirds of the 141 service users were male and their mean age was 40 years. Most (91%) had a diagnosis of schizophrenia or schizoaffective disorder and 7% had a comorbid substance misuse problem. The majority were referred to rehabilitation services from acute admission wards and moved through the care pathway from in-patient to community units over a number of years. Over half had at least one challenging behaviour that was difficult to manage or occurred frequently. The most common unmet needs involved ongoing psychotic symptoms (18%), accommodation (16%), daytime activities (16%) and money (16%). Those in the complex care units had poorer social function and greater numbers of needs than those in the other three types of setting.

A survey of the users of mental health rehabilitation services in the West Midlands area of England found similar results: two-thirds were male, their mean age was 45 years, the majority had a diagnosis of schizophrenia, schizoaffective disorder or bipolar affective disorder and the vast majority were assessed as having a high level of impairment in social functioning (Cowan *et al*, 2012).

The north London cohort was followed-up 5 years later, at which time 124 were still alive (Killaspy & Zis, 2013). Two-thirds had a positive outcome: 40% had moved on from hospital to supported community accommodation successfully (or from a higher to lower supported accommodation in the community if they were community patients at the time of the original survey in 2005), without requiring readmission to hospital and without any placement breakdown; one-quarter of those who were community patients in 2005 had remained in the same placement without needing any readmission to hospital. Overall, 13 (10%) progressed to living in independent (unsupported) accommodation successfully over the 5 years. However, 38% had either moved to a more supported placement or had been readmitted to hospital. The only factor found to be associated with outcome was medication adherence: those who were noted to have any episodes of non-adherence to medication during the 5 years were eight times more likely not to progress to a less supported setting or to be readmitted to hospital (Killaspy & Zis, 2013).

While giving some idea of the proportion of people likely to progress successfully along the rehabilitation care pathway, this study was obviously limited, in terms of providing evidence for the effectiveness of rehabilitation services, by the lack of a comparison group. A larger, multicentre study carried out in Ireland attempted to address this limitation (Lavelle *et al*, 2011). It compared outcomes over 18 months for people receiving mental health rehabilitation services with those wait-listed for these services. Two hundred participants were recruited from five centres across Ireland, 124 of whom were receiving rehabilitation services. The two groups were similar in characteristics: two-thirds of participants were male, their mean age was 40 years, the vast majority had a diagnosis of schizophrenia or schizoaffective disorder and the average length of illness was over 20 years. Outcomes assessed included successful community discharge and improvement in social functioning. Those receiving rehabilitation were eight times more likely than those awaiting rehabilitation to be discharged from hospital and to sustain their community placement (if they were in-patients at recruitment) or to maintain their community placement (if they were living in the community at recruitment). They also showed a statistically significant improvement in social function. However, no specific rehabilitative interventions (including hours of vocational rehabilitation received, number of sessions of cognitive–behavioural therapy or family therapy, the dose of antipsychotic medication prescribed or whether receiving clozapine) were found to predict better outcomes. Those with greater unmet needs, substance misuse and more challenging behaviours at recruitment were less likely to do well.

The Rehabilitation Effectiveness for Activities for Life (REAL) study

Building on these previous studies, an ambitious 5-year programme of research into in-patient mental health rehabilitation services in England began in 2009, funded by the National Institute of Health Research. This programme, the Rehabilitation Effectiveness for Activities for Life (REAL) study, comprises four parts: a detailed national survey of all in-patient mental health rehabilitation services in England; the development of a staff training intervention that aims to increase staff skills and confidence in engaging service users in activities; evaluation of the staff training programme through a cluster randomised controlled trial; and a naturalistic cohort study investigating outcomes over 12 months for users of in-patient mental health rehabilitation services.

The REAL study uses a standardised quality assessment tool, the Quality Indicator for Rehabilitative Care (QuIRC), which was developed through a separate, pan-European study and is described in more detail in Chapter 17, 'Rehabilitation in hospital settings'. The QuIRC is completed by the rehabilitation unit manager and provides ratings of the unit's performance on seven domains: living environment; therapeutic environment; treatments and interventions; promotion of self-management and autonomy; promotion of social integration; human rights; and recovery based practice. The tool produces a printable report for each unit showing its scores (as percentages) on the seven domains in a 'spider web' diagram which also shows the national average scores for similar units.

At the time of writing, the first part of the REAL study, the national survey, has been completed (Killaspy *et al*, 2013). A total of 133 NHS rehabilitation units participated from 52 of the 60 (87%) NHS mental health trusts across England. All 133 service managers and 739 (62%) service users were interviewed. On average, these units had 14 beds, 59% were based in the community rather than in a hospital and most employed a multidisciplinary team comprising psychiatrists, psychologists, nurses and occupational therapists, with an average ratio of staff to service users of 1:1.58. All units had access to social workers, usually through the local community mental health services, and a minority of units also provided art therapy. In around one-third of units, ex-service users were also employed on the staff. Over half the service managers interviewed reported that their trust had a community rehabilitation team which provided support and/or care coordination (under the auspices of the national framework of the Care Programme Approach) to service users discharged from the in-patient rehabilitation service to supported accommodation. The characteristics of service users were similar to the previous studies reported above: two-thirds were male, the average age was 40 years and the mean length of contact with mental health services was 13 years. The majority had a primary diagnosis of schizophrenia (73%), schizoaffective disorder (8%) or bipolar affective disorder (8%). Two-thirds had been detained under the Mental Health Act during their current admission, one-third were currently detained and around 20% had previously been treated in a secure mental health unit of some kind. Over half (58%) had a history of assaulting others at some time. This had occurred within the past 2 years for 21% and was considered a serious assault for 8%. Many service users had a history of self-neglect (49%), self-harm (45%) or vulnerability to exploitation by others (25%).

The national survey facilitated collection of national quality benchmarking data for in-patient mental health rehabilitation units in England using the QuIRC. Further analyses were carried out to investigate the factors associated with quality of care and its relationship with service user outcomes. It was found that service user characteristics (age, functioning, the proportion of detained patients and the proportion of male patients per unit) had little influence on the seven QuIRC domains, but the deprivation of the local area had a significant influence on one domain, the quality of the built environment of the unit. Interestingly, there was little difference in the assessment of quality in hospital-based and community-based units; the community-based units fared slightly better on only one domain, the therapeutic environment. A positive association was found between quality of care and service user outcomes, where improving performance on any of the seven QuIRC domains had a positive effect on service users' autonomy, experiences of care and ratings of the therapeutic milieu of the unit. These

443

findings strongly support investment in interventions that improve the quality of care in in-patient rehabilitation services.

Part 2 of the REAL study involved the development and piloting of a 'hands-on' staff training intervention designed to facilitate service users' involvement in activities both on and off the unit. The focus on an intervention aimed at increasing service users' activities was informed by the knowledge that service users in acute and longer-term in-patient units often spend a great deal of time doing very little. One audit of an acute ward in a south London mental health trust found that service users spent fewer than 17 minutes per day doing something other than eating, sleeping or watching television (South London and Maudsley NHS Trust, 2004). Wing & Brown (1970) had previously described the association between under-stimulating hospital environments and negative symptoms of schizophrenia, a finding replicated over two decades later by Curson *et al* (1992). There is some evidence that interventions aimed at improving service users' engagement in activities through occupational therapy might lead to improvements in social function (Buchain *et al*, 2003; Oka *et al*, 2004).

The development of the intervention for the REAL study was led by an occupational therapist and an organisational psychologist in consultation with mental health occupational therapists at a national event with service users and rehabilitation practitioners. It was then piloted in two mental health rehabilitation units. An intervention manual was developed that provides a comprehensive yet flexible training programme to suit each service's particular resources and context. It includes a 1-day course for staff focusing on the importance of engaging service users in activities, delivered by the intervention team (comprising an occupational therapist, activity worker and service user), followed by 4 weeks of hands-on training where the intervention team's occupational therapist and activity worker support the unit staff to try these out in their everyday clinical practice. This 'hands-on' training approach is rounded off with a final training day to reflect on which aspects have worked best, to consolidate knowledge and to agree an action plan to encourage the team to continue to use the techniques and strategies they have learnt or enhanced during the intervention period to continue to support service users' activities on and off the unit.

In part 3 of the REAL study the intervention is being evaluated through a cluster randomised controlled trial involving 40 in-patient mental health rehabilitation units across England, 20 of which receive the intervention. Outcomes are being assessed 12 months later, the main one being the degree to which service users in the unit are engaged in activities. Social functioning is also being assessed.

Part 4 of the REAL study is being carried out at the same time as part 3. Over 350 service users of 50 in-patient mental health rehabilitation units across England are being followed up over 12 months to investigate whether they achieve and sustain community discharge and whether there are improvements in their social function. Parts 3 and 4 of the REAL study will build on the results from part 1 by exploring the aspects of in-patient mental health rehabilitation care and the specific interventions that are associated with better longitudinal outcomes for service users.

The Boston model of mental health rehabilitation

One approach to mental health rehabilitation that has attracted interest internationally is the Illness Management and Recovery programme developed in Boston, Massachusetts, in the USA (Gingerich & Mueser, 2005). It provides a 9-month integrated programme of evidence-based individual and group-based psychosocial interventions for individuals with a diagnosis of schizophrenia or schizoaffective disorder living in the community in non-residential settings. The programme aims to improve self-management and the interventions focus on psychoeducation, cognitive–behavioural techniques to improve medication adherence, training in social skills and coping skills, and relapse prevention planning. A preliminary evaluation involving 24 clients who had participated in the programme in the USA or Australia found high levels of satisfaction 3 months after completion, with most people reporting they had found the programme useful, helpful for managing their symptoms and beneficial in making progress towards their goals. Clinicians' ratings of global functioning also improved (Mueser et al, 2006).

The programme has been replicated in the Netherlands and evaluated through a multicentre, randomised controlled trial involving 156 participants (Swildens et al, 2011). The primary outcome was the attainment of personal rehabilitation goals and secondary outcomes included empowerment, needs, social participation (assessed by a positive change in work situation or independence of living environment) and quality of life. The authors reported that a higher proportion of participants in the intervention group achieved their personal rehabilitation goals compared with the comparison group at 24 months and achieved greater societal participation. The 'number needed to treat' for both these outcomes was reported as five. However, gains were not seen in the other secondary outcomes. One problem in interpreting the findings of these two studies in the context of mental health rehabilitation services in the UK is that many of the participants were already living in independent accommodation and are likely to be considerably less affected by their illness than users of rehabilitation services in the UK.

Evaluating community rehabilitation services

There have been no rigorous studies of the effectiveness of community rehabilitation teams in the UK. Numerous trials of other types of community mental health services (early intervention, assertive outreach, crisis resolution and home treatment teams) have been carried out both in the UK and abroad. Overall, the results of these studies show that crisis services can provide an effective alternative to in-patient admission for people in acute mental health crisis, and that early-intervention services can intervene quicker than standard community services for those experiencing their first episode of psychosis. However, the evidence for assertive outreach for people with complex psychosis has been much less impressive in the UK than in the USA and Australia. This may be because of the relatively high calibre of the comparison services in the UK (community mental health teams) compared with those used in the US trials and a lack of fidelity such that key components of assertive outreach were not delivered consistently (Rosen *et al*, 2013). However, it may simply reflect the difficulty of delivering complex interventions for people with highly complex needs. Any evaluation of community rehabilitation teams, the logical next step from the ongoing in-patient studies described above, will need to build on the existing evidence base, incorporating the key components of assertive outreach to deliver the evidence-based interventions that specifically target service users' different needs.

Conclusions

Attempts to evaluate what are widely recognisable as rehabilitation services have been underway for over 200 years. Mental health rehabilitation services are complex and multimodal, as would be expected for services treating patients with multiple needs and enduring illnesses. The past decade in particular has seen the development of a clearer understanding of what rehabilitation services comprise in the UK and Europe. This has been developed into a robust quality assessment tool, QuIRC, which has been utilised both to measure quality in in-patient services across England and, importantly, to relate quality to positive outcomes for patients (an uncommon achievement across medicine as a whole). Studies are now underway to evaluate training packages to enhance the effectiveness of in-patient services, with promising early results. Future areas for evaluation are longer-term outcomes and community rehabilitation services. Despite this progress, there are growing challenges for rehabilitation services in evidencing their clinical effectiveness and cost-effectiveness in the context of economic austerity and the increasing complexity of cases referred. Nevertheless, the evidence base for rehabilitation services, along with the policy recognition of their significance as elements of comprehensive mental health services, has advanced hugely over the past decade and looks likely to continue this progress over the next.

References

Buchain PC, Vizottom AD, Netom JH, *et al* (2003) Randomized controlled trial of occupational therapy in patients with treatment-resistant schizophrenia. *Revista Brasileira de Psiquiatria*, **25**: 26–30.

Clarke M, Duggan C, Hollin CR, *et al* (2013) Readmission after discharge from a medium secure unit. *The Psychiatrist*, **37**: 124–9.

Cowan C, Meaden A, Commander M, *et al* (2012) In-patient psychiatric rehabilitation services: survey of service users in three metropolitan boroughs. *The Psychiatrist*, **36**: 85–9.

Craig T, Garety P, Power P, *et al* (2004) The Lambeth Early Onset (LEO) Team: randomised controlled trial of the effectiveness of specialised care for early psychosis. *BMJ*, **329**: 1067–71.

Curson DA, Pantelis C, Ward J, *et al* (1992) Institutionalism and schizophrenia 30 years on. Clinical poverty and the social environment in three British mental hospitals in 1960 compared with a fourth in 1990. *British Journal of Psychiatry*, **160**: 230–41.

Davies S, Clarke M, Hollin C, *et al* (2007) Long-term outcomes after discharge from medium secure care: a cause for concern. *British Journal of Psychiatry*, **191**: 70–4.

Department of Health (1999) *National Service Framework for Mental Health*. Department of Health.

Department of Health (2001) *Mental Health Policy Implementation Guide*. Department of Health.

Gingerich S, Mueser KT (2005) Illness management and recovery. In *Evidence-based Mental Health Practice: A Textbook* (eds R Drake, M Merrens, D Lynde): 395–424. Norton.

Goffman E (1961) *Asylums: Essays on the Social Situation of Mental Patients and Other Inmates*. Doubleday/Anchor Books.

Harding CM, Brooks GW, Asolaga TS, *et al* (1987a) The Vermont longitudinal study of persons with severe mental illness. I. Methodology, study sample, and overall status 32 years later. *American Journal of Psychiatry*, **144**: 718–26.

Harding CM, Brooks GW, Asolaga TS, *et al* (1987b) The Vermont longitudinal study of persons with severe mental illness. II. Long-term outcome of persons who retrospectively met DSM-III criteria for schizophrenia. *American Journal of Psychiatry*, **144**: 727–35.

Harrison G, Hopper K, Craig T, *et al* (2001) Recovery from psychotic illness: a 15- and 25-year international follow-up study. *British Journal of Psychiatry*, **178**: 506–17.

Holloway F (2005) *The Forgotten Need for Rehabilitation in Contemporary Mental Health Services: A Position Statement from the Executive Committee of the Faculty of Rehabilitation and Social Psychiatry*. Royal College of Psychiatrists.

Johnson S, Gilburt H, Lloyd-Evans B, *et al* (2009) Inpatient and residential alternatives to standard acute psychiatric wards in England. *British Journal of Psychiatry*, **194**: 456–63.

Killaspy H, Zis P (2013) Predictors of outcomes of mental health rehabilitation services: a 5-year retrospective cohort study in inner London, UK. *Social Psychiatry and Psychiatric Epidemiology*, **48**: 1005–12.

Killaspy H, Harden C, Holloway F, *et al* (2005) What do mental health rehabilitation services do and what are they for? A national survey in England. *Journal of Mental Health*, **14**: 157–66.

Killaspy H, Rambarran D, Bledin K (2008) Mental health needs of clients of rehabilitation services: a survey in one trust. *Journal of Mental Health*, **17**: 207–18.

Killaspy H, Marston L, Omar R, *et al* (2013) Service quality and clinical outcomes: an example from mental health rehabilitation services in England. *British Journal of Psychiatry*, **202**: 28–34.

Lavelle E, Ijaz A, Killaspy H, *et al* (2011) *Mental Health Rehabilitation and Recovery Services in Ireland: A Multicentre Study of Current Service Provision, Characteristics of Service Users* and Outcomes for Those With and Without Access to These Services. Final Report for the Mental Health Commission of Ireland. Mental Health Commission of Ireland.

Leff J, Trieman N (2000) Long stay patients discharged from psychiatric hospitals. Social and clinical outcomes after five years in the community. TAPS Project 46. British Journal of Psychiatry, 176: 217–23.

Mental Health Strategies (2010) The 2009/10 National Survey of Investment in Mental Health Services. Department of Health.

Mueser KT, Meyer PS, Penn DL, et al (2006) The illness management and recovery program: rationale, development, and preliminary findings. Schizophrenia Bulletin, 32: S32–S43.

National Institute for Clinical Excellence (2002) Schizophrenia: Core Interventions in the Treatment and Management of Schizophrenia in Primary and Secondary Care (Clinical Guideline 1). NICE.

National Institute for Health and Clinical Excellence (2011) Schizophrenia: Core Interventions in the Treatment and Management of Schizophrenia in Primary and Secondary Care (Update) (Clinical Guideline 82). NICE.

Oka M, Otsuka K, Yokoyama N, et al (2004) An evaluation of a hybrid occupational therapy and supported employment program in Japan for persons with schizophrenia. American Journal of Occupational Therapy, 58: 466–75.

Rosen A, Killaspy H, Harvey C (2013) Specialisation and marginalisation: how the worldwide experience with assertive community treatment demonstrates how the interpretation of evidence can impact adversely on investment for those with the most complex needs. The Psychiatrist, 37: 345–8.

South London and Maudsley NHS Trust (2004) Patient Social Engagement and Attendance at Organised Activities on Acute Psychiatric Wards Within the South London and Maudsley Trust: An Observational Study and Audit of 16 Acute Wards. South London and Maudsley NHS Trust.

Swildens W, van Busschbach JT, Michon H, et al (2011) Effectively working on rehabilitation goals: 24-month outcome of a randomized controlled trial of the Boston psychiatric rehabilitation approach. Canadian Journal of Psychiatry, 56: 741–60.

Trieman N, Leff J (2002) Long-term outcome of long-stay psychiatric in-patients considered unsuitable to live in the community: TAPS Project 44. British Journal of Psychiatry, 181: 428–32.

Tuke S (1813) Description of The Retreat, An Institution Near York for Insane Persons of the Society of Friends. Process Press (1996).

Warner R (2004) Recovery from Schizophrenia: Psychiatry and Political Economy. Routledge.

Wing JK, Brown GW (1970) Institutionalism and Schizophrenia: A Comparative Survey of Three Mental Hospitals 1960–1968. Cambridge University Press.

Part 5

Future directions

CHAPTER 30

Psychiatric rehabilitation: future directions in policy and practice

Helen Killaspy, Sridevi Kalidindi, Glenn Roberts and Frank Holloway

Introduction

It is a truism to state that mental health services operate within the context of policy. While health policy has, at various times, gone through cycles of support for growth and investment in mental health services, mental health rehabilitation services have repeatedly had to state the case for their continued existence. In this chapter, we describe this process, focusing on the past decade or so. At its core, this narrative has an unsettling message for rehabilitation practitioners: that policy-makers are only too ready to marginalise people with the most complex mental health problems in the mistaken belief that the latest approach to reorganising services will magically negate the need for mental health rehabilitation. Understanding how to influence policy is a key skill for clinical leaders in mental health rehabilitation and we hope that this chapter will provide an insight and resources into how this can be achieved.

A brief history

Earlier chapters have described in some detail the process of deinstitutionalisation of mental health services in England and Wales in the latter half of the 20th century, and similar activities were carried out in many other high-income countries across the world around the same time. This was a period of relative 'boom' for rehabilitation services, with many of those practising in this discipline being heavily involved in the process of assessment and the 'resettling' of patients in supported accommodation in the community. The first community rehabilitation teams developed around this time to provide ongoing support to this cohort of patients. The outcomes reported by the Team for the Assessment of Psychiatric Services (TAPS) were very positive; most of those who had been long-stay patients in an institution who moved to a community placement did not relapse or require readmission to hospital (Leff & Trieman, 2000) and around two-thirds of those considered the least suitable for community placement not only remained stable in the community but were able to move on to less supported accommodation within 5 years (Trieman & Leff, 2002). Over the past 15 years or so, as described in Chapter 19, 'Housing: a place to live', more refined supported accommodation pathways have been developed, often provided by the third sector, to facilitate people's usual goal of achieving independent living through incremental moves every few years from higher to less supported accommodation.

Consequences for rehabilitation services of the National Service Framework for Mental Health

In 1999, the UK government published the *National Service Framework for Mental Health* (Department of Health, 1999), which set out a national configuration for community mental health services for England, comprising specialist teams to work alongside the community mental health teams (CMHTs) that had evolved since deinstitutionalisation. These specialist teams included: crisis resolution/home treatment teams, whose aim was to provide appropriate support to people in acute crisis in their own homes, thereby avoiding the need for admission; early-intervention teams to focus on people experiencing a first episode of psychosis; and assertive community treatment teams (or assertive outreach teams as they are known in the UK) to work with people with longer-term psychosis who have difficulties engaging with treatment, resulting in recurrent relapse and readmission. This initiative represented a major investment in community mental health services, with a target of 335 crisis teams, 50 early-intervention services and 220 assertive community treatment teams to be in place across the country within 5 years. In fact, only assertive community treatment teams met this target, or, rather, over-met it, with 263 teams in operation by 2004 (Department of Health, 2005).

While the international evidence supporting the potential clinical and cost-effectiveness of these new types of team was relatively strong at the time, especially for assertive community treatment, trials in the UK reported rather mixed findings. Crisis resolution teams were found to be cost-effective through their ability to prevent the need for admission (Johnson *et al*, 2005) but, in keeping with previous studies of different models of intensive case management in the UK, an important trial of assertive community treatment (Killaspy *et al*, 2006) did not find it to have clinical (or cost) advantage over standard care provided by CMHTs, although the model was more acceptable to 'difficult to engage' patients. While a full discussion of the implications of these findings is beyond the scope of this chapter, an important point often missed by service managers and policy-makers is that one-quarter of community rehabilitation teams were simply rebadged as assertive community treatment teams in order to meet the government target for implementation. In fact, a survey by Mountain *et al* (2009) found that over half the mental health rehabilitation services in the UK underwent some form of disinvestment during this period of major investment in community mental health services (2004–07). Of note, some of this represented 'reconfiguration', with a doubling in the provision of local low-secure units during this time (the proportion of National Health Service trusts providing a low-secure unit increased from 15% to 30%). The result of this disinvestment in rehabilitation services was a huge increase in the use of beds in the independent sector – in private hospitals, low-secure units, and nursing and residential homes. Usually these placements were some distance from the person's home – so-called 'out of area' treatments (OATs). This phenomenon was not restricted to the UK. Priebe *et al* (2005) described a similar process across deinstitutionalised European countries and commentators began to refer to this as a 'virtual asylum' (Poole *et al*, 2002). Concerns were raised about the quality of care and lack of rehabilitative ethos in many such settings and the social dislocation involved in being placed far from home (Ryan *et al*, 2004).

Using the phenomenon of out-of-area treatment to make the case for rehabilitation services

Over the past decade or so, the Rehabilitation and Social Psychiatry Faculty of the Royal College of Psychiatrists has used the OATs story to make the case for continued investment in local mental health rehabilitation services. In 2005, the Faculty published a report called *The Forgotten Need for Rehabilitation in Contemporary Mental Health Services*, which described the client group that rehabilitation services work with and the risks, both clinical and economic, of failing to provide local services for people with complex mental health problems (Holloway, 2005). This case has been somewhat easier to make, or at least fallen on more fertile ground, in the context of the economic downturn, since there is a clear financial argument for avoiding the outflow of resources to OATs. Starting with a freedom-of-information enquiry to all National Health Service trusts and local authorities across England in 2010, the Faculty was able to show that 21% of all funded placements for people with complex needs were made out of area and that these placements cost, on average, 64% more than a similar local rehabilitation bed. This proportion is much higher than the proportion of people with very complex needs who require a very specialist service that could be provided only at a regional or national level. The total excess cost to the public purse of these OATs was estimated at over £1.3 million (Killaspy & Meier, 2010). Some areas had already set up processes for reviewing and repatriating some patients to appropriate local services and reinvesting the financial flows into the local pathway for mental health and supported accommodation (Killaspy *et al*, 2009).

A high-level event hosted by the Royal College of Psychiatrists and attended by other relevant groups, including the NHS Confederation and London School of Economics and Political Science, considered the

OATs issue in the context of the response of mental health services to the economic downturn. The ensuing Occasional Paper from the Royal College of Psychiatrists *et al* (2009) stated:

> The large amount of money spent by some Primary Care Trusts (PCTs) on out-of-area treatments is an expense that should be addressed. Doing so, where appropriate in individual cases, will enable the delivery of appropriate services nearer to a patient's home area, which will provide better care at a lower overall cost.... Consequently, some rehabilitation services and PCTs have set up systems to review and 'repatriate' people placed in OATs to their area of origin, usually to less restricted settings such as supported tenancies. In doing so, one PCT was able to 'repatriate' 17 of its 40 clients in OATs, at a saving of £1 million per year, giving an indication of the size of the potential savings to be made (p. 20–21).

This economic argument has been a very important part of making the case for ongoing investment in mental health rehabilitation services. As well as ensuring that it is included in policy documents, it has also been necessary to use media contacts to disseminate the message. In 2010, the Faculty briefed journalist David Brindle to write an article on the OATs problem for the *Guardian*:

> Although not all OATs are deemed replaceable, a significant proportion are and much of the £134m extra cost could be saved.... A major obstacle to this, however, is the lack of availability of rehabilitation services in many areas. Psychiatric rehabilitation is an unfashionable concept in a sector where the dominant model of care has come to be seen as pushing the individual along a time-limited care pathway. Service users with longer-term needs do not easily fit this approach. (Brindle, 2010)

The case appears, finally, to have been heard. In 2010, the Faculty was invited to contribute to the National Mental Health Development Unit's working group on OATs, commissioned by the Department of Health. This group developed an online toolkit for mental health commissioners to minimise the use of OATs and repatriate and reinvest in local mental health rehabilitation services and supported accommodation (National Mental Health Development Unit, 2011).

The 2011 mental health policy document *No Health Without Mental Health* (Department of Health, 2011) was explicit in its support for local rehabilitation services, specifically in its call for 'appropriate and balanced capacity across the various elements of inpatient provision, e.g. acute wards, psychiatric intensive care units, low secure beds, and rehabilitation services'. It went on:

> Being placed out of area can mean that individuals receive care far from their families, friends and familiar surroundings. Lengths of stay may be longer as there is less continuity of care and it can be harder to arrange discharge, so costs can be higher. A number of areas have undertaken work to improve local systems and prevent people having to leave their area to access services (p. 13–14).

No place for complacency

While this clear support for rehabilitation services has now been incorporated into policy, it would be foolish to become complacent. The National Health Service is constantly changing and the politics of healthcare frequently make the news. Currently we are experiencing in England a total reorganisation of the way in which our services are commissioned. We are struggling to understand how the spectre of a tariff-based system will impact on our services and those who use them, and whether the increasing focus on 'personalisation', however vague at present, could transform the way we agree and deliver support to our patients. It is simply too early to do more than hypothesise about the potential challenges and opportunities that these paradigm shifts in policy could bring (see Chapter 31, 'Rehabilitation and recovery in the 21st century'). However, what is increasingly clear is that policy-makers and service commissioners expect us to be more accountable for the services we run and the interventions we deliver. They want to see evidence that the money spent on mental health services is a good investment, delivering good outcomes for patients.

With this in mind, the Faculty of Rehabilitation and Social Psychiatry of the Royal College of Psychiatrists has published a suite of documents detailing what is meant by a 'whole-system care pathway for people with complex needs'. The most important of these documents is the *Guide for Commissioners of Rehabilitation Services for People with Complex Mental Health Needs* (Joint Commissioning Panel for Mental Health, 2012), which gives a fairly detailed overview of the components of the whole-system care pathway, including the different types of in-patient rehabilitation unit that may be required, as well as the specific interventions delivered by the various in-patient and community rehabilitation teams. This document has been sent to every National Health Service chief executive, rehabilitation psychiatrist and mental health commissioner in England. Accompanying the commissioning guide are Faculty reports for practitioners that detail the resources required and interventions that should be delivered by in-patient and community mental health rehabilitation services (Edwards *et al*, 2011; Kalidindi *et al*, 2012; Wolfson *et al*, 2012).

Finally, the ongoing case for investment in mental health rehabilitation services has to be supported by evidence of their effectiveness and quality. Chapter 29, 'Expanding the evidence base', provides a comprehensive description of the current evidence base for contemporary mental health rehabilitation services. However, beyond specific research studies, increasingly, commissioners and service managers will expect all services, including rehabilitation services to produce routine data on their activity, outcomes and quality. Alongside the soon to be mandated Health of the National Outcome Scale, the Faculty of Rehabilitation and Social Psychiatry recommends the addition of a standardised measure of social function and of needs, along with metrics such as length of stay, numbers of readmissions and engagement in meaningful occupation. More details are available in the Royal College of Psychiatrists' Occasional Paper 78 (2011). The most comprehensive approach to quality assessment is provided through the AIMS-Rehab programme run by the College Centre for Quality Improvement (see Chapter 17, 'Rehabilitation in hospital settings'). The authors recommend this programme strongly for the assessment of in-patient rehabilitation services in the UK.

Conclusions

Despite the investment in specialist community mental health services in recent years, there remains a group of service users with very complex needs who require lengthy hospital treatment and high levels of support on discharge to the community. This group are the clients of mental health rehabilitation services. The ongoing need for mental health rehabilitation services has been proven in recent years in the UK through the negative consequences of disinvestment, leading to expansion of the OAT sector. Rehabilitation practitioners must be ready to make the case for their services, using the resources referenced in this chapter and routine outcome data to ensure ongoing investment in a local whole-system care pathway for this group of patients.

References

Brindle M (2010) Millions wasted on treating mentally ill away from their communities. *Guardian*, 14 April. At http://www.theguardian.com/society/2010/apr/14/non-local-mental-health-treatment-wasting-millions (accessed December 2014).

Department of Health (1999) *National Service Framework for Mental Health*. Department of Health.

Department of Health (2005) *National Service Framework for Mental Health – 5 Years On*. Department of Health.

Department of Health (2011) *No Health Without Mental Health. A Cross Government Mental Health Outcomes Strategy for People of All Ages. Supporting Document – The Economic Case for Improving Efficiency and Quality in Mental Health*. DH.

Edwards T, Meier R, Killaspy H (2011) *Making the Case for a Rehabilitation Facility* (FR/RS/05). Faculty of Rehabilitation and Social Psychiatry, Royal College of Psychiatrists.

Holloway F (2005) *The Forgotten Need for Rehabilitation in Contemporary Mental Health Services* (Position Statement from the Executive Committee of the Faculty of Rehabilitation and Social Psychiatry). Royal College of Psychiatrists. At http://www.rcpsych.ac.uk/pdf/frankholloway_oct05.pdf (accessed December 2014).

Johnson S, Nolan F, Pilling S, *et al* (2005) Randomised controlled trial of acute mental health care by a crisis resolution team: the North Islington Crisis Study. *BMJ*, **331**: 599.

Joint Commissioning Panel for Mental Health (2012) *Guidance for Commissioners of Rehabilitation Services for People with Complex Mental Health Needs*. Royal College of Psychiatrists.

Kalidindi S, Edwards T, Killaspy H (2012) *Community Psychosis Services: The Role of Community Mental Health Rehabilitation Teams* (FR/RS/07). Faculty of Rehabilitation and Social Psychiatry, Royal College of Psychiatrists.

Killaspy H, Meier R (2010) A fair deal for mental health rehabilitation services. *The Psychiatrist*, **34**: 265–7.

Killaspy H, Bebbington P, Blizard R, *et al* (2006) REACT: A Randomised Evaluation of Assertive Community Treatment in north London. *BMJ*, **332**: 815–9.

Killaspy H, Rambarran D, Harden C, *et al* (2009) A comparison of service users placed out of their local area and local rehabilitation service users. *Journal of Mental Health*, **18**: 111–20.

Leff J, Trieman N (2000) Long stay patients discharged from psychiatric hospitals. Social and clinical outcomes after five years in the community. TAPS Project 46. *British Journal of Psychiatry*, **176**: 217–23.

Mountain D, Killaspy H, Holloway F (2009) Mental health rehabilitation services in the UK in 2007. *Psychiatric Bulletin*, **33**: 215–18.

National Mental Health Development Unit (2011) *In Sight and in Mind: A Toolkit to Reduce the Use of Out of Area Mental Health Services*. Royal College of Psychiatrists. At http://www.rcpsych.ac.uk/PDF/insightandinmind.pdf (accessed December 2014).

Poole R, Ryan T, Pearsall A (2002) The NHS, the private sector, and the virtual asylum. *BMJ*, **325**: 349–50.

Priebe S, Badesconyi A, Fioritti A, *et al* (2005) Reinstitutionalisation in mental health care: comparison of data on service provision from six European countries. *BMJ*, **330**: 123–6.

Royal College of Psychiatrists (2011) *Outcome Measures Recommended for Use in Adult Psychiatry* (Occasional Paper 78). Royal College of Psychiatrists.

Royal College of Psychiatrists, Mental Health Network, NHS Confederation & London School of Economics and Political Science (2009) *Mental Health and the Economic Downturn: National Priorities and NHS Solutions* (Occasional Paper 70). Royal College of Psychiatrists.

Ryan T, Pearsall A, Hatfield B, *et al* (2004) Long term care for serious mental illness outside the NHS: a study of out-of-area placements. *Journal of Mental Health*, **13**: 425–9.

Trieman N, Leff J (2002) Long-term outcome of long-stay psychiatric inpatients considered unsuitable to live in the community: TAPS Project 44. *British Journal of Psychiatry*, **181**: 428–32.

Wolfson P, Edwards T, Killaspy H (2012) *A Guide to Good Practice in the Use of Out-of-Area Placements* (FR/RS 06). Faculty of Rehabilitation and Social Psychiatry, Royal College of Psychiatrists.

CHAPTER 31

Rehabilitation and recovery in the 21st century

Helen Killaspy, Sridevi Kalidindi, Glenn Roberts and Frank Holloway

Introduction

This book has provided a detailed description of current practice, policy, services and research in the field of mental health rehabilitation. In this concluding chapter, we attempt to draw out the main themes that are most likely to influence practice in the future and highlight areas where rehabilitation clinicians need to remain alert to the conscious and unconscious biases and drivers that can influence disinvestment in specialist services for people with complex mental health needs.

Rehabilitation and recovery – making the distinction

In Chapter 2, 'What is psychiatric rehabilitation?', mental health rehabilitation was defined as requiring a whole system of services that aim to promote an individual's recovery and social inclusion. The two concepts, rehabilitation and recovery, are often referred to together, since they both emphasise the goal of maximising autonomy and independence. Rehabilitation practitioners were early adopters and champions of recovery-oriented services in the UK, perhaps because of a synergy of values (described in more detail in Chapter 3, 'Rehabilitation as a values-led practice'). Both rehabilitation and recovery emphasise collaborative practice and therapeutic optimism, among other things. However, the principles of recovery apply across all mental health services, not just rehabilitation services. While their adoption by generic mental health services is to be welcomed, this can also present something of a threat to rehabilitation services. When services are renamed 'recovery' services, the importance of providing specialist services for people with complex mental health needs can be lost. As we have seen in Chapter 30, 'Psychiatric rehabilitation: future directions in policy and practice', historically, policy-makers, commissioners and service planners seem recurrently to marginalise people with the most severe mental health problems. The conflation of recovery and rehabilitation can feed into this process, either unwittingly or through the mistaken belief that the latest trend in mental health practice can magically transform outcomes for everyone, negating the need for longer-term, more expensive services. In addition, protagonists of the recovery approach can sometimes present the false and unrealistic polarisation of recovery as a positive 'social model' and psychiatry as a negative 'medical model'. This unhelpful positioning has been challenged by two well-respected rehabilitation psychiatrists, both champions of recovery:

> It is a largely non-medical assertion that medical practice is governed by something called 'the medical model', and the largely non-medical recovery literature yields a strong view that psychiatric thought and practice are almost entirely hostage to it. (Roberts & Wolfson, 2004: p. 39)

It is therefore important that rehabilitation practitioners are clear about the distinction between rehabilitation and recovery in order to challenge these issues. While rehabilitation services operate with a recovery orientation, they focus on people with the most complex mental health needs in the system. The time frame that they need to support people through the process of recovery is years rather than weeks or months. Earlier chapters have described the patient group (Chapter 2, 'What is psychiatric rehabilitation?') and the specific treatments, interventions and skills required to do this effectively (Part 2, 'Treatment approaches'). In Part 3 of this book, 'Key elements', the essential components of the whole system that constitutes a rehabilitation service were detailed. Rehabilitation practitioners need to be able to describe this system and justify the need for investment in such a system at a local level on the basis of clinical and economic arguments (described in Chapter 30, 'Psychiatric rehabilitation: future directions in policy and practice'). Evidence of the effectiveness of rehabilitation services strengthens the argument and is presented in Chapter 29, 'Expanding the evidence base'.

Multiple providers of the whole system approach

As we have seen in Chapter 3, 'Rehabilitation as a values-led practice' and Chapter 30, 'Psychiatric rehabilitation: future directions in policy and practice', current health and social care policy in the UK is relatively positively inclined to investment in mental health rehabilitation services and services that are congruent with the principles of recovery. What is less clear is the way in which these will be provided and by whom.

From the national programme of research into mental health rehabilitation services in England (see Chapter 29, 'Expanding the evidence base'), we know that almost all National Health Service (NHS) trusts provide at least one mental health rehabilitation unit (the average is two per trust) and over half also provide a community rehabilitation team whose staff work with people in specialist mental health supported accommodation (see Chapter 18, 'Community-based rehabilitation and recovery'). However, the current provision of specific components of the whole-system rehabilitation care pathway in different areas is unknown. There is also very little information available at a national level on the number of rehabilitation beds in the private sector, although we know from a freedom-of-information enquiry carried out by the Faculty of Rehabilitation and Social Psychiatry of the Royal College of Psychiatrists (referred to in Chapter 30) that around one-fifth of people with complex mental health needs are placed out of area in hospital, nursing and residential care homes, most of these being provided by the independent sector. More recently, a new variety of out-of-area placement has appeared, in the form of 'locked rehabilitation' units. This type of unit does not appear in the *Guidance for Commissioners of Rehabilitation Services for People with Complex Mental Health Needs* (Joint Commissioning Panel for Mental Health, 2012) and is not recognised by the Faculty of Rehabilitation and Social Psychiatry. It appears to be a response to recent changes to commissioning structures in England which have made it increasingly difficult to access low-secure rehabilitation beds for people with challenging behaviours and severe mental health problems. The independent sector has seen this 'gap in the market' and filled it, illustrating how responsive the sector is to market forces. As described in Chapter 30, the expansion of out-of-area placements represents a serious threat to the provision of a coherent, local whole system of rehabilitation services and risks social dislocation of people with complex mental health problems. The expansion of the independent sector seems to be a covert aim of the current government's health policy. Assuming that this trend continues, it brings specific challenges for rehabilitation practitioners and services.

Different components of the whole-system rehabilitation pathway can be (and usually are) delivered by different providers, including the NHS, the independent sector, social services and the third (not for profit) sector. The NHS tends to focus on provision of in-patient rehabilitation units and community rehabilitation teams. The independent sector tends to provide secure and non-secure in-patient rehabilitation units and, increasingly, different levels of supported accommodation. Social services and the third sector provide more community-based care, including nursing and residential care homes, supported accommodation, vocational rehabilitation services and peer-support services.

In addition, increasingly, and as part of the policy agenda on personalised care, individual, tailored 'care packages' (specific treatment, support and activities) are funded by health and social care through a system known as personal budgets. These can be managed by the individual or someone appointed to manage them for the person (such as a relative or care coordinator). This personalised approach to the provision of care is currently at a relatively early stage of development. The evidence from pilots of this system across a range of health conditions (not just mental illness) in England have found that people rarely abuse the funds allocated and, overall, they appear to be associated with positive outcomes in terms of health-related quality of life and psychological well-being (Forder *et al*, 2012). This shift away from more institutionalised to more individualised care may, if it continues to show positive benefits, become a 'quiet revolution' in the way in which care is provided, particularly in the community. However, how far these initiatives can be used successfully by people with complex mental health problems has yet to be tested. The broader issues relevant to rehabilitation services related to the increased personalisation of mental healthcare are covered in more depth in Chapter 3, 'Rehabilitation as a values-led practice'.

Different providers bring different strengths and perspectives to the complex whole system of mental health rehabilitation. Those working across the system, such as mental health practitioners, need to be aware of the specific challenges. An obvious one is the importance of holding an overview and providing continuity for individuals as they transit between different services over the course of their recovery. The care coordinator or rehabilitation psychiatrist may well be the person working within the system who has known the individual longest and seen him or her when most unwell and through periods of recovery. Communicating important information to others involved in people's care (such as their individual strengths, interests, relapse indicators, and previous response to treatment) is vital. Involvement in people's care across the whole care pathway is particularly key when decisions are being made to place them out of area. If such a placement is deemed necessary because of a lack of suitable local provision, the rehabilitation practitioner must remain involved to ensure that there are systems in place for regular review of the person's needs in order to facilitate a move back to the local service as soon as possible (Edwards *et al*, 2012).

Working in partnership with other providers can be difficult but will be increasingly required as the system continues to be delivered by multiple agencies. Indeed, the socioeconomic and political drive to reduce in-patient mental health bed numbers to the absolute minimum encourages the expansion of community-based care through hybrid provider formats (such as co-provision by NHS and non-statutory providers) to gain commissions in a competitive tendering environment. This can provide a refreshing opportunity to work with other professionals from other organisations who hold a different perspective and have different ideas on what may help an individual in recovery. Nevertheless, there may be an increasing strain on the capacity of functionally divided services to offer the sort of committed relationships people need to support them through their recovery from complex and long-term mental health problems. Peer-support services (see Chapter 21, 'Peer support in mental health services') may, in the future, develop to become an important provider of this longer-term continuity and support.

Tariff-based mental health services

In England, there are plans to extend the current tariff-based funding system of other secondary health services to mental health services. This system is already in operation in other parts of the world (such as Australia) and, although there has been some opposition to and delays in its adoption in England, some version of this approach is likely to be implemented soon. In essence, government funding of services will be based on specific tariffs awarded according to the number of individuals with a condition of a particular level of complexity treated during a specific time period. Many NHS mental health trusts have reconfigured their services in recent years in preparation for the new system, using 'care clustering' and 'service line management'. Treatment and care will be delivered according to the care cluster a patient is allocated to, through the appropriate service line for that cluster. While this has some logic, in that staff working in a particular service line can gain enhanced skills to deliver evidence-based interventions specific to their patients, there are many unanswered questions and concerns about whether such a system can really work effectively for people with mental health problems, given that many cannot be easily allocated to a specific cluster owing to comorbidities and many do not accept or respond well to evidence-based treatments.

For people with the most complex problems, this issue is highly pertinent. Mental health rehabilitation services work with people allocated to a range of clusters, including developmental disorders such as those on the autism spectrum (cluster 0), psychoses (clusters 11, 12 and 13), those who are difficult to engage and have comorbid problems with substance misuse (clusters 16 and 17) and those with personality disorder (cluster 7). There is no process for identifying which of the individuals within any of these clusters are those with the most complex problems. It therefore seems likely that the tariff allocated to each cluster will underestimate the actual costs for this group. This is a serious concern, as it could lead to major underfunding of mental health rehabilitation services and a lack of specialist provision for those with the most complex needs. Since the actual patients will still exist, the consequences could be a replication of those seen during the last period of disinvestment in rehabilitation services, during the implementation of the *National Service Framework for Mental Health* (Department of Health, 1999), as described in Chapter 30. In order to address this concern, data are currently being collated to try to identify the proportion of people in each cluster who are under the care of mental health rehabilitation services and the associated costs of their care. As the tariff-based system develops, specific indicators and measures will be used to reward services for appropriate outcomes over a specific period. This is also of concern given the lack of robust data available on the sensitivity to change of these measures for people with complex needs and the lengthy periods required for their treatment. This issue is being discussed with the Department of Health.

The renaissance of rehabilitation services

Despite the challenges described in this chapter, the past 5 years or so has been a period of relative renaissance for mental health rehabilitation services. The economic downturn provided a fertile context to make the case for local reinvestment in rehabilitation services, as described in Chapter 30. Most NHS trusts continue to provide in-patient rehabilitation services of various types, and there has been an expansion in the number of community rehabilitation teams across England in recent years. There is also anecdotal evidence of increasing investment in supported accommodation in many areas for people to move on to from hospital in many areas. However, the general trend towards more business-type models of healthcare provision operating in increasingly competitive environments means that rehabilitation practitioners will need to be well placed and well informed in order to argue successfully for appropriate investment in rehabilitation services, describing their role and purpose, values, clinical effectiveness and cost-effectiveness. Encouragingly, the investment by the Department of Health in national programmes of research in this field points to an increasing awareness of the importance of rehabilitation services as part of the wider constellation of mental health services. The results of these studies will help to inform the evidence base in this little-researched area and guide practitioners and service planners as to how to focus their energies and resources.

This is a good time to be a rehabilitation practitioner. After many years as the unfashionable arm of psychiatry, rehabilitation appears now to be acknowledged as an essential part of the mental health system. Rehabilitation remains one of the most rewarding areas of psychiatry and is one of the few specialties where it is still possible to work with patients over the longer term. It is a growing field and an exciting area in which to work. We hope that, after finishing this book, our readers feel the same.

References

Department of Health (1999) *National Service Framework for Mental Health*. London: Department of Health.

Edwards T, Wolfson P, Killaspy H (2012) *A Guide to Good Practice in the Use of Out-Of-Area Placements* (FR/RS/06). Royal College of Psychiatrists.

Forder J, Jones K, Glendinning C, *et al* (2012) *Evaluation of the Personal Health Budget Pilot Programme*. PSSRU University of Kent.

Joint Commissioning Panel for Mental Health (2012) *Guidance for Commissioners of Rehabilitation Services for People with Complex Mental Health Needs*. Royal College of Psychiatrists.

Roberts G, Wolfson P (2004) The rediscovery of recovery: open to all. *Advances in Psychiatric Treatment*, **10**: 37–48.

Index

Compiled by Linda English

465

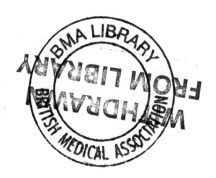